Evidence-Based Rehabilitation
A Guide to Practice

THIRD EDITION

EDITED BY

Mary Law, PhD, OT Reg (Ont), FCAHS
School of Rehabilitation Science
McMaster University
Hamilton, Ontario, Canada

Joy C. MacDermid, PhD, PT Reg (Ont), FCAHS
School of Rehabilitation Science
McMaster University
Hamilton, Ontario, Canada

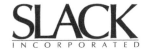

www.Healio.com/books

ISBN: 978-1-61711-021-4

Instructors: *Evidence-Based Rehabilitation: A Guide to Practice, Third Edition Instructor's Manual* is also available from SLACK Incorporated. Don't miss this important companion to *Evidence-Based Rehabilitation: A Guide to Practice, Third Edition.* To obtain the Instructor's Manual, please visit http://www.efacultylounge.com

The procedures and practices described in this publication should be implemented in a manner consistent with the professional standards set for the circumstances that apply in each specific situation. Every effort has been made to confirm the accuracy of the information presented and to correctly relate generally accepted practices. The authors, editors, and publisher cannot accept responsibility for errors or exclusions or for the outcome of the material presented herein. There is no expressed or implied warranty of this book or information imparted by it. Care has been taken to ensure that drug selection and dosages are in accordance with currently accepted/recommended practice. Off-label uses of drugs may be discussed. Due to continuing research, changes in government policy and regulations, and various effects of drug reactions and interactions, it is recommended that the reader carefully review all materials and literature provided for each drug, especially those that are new or not frequently used. Some drugs or devices in this publication have clearance for use in a restricted research setting by the Food and Drug and Administration or FDA. Each professional should determine the FDA status of any drug or device prior to use in their practice.

Any review or mention of specific companies or products is not intended as an endorsement by the author or publisher.

SLACK Incorporated uses a review process to evaluate submitted material. Prior to publication, educators or clinicians provide important feedback on the content that we publish. We welcome feedback on this work.

Published by: SLACK Incorporated
                     6900 Grove Road
                     Thorofare, NJ 08086 USA
                     Telephone: 856-848-1000
                     Fax: 856-848-6091
                     www.Healio.com/books

Contact SLACK Incorporated for more information about other books in this field or about the availability of our books from distributors outside the United States.

Library of Congress Cataloging-in-Publication Data

Evidence-based rehabilitation : a guide to practice / [edited by] Mary Law, Joy MacDermid. -- Third edition.
      p. ; cm.
   Includes bibliographical references and index.
   ISBN 978-1-61711-021-4 (alk. paper)
   I. Law, Mary C., editor of compilation. II. MacDermid, Joy, editor of compilation.
   [DNLM: 1. Rehabilitation--methods. 2. Evidence-Based Medicine--methods. 3. Treatment Outcome. WB 320]
   RM930
   617'.03--dc23
                              2013027660

Printed in the United States of America.

Last digit is print number: 10   9   8   7   6   5   4   3   2

DEDICATION

This book is dedicated to my Mom who died in April 2013 at the age of 93 years. I thank her for her love and wisdom, and will always remember her pride in her children and grandchildren and her ability to make friends across the generations.

Mary Law, PhD, OT Reg (Ont), FCAHS

This book is dedicated to my brother Stephen who has my great respect and love. He lived with immense dedication to family and community and brought a sense of humor and calm to everything he did. I treasure my memories of our time together and miss him every day.

Joy C. MacDermid, PhD, PT Reg (Ont), FCAHS

CONTENTS

Instructors: *Evidence-Based Rehabilitation: A Guide to Practice, Third Edition Instructor's Manual* is also available from SLACK Incorporated. Don't miss this important companion to *Evidence-Based Rehabilitation: A Guide to Practice, Third Edition*. To obtain the Instructor's Manual, please visit http://www.efacultylounge.com

ACKNOWLEDGMENTS

In writing this book, we appreciate the excellent authors who have willingly shared their knowledge by writing chapters of this book. We thank each of them for their thoughtful and comprehensive contributions. Our work in evidence-based rehabilitation has been stimulated and supported by colleagues and students at McMaster University, Canada. We are grateful to work in an environment where new ideas are explored, challenged, and developed.

ABOUT THE EDITORS

Mary Law, PhD, OT Reg (Ont), FCAHS is a professor at the School of Rehabilitation Science and CanChild Centre for Childhood Disability Research at McMaster University, Canada. She holds the John and Margaret Lillie Chair in Childhood Disability Research. Mary, an occupational therapist by training, is cofounder of CanChild Centre for Childhood Disability Research, a multidisciplinary research centre at McMaster University. Mary's research centers on the development and validation of client-centered outcome measures, evaluation of occupational therapy interventions with children, the effect of environmental factors on the participation of children with disabilities in day-to-day activities, and transfer of research knowledge into practice. In her educational activities, Mary is involved in teaching the theoretical basis of occupational therapy practice and evidence-based occupational therapy practice in the occupational therapy program as well as supervising graduate students. Mary is the lead author of the Canadian Occupational Performance Measure, a client-centered outcome measure for occupational therapy, and has written books on client-centered occupational therapy and measurement of occupational performance.

Joy C. MacDermid, PhD, PT Reg (Ont), FCAHS is a physical therapist, hand therapist, and clinical epidemiologist. She is a professor at the School of Rehabilitation Science and Assistant Dean of Rehabilitation Science Graduate Programs at McMaster University. Joy is also codirector of the Hand and Upper Limb Centre (HULC) Clinical Research Lab. She is cross-appointed into Health Research Methodology at McMaster University and the Departments of Surgery at both McMaster University and the University of Western Ontario. Her teaching and research emphasizes evidence-based practice, clinical measurement, and knowledge translation. Joy's research focuses on developing and transferring into practice the best evidence for prevention, assessment, and management of musculoskeletal injuries and disorders including musculoskeletal health (upper extremity/neck); rehabilitative and surgical interventions for bone, joint, nerve, muscle, and tendon disorders; design and conduct of randomized clinical trials and cohort studies; clinical measurement of pain and disability (performance and self-report); and work-related risks, interventions, and work disability.

Contributing Authors

Laura Bradley, MSc OT, OT Reg (Ont) (Chapter 7)
Clinician
Early Childhood Program
Ottawa Children's Treatment Center
Ottawa, Ontario, Canada

Winnie Dunn, PhD, OTR, FAOTA (Chapter 2)
Professor and Chair
Department of Occupational Therapy
    Education
University of Kansas Medical Center
Kansas City, Kansas

Paola Durando, BA, MLS (Chapter 5)
Public Services Librarian
Bracken Health Sciences Library
Queen's University
Kingston, Ontario, Canada

Jill E. Foreman, BP, BHScOT (Chapter 2)
OT Practitioner
Calgary, Alta, Canada

Jocelyn Harris, PhD, OT Reg (Ont) (Chapter 13)
Assistant Professor
School of Rehabilitation Science
McMaster University
Hamilton, Ontario, Canada

Michael Law, PhD (Chapter 8)
Assistant Professor
School of Public Health
University of British Columbia
Vancouver, British Columbia, Canada

Jennie Q. Lou, MD, MSc, OTR (Chapter 5)
Director, Master of Science in Biomedical
    Informatics Program
Professor of Public Health & Internal Medicine
College of Osteopathic Medicine
Nova Southeastern University
Ft. Lauderdale, Florida

Annie McCluskey, PhD, MA, DipCOT (Chapter 3)
Faculty of Health Sciences
The University of Sydney
Sydney, Australia

Saurabh Mehta, PT, PhD (Chapter 13)
Assistant Professor
School of Physical Therapy
Marshall University
Huntington, West Virginia

Susan L. Michlovitz, PT, PhD, CHT (Chapter 4)
Adjunct Associate Professor, Rehabilitation
    Medicine
Program in Physical Therapy
Columbia University
New York, New York

Linda Tickle-Degnen, PhD, OTR/L, FAOTA
    (Chapter 12)
Professor and Chair
Department of Occupational Therapy
Director
Health Quality of Life Lab
Tufts University
Medford, Massachusetts

Aliki Thomas, PhD, OT(c), Erg (Chapter 3)
Assistant Professor and Associate Director
Occupational Therapy Program
School of Medicine and Occupational Therapy
Montreal, Quebec, Canada

Diane Watson, PhD (Chapter 8)
Faculty, Centre for Health Services and Policy
    Research
University of British Columbia
Director of Research and Analyses
Health Council of Canada
Toronto, Ontario, Canada

PREFACE

"Science is not formal logic—it needs the free play of the mind in as great a degree as any other creative art. It is true that this is a gift which can hardly be taught, but its growth can be encouraged in those who already posses it."

—Max Born (1882–1970)

Evidence-based practice continues to be one of the most discussed and debated topics in health care over the past decade. Initially described and developed in area of medicine, evidence-based practice is now part of every health care discipline and professional education program. While everyone agrees that it is important to use evidence in practice, the challenges of finding, evaluating, and using evidence are substantial. For rehabilitation, our evidence base is growing rapidly but moving these findings into practice remains a substantial challenge. Integrating research findings with clinical wisdom and clients' preferences and values is the goal of evidence-based rehabilitation. Our aim in editing this text is to provide information to students and practitioners in rehabilitation to aid in the development and use of evidence-based practice.

The book is designed to outline the concepts, methods, and strategies underpinning evidence-based rehabilitation. We begin the book with an introduction to evidence-based practice where we describe the basic concepts of evidence-based rehabilitation and discuss how knowledge is developed within a discipline. The role of reflective practice in supporting evidence-based practice is outlined. We then move on to chapters focused on finding that evidence, which detail outcomes in evidence-based rehabilitation and methods to search for evidence. Evaluation, critical appraisal, and systematic review of evidence are then highlighted. Finally, a series of chapters focus on using the evidence. We discuss strategies to build evidence in practice and communicate evidence to clients, managers, funders, and practitioners. The relationship between practice guidelines and evidence-based practice is described in the chapter outlining the use of guidelines. Information about knowledge exchange and transfer is discussed.

We have benefited greatly from feedback concerning the first and second editions of this book. We hope that rehabilitation students, practitioners, and educators will explore the issues and methods in this book and find it useful to build professional knowledge. We welcome your thoughts and comments about the content of this new edition.

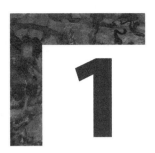

INTRODUCTION TO EVIDENCE-BASED PRACTICE

Mary Law, PhD, OT Reg (Ont), FCAHS and
Joy C. MacDermid, PhD, PT Reg (Ont), FCAHS

LEARNING OBJECTIVES

After reading this chapter, the student/practitioner will be able to:

- Understand the origins and definitions of evidence-based practice (EBP) and recognize the key elements.
- Critically discuss the concepts and misconceptions surrounding EBP.
- Recognize the nature of EBP in rehabilitation.
- Understand and explain the key characteristics of evidence-based rehabilitation (EBR), including awareness, consultation, judgment, and creativity.

"I have used this intervention for many years, and now researchers have shown that it is not effective. How do I know whether I should believe them and stop using this approach?"

"The program in which I work is starting a new service designed to improve the work tolerance and function of injured workers. We will need to demonstrate that the outcomes of this new program are excellent. How do I identify assessment tools to evaluate client outcomes after receiving the program?"

"Several studies have shown that a short, intensive therapy intervention may be more effective than therapy for a longer period of time. What are the cost implications of this type of service delivery?"

EVIDENCE-BASED REHABILITATION

Any rehabilitation practitioner could ask these questions. For occupational therapists, physical therapists, speech pathologists, and other rehabilitation health professionals, there is a need for high-quality information on which to base clinical and managerial decisions. These issues point to

Law M., & MacDermid, J. C.
Evidence-Based Rehabilitation: A Guide
to Practice, Third Edition (pp 1–14).
© 2014 SLACK Incorporated.

the need for practice based on available evidence. EBP in rehabilitation has emerged as one of the most influential concepts in the past decade.

The very mention of EBP brings out different reactions from rehabilitation practitioners. The concept of such practice may seem daunting to the beginner—finding applicable evidence, evaluating it, and putting its recommendations into practice is no small feat! However, if done right, EBP is not a burden but a very powerful tool that helps practitioners provide higher-quality services for their clients and families.

Over the past 15 years, rehabilitation practitioners have become more aware of and comfortable with the concept of EBP. In effect, research evidence indicates that the majority of rehabilitation practitioners hold positive attitudes toward the use and implementation of EBP (Bennett et al., 2003; Humphries et al., 2000; Iles & Davidson, 2006; Jette et al., 2003; Metcalfe et al., 2001; Upton & Upton, 2006). Though there are still misconceptions about what EBP means on a day-to-day basis, rehabilitation practitioners have demonstrated a positive commitment to ensuring that their practice is up to date and based on the best information available.

EBP is often perceived as an all-or-nothing approach but, in reality, it can be put into practice in stages through setting priorities for action. Learning about and implementing EBP is best done one step at a time. The fears that surround EBP are largely unfounded and are based on a misunderstanding of the concept. Indeed, EBP is probably one of the most misunderstood concepts in health care because of its relative newness, the degree to which it breaks from tradition, and the amount of information available today. This chapter aims to provide a number of working definitions of EBP and to debunk the myths surrounding it.

THE ORIGINS OF EVIDENCE-BASED PRACTICE

EBP emerged in medicine due to a clear need for a better way to make clinical decisions and was fueled by developments in the field of clinical epidemiology. Although a number of scientists were active in moving the emerging field of clinical epidemiology forward at different institutions in Canada and Europe, McMaster University in Canada has been recognized as the birthplace of evidence-based medicine (EBM). This credit is largely attributable to the original work of Dr. David Sackett, who collaborated with colleagues in the new and innovative "problem-based" medical program established at McMaster University in 1970. The first textbook on clinical epidemiology Dr. Sackett published with his colleagues in the Department of Clinical Epidemiology at McMaster University (Sackett, Haynes, & Tugwell, 1985) contained many of the core concepts of EBM. Colleagues such as Bryan Haynes and Gord Guyatt continued to develop and disseminate the key principles and methods of EBM, the latter often credited with coining the term *evidence-based medicine*. Despite its relative youth, this concept has infiltrated many different disciplines and is now recognized worldwide. In fact, it was named one of the top 10 developments in medicine (Dickersin, Straus, & Bero, 2007). As concepts dissipate, they can be adapted for greater impact but also misused and misunderstood, so it is important to retain the key principles.

DEFINING EVIDENCE-BASED PRACTICE

"What does the evidence say?"
"Have you looked at the evidence?"
"Based on the evidence, I recommend ..."
Sound familiar? The term *evidence-based practice* is appearing more and more frequently in the literature, educational programs, client groups, and job descriptions in health care. Numerous

attempts have been made to conclusively define EBP, and these variants reflect the necessary process of adapting and refining the classic definition to different environments. EBM and EBP are often used interchangeably to mean the same thing. Technically, EBM refers only to the medical field, whereas EBP encompasses more aspects of health care, including rehabilitation.

As EBP has developed, a number of different definitions have been proposed. EBM, as first described by researchers and practitioners at McMaster University, was described as "a new paradigm for medical practice" (Guyatt et al., 1992, p. 2420). In this first article outlining EBM, Guyatt and colleagues wrote about the need for physicians to develop skills in critical appraisal and the application of evidence guidelines to the provision of care. In that paper, EBM was not given a formal definition. A later paper defined EBM as the "conscientious, explicit, and judicious use of current best evidence in making decisions about the care of individual patients/clients" (Sackett, Rosenberg, Gray, Haynes, & Richardson, 1996, p. 71). As EBM was more widely adopted, the role of clinical expertise was becoming integral in the understanding of best practice. EBP was becoming known as a framework for answering clinical questions by evaluating and incorporating the best clinical knowledge related to the patient's state, the clinical setting, and clinical circumstances present (Haynes, Deveraux, & Guyatt, 2002). The practice of EBM means integrating individual clinical expertise with the best available external clinical evidence from systematic research. This definition has been carefully worded to strike a fine balance between clinical expertise and external clinical evidence.

One of the greatest obstacles to the spread of EBP is that some established practitioners are opposed to it on ideological grounds. They object to EBP because they claim it pays no heed to the experience and expertise that professionals have been developing throughout their entire careers. This is one of the main misconceptions about EBP. The EBP framework does not ignore clinical skill; in fact, it welcomes it. EBP tries to root out assessment procedures and interventions that have worked their way into accepted practice but that may not be the most beneficial for the client.

The argument for EBP is simple: If there is a better way to practice, therapists should find it. This means critically evaluating what is already done to see whether it could be improved, which makes EBP a heavily client-centered approach to providing care. However, EBP in no way advocates throwing the clinical experience of established practitioners out the window. If anything, the practitioner's experience is more important, because knowledgeable practitioners are the ones who will know how best to implement EBP's findings. EBP's central message here is one of flexibility and of being able to blend the old ways with the fruits of research and new knowledge. As Sackett et al. (1996) went on to say, "By individual clinical expertise we mean the proficiency and judgment that individual clinicians acquire through clinical experience and clinical practice" (p. 71).

As the idea of EBP unfolded, the definition began to expand to include components other than current literature. Soon, EBP was seen as an approach to decision making that used the best evidence available in conjunction with client choices to decide on an option that suits the client best (Muir Gray, 1998). Initially, EBP reduced the emphasis on clinical judgment, instead favoring research studies. Now there appears to be more of a balance between research and clinical judgment, recognizing that clinicians and their colleagues bring valuable information to client choices (Guyatt, 2004).

EBP is seen as a process that begins with clinical questions, appraisal of the evidence, application of the evidence considering the client's wishes and needs, and finishing with an evaluation of the clinical outcomes (Haynes, 2002). The Canadian Health Services Research Foundation adds that evidence-based practitioners not only combine research evidence but also political and organizational evidence to arrive at clinical decisions. EBP has also been described as a total process, beginning with knowing what clinical questions to ask, how to find best practice, and how to appraise evidence for validity and applicability to a particular care situation. The best evidence then must be applied by a practitioner with expertise in considering the patient's unique values and needs. The final aspect of this process is the evaluation of the effectiveness of care and the continual improvement of this process (DePalma, 2000).

Recently, the Sicily statement (Dawes et al., 2005) was developed by a group of EBP educators to provide a clear statement of the core principles of EBP. In the statement, Dawes et al. (2005) outlined the requirements for EBP as the following:

> Evidence-Based Practice requires that decisions about health care are based on the best available, current, valid, and relevant evidence. These decisions should be made by those receiving care, informed by the tacit and explicit knowledge of those providing care, within the context of available resources. (p. 4)

During the past few years, research evidence has also played a larger role in informing policy initiatives. For policy, the use of evidence has been termed *evidence-informed practice*, in light of the fact that policy decisions are influenced by other factors beside research evidence (e.g., budgets and political decisions).

In essence, EBP is based on a self-directed learning model, whereby practitioners must not only continue learning but also continue evaluating their techniques and practice in light of this learning to see what can be improved. This is, in the truest sense of the form, the ability to critically examine, evaluate, and apply knowledge and then assess one's own findings. Strange as it may sound, practitioners must maintain a humble attitude about their own practice patterns to excel at EBP. The ability to admit one's own errors and oversights and to critically assess one's own prior work is crucial because knowing one's own limitations (and when to look for help) is the basis of EBP. If you maintain this attitude, EBP's use of the best external evidence allows you to tap into the work of thousands of professionals around the world in order to find the best possible interventions for your clients. As Sackett et al. (1996) said, "By best available external clinical evidence we mean clinically relevant research, often from the basic sciences of medicine, but especially from patient-centered clinical research" (p. 71).

Thus, the definition offered by Sackett et al. (1996) is an acknowledgment that health care is an imperfect science that requires both overarching clinical guidelines and individual judgment in equal parts. EBP works with the interplay of these two factors, making it a powerful tool that practitioners can use to guide their clinical decisions. EBP uses research evidence, but not in isolation.

Another useful definition of EBP comes from another expert in the field, Dr. Trisha Greenhalgh. She offered a simple definition of EBP: "Evidence-based medicine requires you to read the right papers at the right time and then to alter your behavior (and, what is often more difficult, the behavior of other people) in light of what you have found" (Greenhalgh, 1997, p. 2). A more detailed definition comes from Rosenberg and Donald (1995) in their paper, "Evidence-Based Medicine: An Approach to Clinical Problem Solving." They wrote that EBM/EBP is "the process of systematically finding, appraising, and using contemporaneous research findings as the basis for clinical decisions. Evidence-based medicine asks questions, finds and appraises the relevant data, and harnesses that information for everyday clinical practice" (p. 1122).

The definition offered by Rosenberg and Donald (1995) not only outlines EBP but also provides a step-by-step method of going about it. The four steps are questioning, searching, evaluating, and implementing and should be used in a constant cycle for the dedicated practitioner of EBP. At any moment, practitioners will likely be faced with a number of problems to which they must apply EBP, and they will be at various stages of the process at different times.

Recent literature has emphasized an expanded definition and scope for EBP. Haynes (2002) stated that "EBM advocates want patients, practitioners, health care managers and policy makers to pay attention to the best findings from health care research that meet the dual requirements of being both scientifically valid and ready for clinical application" (p. 2). The goal of EBP is to create strategies and tools for practitioners to access, understand, and use the latest research knowledge to improve services for clients. Much work has been done to increase the accessibility of research knowledge through the development of critical review guides, systematic reviews, and easy-to-understand knowledge transfer materials.

There is now a recognition among EBP proponents that research knowledge is only one of several factors that is considered in clinical decision making (Haynes, 2002; Law, Pollock, & Stewart, 2004).

> In fact, evidence-based practice can be considered to be a combination of information from what we know from research, what we have learned from clinical wisdom, and what we learned from information from the client and their family. This combination of information enables us to work together with clients and families to make the best use of knowledge. (Law, Pollock, & Stewart, 2004, p. 14)

Despite the different word choices in the many definitions of EBP, therapists use a combination of many facets of current literature, client choice, expertise, and clinical judgment to best serve the clients in their practice.

CONTROVERSY IN EVIDENCE-BASED REHABILITATION

Knowing that EBR is the standard we must reach is not enough. How, then, do we become evidence-based practitioners? At the outset, this seems a simple process. Discover what your client's wishes are, research different alternatives, appraise the evidence available, confer with colleagues, weigh the pros and cons of each option, and come to a choice. In practice, some feel that this is not as easy as it appears. Clinicians report several challenges associated with becoming and remaining effective evidence-based practitioners.

There is a heavy cost associated with generating high-level, good-quality studies. Because researchers may be financially limited in what they can produce, consumers of research may be left with fewer choices of evidence. There may be relatively few high-level, quality studies available on a given topic but more research being done at lower, less expensive levels. This will leave clinicians at a loss to find large banks of high-level evidence to support or refute a treatment option (Guyatt, 2004). Clinicians who understand the importance of evidence in practice may feel that although they are encouraged to use evidence, they often feel discouraged from conducting research to produce evidence due to the high costs and time constraints involved (Hart et al., 2008).

Evidence of all qualities is being generated and indexed in the databases at an astounding rate. Many practitioners feel that this is simply too much to contend with and are not able to effectively create summaries that are current. Because of the influx of information, past systematic reviews are often not updated, leaving clinicians with "older" evidence (Guyatt, 2004).

Practitioners incorporating research into current clinical practice can run into problems due to the design of studies. Evidence-based practitioners must incorporate research into their current therapies to ensure best practice. However, methodological differences in current studies may affect the clinician's ability to use them. For example, randomized control trials (RCTs) and meta-analyses are considered the highest level of quantitative evidence, but many of them cannot be generalized due to subgroup makeup, clinical size of effect, or quality of outcome measures used. This will limit the practitioner's ability to use the conclusions clinically (Grimmer, 2004).

Presentation of evidence can also impede the ability of clinicians to incorporate it into practice. Research is often presented in a language that clinicians have difficulty understanding, with the implications to current practice not always outlined. Certain health professions can also feel less at ease with research language, making it more difficult for certain allied health groups to access the information (Upton & Upton, 2006). Without someone to help translate the findings into a format

Table 1-1	
Myths of Evidence-Based Practice	
MYTH	**REALITY**
• Evidence-based practice already exists	• Many practitioners take little or no time to review current medical findings
• Evidence-based practice is impossible to put into place	• Even extremely busy practitioners can initiate evidence-based practice through little work
• Evidence-based practice is cookie-cutter medicine	• Evidence-based practice requires extensive clinical expertise
• Evidence-based practice is a cost-cutting mechanism	• Evidence-based practice emphasizes the best available clinical evidence for each client's situation

that clinicians can understand and apply, the research has often not reached its intended audience and clients are not able to benefit from it (Sudsawad, 2005).

Finally, clinicians feel that there is often a lack of time and resources which prevents them from becoming effective evidence-based practitioners (Curtin & Jaramazovic, 2001; Upton & Upton, 2006). Many feel that they are not skilled in effectively searching the evidence and, when they do, the studies they wish to access are not available due to access issues, publication bias, or incomplete databases (Bennett et al., 2003; Curtin & Jaramazovic, 2001; Maher et al., 2004; Metzler & Metx, 2010). There can be a perception that EBP is something to be done on top of clinical work, rather than as an integral part of a complete practice (Caldwell, Whitehead, Fleming, & Moes, 2008).

Despite these concerns, rehabilitation clinicians have a positive attitude about using evidence in their practice (Curtin & Jaramazovic, 2001; Hart et al., 2008), and a recent Australian survey suggests that 96% of practitioners say that EBP is important to therapists (Bennett et al., 2003), and therapists, academics, researchers, and managers can all work together to incorporate research into clinical settings (Tse, Lloyd, Penman, King, & Bassett, 2004). With this in mind, how can we become (and remain) effective evidence-based practitioners?

If client values and therapist values are not the same, we can research all options and present graded recommendations based on all available options (Guyatt, 2004). Researchers can liaise with clinicians to ensure that clinically relevant information is being presented in a way that practitioners can understand (Grimmer, 2004). Companies and hospitals can offer practical incentives of time to therapists, as well as targeted educational initiatives around search strategies to assist the implementation of research into current practice (Bennett et al., 2003; Curtin & Jaramazovic, 2001; Caldwell et al., 2008).

MYTHS SURROUNDING EVIDENCE-BASED PRACTICE

Despite attempts to publicize the realities surrounding EBP, there continue to be some myths surrounding it (Table 1-1), which Sackett et al. (1996) and Haynes (2002) discussed in their articles. The misconception that EBP is either already in place or impossible to practice is their first target. Addressing the first point, Sackett et al. (1996) pointed out that though completely keeping up with the health research literature is impossible for any person, many practitioners take little or no time in their weekly routine to examine journals and publications, preferring instead to rely completely on their initial training to guide their practice.

EBP does not mean that every clinical situation will send a practitioner slavishly running to the library, but it does mean that when a new situation presents itself, a clinician should employ research skills to find an answer and pass this information on to colleagues. Unfortunately, this is not always the case; many clinicians rely solely on the expertise of others, which—though it can be helpful—is inherently based on the quirks of individual experience. As previously stated, a balance between the two sources of information can hardly hurt practitioners in making more accurate and more insightful diagnoses.

This argument also coincides with Sackett et al.'s (1996) further point that EBP is not impossible to put into place. In fact, they specifically stated that "studies show that busy clinicians who devote their scarce reading time to selective, efficient, client-driven searching, appraisal, and incorporation of the best available evidence can practice evidence-based medicine." Practicing EBP is not a matter of inundating oneself with evidence; it is a matter of deftly locating and snatching the evidence from the ever-growing pile of research and rehabilitation knowledge. This practice becomes easier as systems are developed to filter or evaluate the wealth of published studies.

Another criticism of EBP is that it is "cookie-cutter" care or devoid of the need for individual clinical judgment. This criticism returns to the earlier fears of EBP making clinicians' expertise irrelevant, and Sackett et al. (1996) again attempted to clarify the goals of EBP. As they stated, "External clinical evidence can inform, but can never replace, individual clinical expertise; this expertise will assist the practitioner in deciding whether the external evidence applies to the individual client at all and, if so, how it should be integrated into a clinical decision." No supporters of EBP have argued for the removal of regular training for practitioners; they have merely suggested that the training include information on how EBP fits into the clinical equation.

Lastly, Sackett et al. (1996) debunked the concept that EBP is merely a malicious tool of health policy makers—either introduced to cut costs or insisting that each clinical intervention be backed by an RCT. Both issues miss the point of EBP, which is to bring the best available clinical evidence to each client's situation. Using the best available evidence does not reduce the need for costly interventions; it simply attempts to ensure that each client gets the treatment appropriate for his or her condition. Furthermore, EBP insists that each case is treated with the best available evidence and is not so haughty that it rejects anything that is not an RCT outright. Because of this strength of EBP, it can be applied now in all forms of health care. This fact was discussed by Dr. Pamela Duncan (1997) in her article on evidence-based physical therapy. Though the health care climate may create a situation where some policy makers misuse the core concepts of EBP, it is clear that EBP definitions do not encourage suspending treatments if there are no RCTs available to support them; they merely suggest that the best available evidence inform the choice.

EVIDENCE-BASED REHABILITATION

One of the goals of this book is to assist students in becoming better practitioners and caregivers by using evidence-based strategies and tools. The previous discussion of EBP provides a theoretical understanding of the concept. The remainder of the chapter focuses on a discussion of EBR, which students may find more applicable and more relevant to their future work. EBR is similar to EBM in that it follows a process toward developing, appraising, and implementing evidence into practice (Cook, Jaeschke, & Guyatt, 1992).

EBR is a subset of evidence-based clinical practice, which has been discussed at length. Let us look at some ideas that will help us to ascertain the key skills that assist clinicians in practicing EBR (Table 1-2).

Table 1-2
Important Concepts in Evidence-Based Rehabilitation

• Awareness	• Judgment
• Consultation	• Creativity

Awareness

The first definition is from the Health Informatics Research Unit (HIRU, 2002) at McMaster University which states, "Evidence-based clinical practice is an approach to health care practice in which the clinician is aware of the evidence that bears on her clinical practice, and the strength of that evidence." The HIRU makes an important point: the clinician must be aware of the evidence related to his or her practice. This does not mean that he or she must read every new journal that comes out cover to cover, but that he or she should find ways of staying up-to-date with new research that is happening in his or her field. There are many ways to do this, such as obtaining journals that specifically summarize research advances or reviewing Web sites that bring information together to online discussion groups and chat forums in which practitioners can interact. Instead of awareness of everything without comprehension, the goal is focused awareness, or knowledge of where to look. Each practitioner must find his or her own natural way to stay current. This is important because striving for excellence means giving the best to each client and his or her family.

Consultation

A second definition comes from J. A. Muir Gray's (1997) book on evidence-based health care, in which he pointed out, "Evidence-based clinical practice is an approach to decision making in which the clinician uses the best evidence available, in consultation with the patient, to decide upon the option which suits that patient best." Muir Gray's (1997) definition is a reminder of one of the most important aspects of health care—transparency. Practitioners have a specialized set of skills and knowledge, and an essential part of their job has always been to communicate well. Their role is to work together with the client to ascertain the problem and how it can be resolved in the easiest possible way. With the advent of EBR, that job remains the same, albeit somewhat more complex. EBP is a method for distilling information from the findings of others and, equally, a vehicle for educating the client. Practitioners who are able to adeptly explain the practice of EBR to their clients, how they have found the clinical data they are using, and what they are doing with it will be the most successful. This opens the process up to the client so that he or she can see what the practitioner is doing. EBP turns the focus toward the community, with the practitioner working as an educator as well as a service provider.

Judgment

Although EBP and EBR represent a major advance in the field of rehabilitation, they should not be embraced blindly. At the 60th Annual Assembly of the American Academy of Physical Medicine and Rehabilitation, keynote speaker Dr. Joel DeLisa (1999) made these remarks about EBP and rehabilitation, "However, there are problems in the 'evidence' of evidence-based medicine … the laudable goal of making clinical decisions based on evidence can be impaired by the restricted quality and scope of what is collected as 'best available evidence'" (p. 7).

The problems or limits to the evidence in EBP cannot and should not be ignored. As DeLisa (1999) pointed out:

> Derived almost exclusively from randomized trials and meta-analysis … the results [of EBP work in rehabilitation] show comparative efficacy of treatment for an "average" randomized patient and are not for pertinent subgroups formed by cogent clinical features such as severity of symptoms, illness, comorbidity, and other clinical nuances. (p. 7)

Practitioners must possess good clinical judgment to differentiate how to apply the recommendations of EBP and how they must be tailored to the specific elements of each client's situation.

Creativity

A final definition of evidence-based health care, which lends itself to EBR, comes from an article in the *Journal of the American Medical Association*, which summarizes a discussion on the practice of EBM. The definition that comes from this round table is that evidence-based health care is "a conscientious, explicit, and judicious use of the current best evidence to make a decision about the care of patients" (Marwick, 1997). Using the best effort in a conscientious, explicit, and judicious way will not always be straightforward, and practitioners will have to use their creative skills to meet the challenges of real life. Learning EBP is both a science and an art and, as such, must be melded to the already existing body of skills that a practitioner has in his or her repertoire. EBR may sound like cookie-cutter practice but, in actuality, it requires a great deal of creativity and insight to work correctly. Ultimately, EBP allows practitioners to write their own textbook, so to speak, and teach themselves what they need to do. This makes creativity essential.

CONCLUSION

EBR is an important part of current practice. Practicing confident, resourceful, and creative rehabilitation is an art and must be developed over time. It is hoped that this book will serve to speed that process for many practitioners as they formulate their own definition of EBR.

TAKE HOME MESSAGES

Evidence-Based Practice

✓ There are misunderstandings of EBP because of the way in which it breaks with traditional practice; it should be seen as a powerful tool, not a burden.

✓ EBP maintains a fine balance between clinical expertise and external clinical evidence.

✓ EBP is based on an ongoing and self-directed learning model.

✓ EBP can support a strongly client-centered approach to rehabilitation.

✓ Clinical experience remains crucial because knowledgeable practitioners will best implement their findings based on the evidence.

✓ EBP makes use of the current best methods of treatment.

Evidence-Based Rehabilitation

✓ EBR is an adaptation of the concepts of EBP to rehabilitation practice and necessitates specific skills that allow clinicians to use evidence within the complex decision making required for rehabilitation practice.

✓ Awareness: The clinician must be aware of the evidence that has to do with practice and maintain focused awareness.

✓ Consultation: Specialized set of skills and knowledge and the ability to communicate well; the practitioner works as an educator/service provider.

✓ Judgment: The practitioner differentiates between cases about how to apply recommendations of EBP; tailored to specifics of each client's situation.

✓ Creativity: EBR requires creativity and insight because the practice and application of the best available evidence is not always straightforward.

WEB LINKS

Definitions of Evidence-Based Practice

www.shef.ac.uk/scharr/sections/ir
This site has an extensive selection of definitions for EBP, including many found in this chapter. It also has links to other resources for learning more about the essential aspects of EBP.

Sicily Statement

www.biomedcentral.com/1472-6920/5/1
A consensus statement developed on EBP and its definition.

California Institute for Mental Health

www.cimh.org/Initiatives/Evidence-Based-Practice/Definitions-Resources.aspx
This site provides a brief definition of EBP and links to other resources.

EVIDENCE-BASED PRACTICE LEARNING RESOURCES

Evidence-Based Informatics

http://hiru.mcmaster.ca/hiru

This page from the HIRU site at McMaster University provides information on the idea of EBR, as well as the preferences and outcomes it has delivered for rehabilitation.

Another similar initiative can be found at The Centres for Health Evidence at the following address: http://cche.net/default.asp.

Evidence-Based Occupational Therapy Web Portal

www.otevidence.info

This site is an internationally developed and supported portal for information on evidence-based occupational therapy. The site development was funded through the Canadian Association of Occupational Therapists and McMaster University School of Rehabilitation Science and is endorsed by the World Federation of Occupational Therapists.

Alberta EBM Toolkit

www.ebm.med.ualberta.ca

This site has tools for identifying and appraising evidence.

OTseeker: Occupational Therapy Systematic Evaluation of Evidence

www.otseeker.com/resources

OTSeeker, developed in Australia, is a database containing abstracts of systematic reviews and RCTs relevant to occupational therapy. All trials cited have been critically appraised and rated regarding their validity.

Physiotherapy Evidence Database

www.pedro.org.au

The Physiotherapy Evidence Database (PEDro), developed in Australia, is a database of abstracts of systematic reviews, RCTs, systematic reviews, and practice guidelines in physiotherapy. All citations have been critically appraised and rated regarding their validity.

American Speech-Language-Hearing Association

www.asha.org/members/ebp/intro.htm

This site from the American Speech-Language-Hearing Association provides a useful overview to EBP, in addition to Web-based tutorial links regarding the application of EBP.

Queensland Government—Occupational Therapy Services

www.learningplace.com.au/deliver/content.asp?pid=32622

This site is a resource that contains introductory materials for the mechanics of EBP.

Centre for Evidence-Based Medicine

http://ktclearinghouse.ca/cebm

This site provides materials about EBM based on the Sackett et al.'s (1985) book.

www.cebm.net/index.aspx?o=1914

This site provides information explaining EBM and providing an overview to EBP.

www.cebm.net/index.aspx?o=1023

This site provides information explaining how to conduct different steps of EBP.

LEARNING AND EXPLORATION ACTIVITIES

The purpose of this segment is to introduce the concept of EBP through the exploration of key definitions found in the literature. The following exercises guide the student through the process of thinking critically about the definition of EBP and applying this knowledge to possible clinical scenarios. The work done in these exercises should be saved by students as a good reference during their study of EBP.

1. Defining EBP

    a. What is your conception of EBP? What was your conception before you read this chapter? Make a chart and list both side by side, then attempt to locate where the gaps were in your knowledge. Then address the follow-up questions by thinking on a wider scale. How could misinformation about EBP be misleading other practitioners? What could be done about it?

    b. Build upon the ideas uncovered in the previous step by writing your own definition of EBP. You can incorporate parts of the definitions given previously if you would like, but make sure that the definition is meaningful and makes sense to you. Keep this definition written down somewhere, and look at it again once you have finished working through this book. Has your definition changed? Why?

    c. In small groups, write out a definition of EBP, listing the most crucial aspects. Prepare a short (5 minute) presentation about your definition and present it to the rest of the class. This can include debate or creative elements (dramatic, artistic, etc.). Your goal is to get the message across and make it stick in the minds of your audience.

    d. Myths surrounding EBP are presented in this chapter, along with the responses from Sackett et al. (1996). What are your assumptions about EBR? Write these down. How do you propose that these myths can be addressed?

2.   Best Practice

    a. What is your definition of *best practice*? How does that definition compare to your thoughts before and after reading this chapter? How does the concept of best practice fit into EBP; are they components of one another or different concepts?

3.   EBR

    a. The four principles of EBR outlined in the chapter—awareness, consultation, judgment, and creativity—serve as good guideposts for practitioners implementing EBR, but they are not perfect. Can you think of any other guideposts for yourself? If not, can you further define what is meant from each of the original guideposts?

    b. List briefly the differences and similarities between how EBM and EBR might be practiced. What are the key dissimilarities? How are EBM and EBR the most different? How are they the most similar? Why?

REFERENCES

Bennett, S., Tooth, L., McKenna, K., Rodger, S., Strong, J., & Ziviani, J., et al. (2003). Perceptions of evidence-based practice: A survey of Australian occupational therapists. *Australian Occupational Therapy Journal, 50*(1), 13–22.

Caldwell, E., Whitehead, M., Fleming, J., & Moes, L. (2008). Evidence-based practice in everyday clinical practice: Strategies for change in a tertiary occupational therapy department. *Australian Occupational Therapy Journal, 55,* 79–84.

Cook, D. J., Jaeschke, R., & Guyatt, G. H. (1992). Critical appraisal of therapeutic interventions in the intensive care unit: Human monoclonal antibody treatment in sepsis. Journal Club of the Hamilton Regional Critical Care Group. *Journal of Intensive Care Medicine, 7,* 275–282.

Curtin, M., & Jaramazovic, E. (2001). Occupational therapists' views and perceptions of evidence-based practice. *British Journal of Occupational Therapy, 64*(5), 214–222.

Dawes, M., Summerskill, W., Glasziou, P., Cartabellotta, A., Martin, J., Hopayian, K., …, Osborne, J. (2005). Sicily statement on evidence-based practice. *BMC Medical Education, 5*(1). doi:10.1186/1472-6920-5-1

DeLisa, J. A. (1999). Issues and challenges for psychiatry in the coming decade. *Archives Physical Medicine & Rehabilitation, 80,* 1–12.

DePalma, J. A. (2000). Evidence-based clinical practice guidelines. *Seminars in Perioperative Nursing, 9*(3), 115–120.

Dickersin, K., Straus, S. E., & Bero, L. A. (2007). Evidence based medicine: Increasing, not dictating, choice. *British Medical Journal, 334*(Suppl. 1), 10.

Duncan, P. W. (1997). Evidence-based medicine. *Physiotherapy Research International, 2,* 271–272.

Greenhalgh, T. (1997). *How to read a paper: The basics of evidence-based medicine.* London, England: BMJ Press.

Grimmer, K. (2004). Implementing evidence in clinical practice: The "therapies" dilemma. *Physiotherapy, 90*(4), 189–194.

Guyatt, G. (2004). Evidence based medicine has come a long way. *British Medical Journal, 329*, 990–996.

Guyatt, G., Cairns, J., Churchill, D., et al. (1992). Evidence-based medicine. A new approach to teaching the practice of medicine. *Journal American Medical Association, 268*, 2420–2425.

Hart, P., Eaton, L. A., Buckner, M., Morrow, B. N., Barrett, D. T., Fraser, D. D., et al. (2008). Effectiveness of a computer based educational program on nurses' knowledge, attitude and skill level related to evidence based practice. *Worldviews on Evidence-Based Nursing, 5*, 75–84.

Haynes, B. (2002). What kind of evidence is it that evidence-based medicine advocates want health care providers and consumers to pay attention to? *BMC Health Services Research, 2*(3), 1–7. Retrieved from http://www.biomedicalcentral.com/1472-6963/2/3

Haynes, B., Devereaux, P. J., & Guyatt, G. H. (2002). Clinical expertise in the era of evidence-based medicine and patient choice. *Evidence Based Medicine, 7*, 36–38.

Health Informatics Research Unit. (2002). How to teach evidence-based clinical practice 2002. Retrieved from http://hiru.mcmaster.ca

Humphries, D., Littlejohns, P., et al. (2000). Implementing evidence-based practice: Factors that influence the use of research evidence by occupational therapists. *British Journal of Occupational Therapy, 63*(11), 516–222.

Iles, R., & Davidson, M. (2006). Evidence based practice: A survey of physiotherapists' current practice. *Physiotherapy Research International, 11*(2), 903–103.

Jette, D. U., Bacon, K., Batty, C., et al. (2003). Evidence-based practice: Beliefs, attitudes, knowledge and behaviors of physical therapists. *Physical Therapy, 83*(9), 786–805.

Law, M., Pollock, N., & Stewart, D. (2004). Evidence-based occupational therapy: Concepts and strategies. *New Zealand Journal of Occupational Therapy, 51*(1), 14–22.

Maher, C., Sherrington, C., Elkins, M., Herbert, R., & Moesley, A. (2004). Challenges for evidence based physical therapy: Accessing and interpreting high quality evidence. *Physical Therapy, 84*, 644–654.

Marwick, C. (1997). Proponents gather to discuss practicing evidence-based medicine. *Journal of the American Medical Association, 278*(7), 531–532.

Metcalfe, C., Lewin, R., Wisher, S., Perry, S., Bannigan, K., & Moffett, J. K. (2001). Barriers to implementing the evidence base in four NHS therapies: dieticians, occupational therapists, physiotherapists, speech and language therapists. *Physiotherapy, 87*(8), 433–441.

Metzler, M., & Metx, G. (2010). Analyzing the barriers and supports of knowledge translation using the PEO model. *Canadian Journal of Occupational Therapy, 77*(3), 151–158.

Muir Gray, J. A. (1997). *Evidence-based health care: How to make health policy and management decisions.* London, England: Churchill Livingstone.

Rosenberg, W., & Donald, A. (1995). Evidence-based medicine: An approach to clinical problem solving. *British Medical Journal, 310*(6987), 1122–1126.

Sackett, D. L., Haynes, R. B., & Tugwell, P. (1985). *Clinical epidemiology: A basic science for clinical medicine.* London, England: Little Brown.

Sackett, D. L., Rosenberg, W. M., Gray, J. A., Haynes, R. B., & Richardson, W. S. (1996). Evidence-based medicine: What it is and what it isn't. *British Medical Journal, 312*(7023), 71–72.

Sudsawad, P. (2005). A conceptual framework to increase usability of outcome research for evidence-based practice. *American Journal of Occupational Therapy, 59*(3), 351–355.

Tse, S., Lloyd, C., Penman, M., King, R., & Bassett, H. (2004). Evidence-based practice and rehabilitation: Occupational therapy in Australia and New Zealand experiences. *International Journal of Rehabilitation Research, 227*, 269–274.

Upton, D., & Upton, P. (2006). Knowledge and use of evidence based practice by allied health and health scientist professionals in the United Kingdom. *Journal of Allied Health, 35*, 127–133.

SUGGESTED READING

Cook, D. J., & Levy, M. M. (1998). Evidence-based medicine: A tool for enhancing critical care practice. *Critical Care Clinics, 14*(3), 353–358.

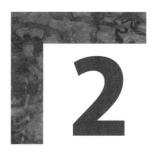

DEVELOPMENT OF EVIDENCE-BASED KNOWLEDGE

Winnie Dunn, PhD, OTR, FAOTA and Jill E. Foreman, BP, BHScOT

LEARNING OBJECTIVES

After reading this chapter, the student/practitioner will be able to:

- Recognize and understand the multiple levels at which knowledge develops within a discipline.
- Define the different periods of development for the practitioner and explain the corresponding relationship with the development of knowledge.
- Understand the subsequent responsibilities and challenges of the practitioner as an individual, a member of a discipline, and a representative of a discipline.
- Understand the challenges in developing evidence for practice.

INTRODUCTION

It is easy to believe that the knowledge of a particular discipline has been there for all time, was established quickly by experts who were defining the discipline, and was carried forth by all subsequent generations as stable and clear factors that characterize the discipline's perspectives and work. With this belief, persons would only have to acquire the knowledge, skills, and viewpoints of the discipline so that they can use the information and then pass it along, with little need for ongoing reevaluation.

Therapists have long recognized the need for ongoing development of knowledge, skills, and associated professional reasoning. For example, high participation rates in continuing education and peer consultation are most commonly used by rehabilitation therapists as a means of gathering and implementing new knowledge (Rappolt & Tassone, 2002).

In fact, knowledge develops at many levels within one's own discipline and in concert with other disciplines that are interested in similar ideas. Additionally, as each new insight emerges, people have the opportunity to understand their profession in a new way and to consider what new dilemmas this insight reveals. There are many issues that people cannot even conceive are present until certain other knowledge becomes clear to them.

Law M., & MacDermid, J. C.
*Evidence-Based Rehabilitation: A Guide
to Practice, Third Edition* (pp 15–35).
© 2014 SLACK Incorporated.

Knowledge is a collection of ideas and facts about a topic. People tend to say that they have knowledge when information and ideas have stood the test of time and experience. *Evidence* is information that makes a conclusion apparent, and it is the accumulation of these conclusions that leads to new insights. The accumulation of evidence typically advances knowledge in a particular area, and knowledge, in turn, introduces other possibilities for gathering evidence. Although people generally refer to formal research as evidence for professional practice, in actuality each professional act provides evidence that accumulates into that professional's knowledge base.

An Example

It was standard practice in the United States during the early 1900s to institutionalize persons with disabilities (i.e., people with disabilities were housed in large government-funded facilities and the staff provided basic care for their survival). This practice was based on the belief that persons who were mentally or physically deficient could not contribute and could not care for themselves; therefore, they need to be isolated from society and cared for.

People then began to demonstrate that individuals with disabilities could learn. This insight led people to question their beliefs about individuals with disabilities: Could these individuals take care of themselves and contribute to society? People began to consider what the possibilities were for persons who could learn; they had to reconsider the standard practice of institutionalization, which by its very nature kept people with disabilities from participating in certain activities including contributing to society and learning to care for themselves. Some members of society began to press for persons with disabilities to be moved out of institutions so that they could become members of communities and realize their potential (i.e., the deinstitutionalization movement).

Deinstitutionalization operationalized the knowledge about persons with disabilities having the potential to learn and, therefore, the possibility to contribute to society. When communities began to move people out of institutions, everyone realized that the communities did not have the infrastructure in place to support these new community members. Communities needed housing for all these persons; this issue had been irrelevant when people with disabilities were housed in large institutions. The community members who had worked in the institutions were now displaced from their work, creating an economic shift in the community. Communities were certainly able to tackle these challenges, but prior to deinstitutionalization there was no opportunity to see these issues; therefore, there was no opportunity to develop knowledge. As each insight occurred, other opportunities for insight presented themselves.

A century later, we see that those who had the courage to challenge institutionalization beliefs and practices began a process of changing services for persons with disabilities forever. In fact, there is a current movement led by people with various conditions (such as autism spectrum disorders) to reject the notion that anything is wrong with them. The movement asserts that people who have a different lived experience and unique interests have something to contribute that no one else can.

Those who provided institutional care could not have conceived of some of our current practices (e.g., buildings that are accessible to everyone) because they did not think about the idea that people with disabilities have unique contributions to make to our communities. This is the nature of knowledge development; that which is inconceivable today becomes accepted practice decades later. It reminds us to ask ourselves what we might be stuck on and what might be possible if we stay open to possibilities.

Evidence-based knowledge serves a generative function in the evolution of information for practice. It invites us to simultaneously gain insight to solve a current problem and see the dilemmas that are only visible from the next vantage point.

PURPOSE

The purpose of this chapter is to introduce the ways in which evidence-based knowledge develops within a discipline. Primarily, there are three vantage points for knowledge development. First, the individual professional travels through a developmental process beginning with preservice educational preparation and continuing through the "expert" phase of the professional career path. Second, professionals develop and share information with each other within their own disciplines. Finally, professionals develop and share information across disciplines to inform a wider circle of thinkers. We will discuss each of these in turn and consider what our responsibilities are in the development of evidence-based knowledge.

THE INDIVIDUAL PROFESSIONAL'S RESPONSIBILITIES

Individual professionals are responsible for facilitating knowledge development as insights emerge in daily practice. In order to accomplish this, professionals must first develop awareness of their own beliefs. It is essential to recognize that knowledge is not a prerequisite for a belief (Quine & Ullian, 1978). Beliefs emerge from experiences, viewpoints of those we trust, and sociocultural influences. Awareness of individual beliefs is important because beliefs form a filter through which professionals view and therefore interpret events and information. When beliefs are undefined, professionals are unaware of the reasons for their choices in practice (i.e., they act on interpretations that are guided surreptitiously by their beliefs), masking alternative interpretations.

For example, therapists may believe in the benefits of a therapeutic modality based on practice experience and a mentor's fervor for the method, though scientific knowledge of how the modality works may be scarce. Conductive education techniques are an example of this. Conductive education has been used with children who have cerebral palsy, although there is little evidence to support its efficacy (Bairstow, Cochrane, & Rusk, 1991; Bochner, Center, Chapparo, & Donelly, 1999; Darrah, Watkins, Chen, & Bonin, 2004; Lonton & Russell, 1989; Reddihough, King, Coleman, & Catanese, 1998). Similarly, manual therapy is an area of physical therapy practice in which practitioners have strong beliefs in hands-on techniques that are commonly passed on by "gurus," frequently before adequate evidence is in place to support their use. Therapists have a belief in the power of movement, hands-on treatment, and therapeutic interaction and have experienced changes in their patients with these types of interventions. Therefore, they have a predisposition toward believing that these techniques are effective, even when research is sparse and varied. Reddihough et al. (1998) studied 34 children with cerebral palsy and found that those receiving conductive education made progress similar to that of children in alternative intervention groups. Bochner et al. (1999) reported that results of conductive education were quite variable with children who have motor disabilities, with some children showing no changes and others learning specific motor skills; however, they also cited lack of generalization of skills as a problem. A recent systematic review by Antilla, Suoranta, Malmivaara, Makela, and Autti-Ramo (2008) found insufficient evidence for the effectiveness of conductive education intervention in comprehensive therapy programs but found some supporting evidence for strength training and constraint-induced movement therapy. Systematic reviews on the use of manual therapy for neck pain indicate that manual therapy is less effective when used alone as compared to exercise, which has the larger impact (Gross et al., 2002).

The example of conductive education and other therapies that have been embraced within rehabilitation without adequate supporting evidence illustrates what Quine and Ullian (1978) described: "The intensity of a belief cannot be counted on to reflect its supporting evidence" (p. 7). When developing evidence-based practice (EBP), professionals must remain aware of the power of personal beliefs, be open to identifying the source and nature of the beliefs, and be willing to search for evidence-based knowledge to inform their practice techniques separate from their personal beliefs. Many professional practices begin with an experienced professional acting out a hunch; this willingness to discover new possibilities is appropriate as long as we take the next steps to evaluate effectiveness.

Evaluating effectiveness is the second responsibility for professionals (Feyerbend, 1993). The ability to continually question current information and seek new answers is often described as life-long learning for the individual; this process forms the basis of EBP for the profession. Developing knowledge about how to search for and critically appraise research studies is an important skill for all rehabilitation practitioners. In the absence of such knowledge, evaluating the outcomes of intervention for each person receiving services is vital. This idea is discussed in more detail later in this section.

The third responsibility is a willingness to use information to abandon ineffective methods and/ or erroneous ideas and beliefs in favor of more effective options. This responsibility is challenging to fulfill because it requires professionals to entertain the possibility that their particular framework for thinking and problem solving needs adjustment. Beliefs and conceptual frameworks are inter-woven; if one's framework does not change, the beliefs within that framework will be difficult to alter (Kuhn, 1996).

For example, rehabilitation professionals educated within a medically based framework may have difficulty abandoning the belief that doing something to or for the patient is best as part of the "pro-fessional as expert" conceptual framework. A client-centered framework suggests that professionals collaborate with the client and family, and it has been shown to be an effective approach (Dunst, 2002; Dunst, Deal, & Trivette, 1996; Rosenbaum, King, Law, King, & Evans, 1998). However, it requires professionals to reconstruct their beliefs to acknowledge the client and family as active participants in planning.

To meet the responsibility of knowledge development for EBP, professionals must also share their emerging insights and broader beliefs with others. Open dialogue and the ability to request feedback in practice encourages the development of efficacious practices. It enables professionals to remain flexible in their approach to practice challenges and facilitates ongoing improvement in practice (Feyerbend, 1993).

Finally, professionals must participate in activities that are effective in their practices. In order to implement effective practices, professionals must conduct critical reviews of the literature, par-ticipate in quality reviews, and/or participate in formal data collection activities. Vigilance in col-lecting data enables patterns to emerge, hypotheses to be tested, and decisions to be made based on information actually available within the practice. There is potential to gather evidence-based data for a variety of audiences (e.g., for the professional's own practice, for the discipline, for the consumer, for the payer). With each audience, the evidence is gathered as a means of convincing the professionals that interventions are effective, providing support for the viability of the discipline, demonstrating changes to consumers, and/or convincing payers that they are using their resources to purchase valuable services.

In summary, several personal responsibilities that facilitate professional knowledge development that we have highlighted, including awareness of personal beliefs, evaluating the effectiveness of current practices, maintaining open dialogue and feedback regarding current practices, and partici-pating in activities, will enhance current practice. Although several personal responsibilities exist, it is important to acknowledge that professionals do not practice in isolation. Responsibilities also exist beyond the individual to include the health care profession, the organization or institution, and the interdisciplinary team to support the acquisition and implementation of knowledge develop-ment within the health care system (Hannes et al., 2005; Ketefian, 2001; Reimer, Sawka, & James, 2005). These influences will be explored further when we examine the challenges in developing evidence in practice.

Table 2-1
Professional Knowledge Development
PRESERVICE EXPERIENCES
• Becomes aware of own beliefs and learns initial strategies for questioning beliefs.
NOVICE PROFESSIONAL PERIOD
• Begins to generalize ideas, determine effective and ineffective methods for practice, and test knowledge and beliefs.
EXPERIENCED PROFESSIONAL PERIOD
• Establishes methods for evaluating effectiveness, hypothesizes successful therapeutic techniques, and shares with colleagues.
EXPERT PROFESSIONAL PERIOD
• Participates in formal methods of collecting data and evaluating interventions, shares knowledge more globally, and critiques the work of others.

Phases of Professional Development

Professionals do not leave their educational preparation and enter work fully equipped to meet all of the responsibilities of serving as evidence-based professionals. The course of one's career affords different possibilities (Table 2-1).

Preservice Experiences

The preservice experience occurs while students learn the knowledge and skills necessary to practice once their educational preparation is complete. Through preservice experiences, students learn the knowledge base of the discipline and are exposed to the available evidence for current interventions. In this initial stage, the professional learns how to use the available evidence to construct preliminary professional reasoning strategies and decision-making guides. The knowledge development for preservice students occurs within the current thought paradigms of the discipline, thereby focusing learning to include current knowledge and evidence (Kuhn, 1996; Schell, 1998; Schell & Schell, 2007). Preservice professionals meet the first and second responsibilities of becoming evidence-based professionals (i.e., they become aware of their beliefs and learn initial strategies for questioning those beliefs in the interest of effectiveness).

Novice Professional Period

The novice professional period usually occurs within the first 5 years of practice. In the novice period, professionals learn how others apply knowledge and evaluate evidence. Novice professionals try ideas and evaluate their effectiveness in individual situations. It is during this period of development that professionals begin to generalize ideas across peoples and settings and determining effective and ineffective methods for practice, thus building a resource of professional experiences that guide future decisions. The novice professional period provides opportunities to test the knowledge and beliefs that professionals have acquired through educational preparation, thereby increasing clarity and generalizability of knowledge for practice. This period provides an opportunity for professional and organizational socialization in which the novice professional experiences the attitudes, values, and beliefs of the profession and the organization in which they work (P. A. Miller, Solomon, Giacomini, & Abelson, 2005; Solomon & Miller, 2005). This period forms the foundation for understanding how professional reasoning occurs within the broader context of work environments.

Therefore, the novice professional period forms the foundation for professional reasoning as knowledge and personal beliefs, now grounded in experience, begin to merge. As the novice identifies challenges, the literature becomes a more functional tool for finding solutions for practice because the novice typically has a particular setting or population as a focus of the professional work.

Experienced Professional Period

The experienced professional period typically occurs within the second decade of practice. With further experience, professionals begin to create a personal "database" from all of their professional experiences and learning. The experienced professional period enables the individual to establish methods for evaluating the effectiveness of selected interventions based on their personal database (Feyerbend, 1993). Professionals working within particular settings will evaluate the effectiveness of therapeutic interventions on functional outcomes that clients achieve in that setting. The experienced professional is better able to hypothesize those therapeutic techniques that will be most successful for clients admitted with particular functional concerns due to the breadth and depth of the professional practice to inform these decisions. Experienced professionals make EBP decisions by weighing multiple factors including their practice context, their practice expertise, the knowledge of expert colleagues, the evidence from relevant literature, and their client's preferences (Wilkins, Jung, Wishart, Edwards, & Gamble-Norton, 2003).

There is also a risk during this period. Because professionals have their own experience to reflect on, it becomes easier to disregard new evidence from the literature, particularly if that evidence challenges current practices. As professionals generate evidence in practice, they also begin to share their personal "evidence" with other professionals; sharing facilitates the development of collective knowledge about effective practices. This collective knowledge can be shared in team meetings, focus groups, and professional conference presentations for specific areas of practice. These types of gatherings need to include published studies to keep everyone in a balanced state between practice insights and new evidence that becomes available.

Expert Professional Period

The expert professional period typically occurs after 2 decades of practice experience. In the expert professional period, professionals participate in more formal methods of collecting data and evaluating effectiveness of interventions. Professionals may solicit funding to conduct research within their service setting or population. For example, professionals may participate in a randomized controlled trial study to try to determine which of two intervention methods is most effective, or they may publish a case study to illustrate a client's experience with a particular disability. The knowledge gained through this research allows professionals to make findings more globally available to other professionals. When expert professionals share in more public forums, they can impact EBP knowledge development by demonstrating the importance of systematically evaluating practice. Experts can also offer to mentor less advanced colleagues. This period also includes critiquing the works and insights of others to advance knowledge for the discipline (Feyerbend, 1993; Quine & Ullian, 1978).

PROFESSIONALS WITHIN A DISCIPLINE

Just as in individual development, professionals within a discipline have collective responsibilities to contribute to evidence-based knowledge. These include challenging current beliefs, sharing information with colleagues, introducing new ideas, and formally testing hypotheses for their new ideas.

The growth of knowledge in a discipline is possible only when the members and interested others challenge current beliefs and theories. By challenging current theory, a discipline ensures thoroughness and refinement and fosters further development of knowledge. Knowledge development within a professional community requires its members to constantly push the limits imposed by current working paradigms. By encouraging professionals to participate in dialogues about how we understand current knowledge development, both the discipline and the individual professionals evolve (Feyerbend, 1993), creating a generative cycle.

Individuals within a discipline relate their practice knowledge base to theories of the profession. Theories within the profession guide practice decisions, and practice experiences, in turn, inform the theory. It is valuable to recognize the challenge that members have when they wish to introduce new ideas to a professional group with established theories that form the basis for research and communication within the profession. One may expect new ideas to be encouraged because new ideas serve to further develop professional knowledge. However, new ideas also challenge the foundation of current activities, which can be threatening to the stability of professional beliefs (Feyerbend, 1993).

Professionals within a discipline are responsible for designing and implementing formal methods for testing hypotheses that grow out of the practice–theory cycle. Professionals need to have current beliefs to begin with, but these ideas need to be challenged in some way to advance professional practice and, ultimately, refine the constructs and beliefs. Thus, tension between research and practice is inevitable and a necessary struggle for the advancement of knowledge (Quine & Ullian, 1978). For researchers to understand how to propose change, they must understand that issues arise in practices that seem contradictory to currently held beliefs. Schachter and Cohen (2005) suggested several factors that enhance the potential of a professional community to adopt a change in practice based on new evidence, including "an on-site champion, staff buy-in, a willingness to see systems change, and the availability of additional resources" (p. 1). New data can be generated to inform more advanced thinking, thus advancing the discipline's body of knowledge. How a professional community adopts or rejects innovative or controversial information determines its evolution and viability (Chinn & Brewer, 1993).

PROFESSIONALS ACROSS DISCIPLINES

Evidence-based knowledge development must also occur in collaboration with other disciplines that are interested in similar ideas. There are many professional practice problems that simply cannot be solved with a single discipline's perspective. When a variety of disciplines share knowledge, many more possibilities emerge. To enable the sharing of knowledge across disciplines, members of professional communities have several responsibilities.

First, professionals must remain open to other points of view. Collaboration among professionals requires teamwork with a desire to share and receive new ideas. Second, it is important to remain aware of how decisions made by a variety of disciplines may impact families and individuals being served. The paradigm of family-centered care provides a good example of this need for collaboration. Professionals employing this paradigm encourage and support family involvement regardless of the expertise of any particular discipline. For family-centered care to be effective, professionals need to identify the unique and complementary knowledge that will enable a family to act on their goals without creating undue burden on the family (e.g., an undue burden would be each discipline designing its own intervention plans, expecting the family to carry out all of them).

The third professional responsibility is to facilitate awareness about the similarities and differences in approaches to problem solving and knowledge development for each discipline. Clear communication between professionals about investigation approaches and methods ensures effective collaboration across disciplines. Awareness about similarities and differences may be enhanced through interdisciplinary training (Clark, 2004; Fertman, Dotson, Mazzocco, & Reitz, 2005;

Rodehorst, Wilhelm, & Jensen, 2005) and collaborative learning facilities (Moore, Vaughan, Hayes, & McLendon, 2005).

The fourth responsibility in advancing collective evidence-based knowledge among disciplines is to conduct collaborative research. Professionals can work together to design and implement formal methods for testing hypotheses that grow out of the interdisciplinary dialogue. Research can focus on problems that are best tested from an interdisciplinary perspective, which draws upon a range of theoretical frameworks, thereby resulting in a comprehensive perspective (Barbour & Barbour, 2003).

For example, several disciplines contribute to knowledge about barrier-free design (sometimes called *universal design* or *universal access;* see www.ncsu.edu/project/design-projects/udi). Individuals with backgrounds in occupational therapy, physiotherapy, architecture, interior design, environmental psychology, human ecology, and urban and regional planning all have knowledge and skills related to barrier-free design. The collective knowledge of these professionals expands the possible solutions for designing a barrier-free environment (Cooper, Cohen, & Hasselkus, 1991; Steinfeld & Shea, 1993).

Finally, professionals from across disciplines must recognize uncomfortable places as opportunities for knowledge development. It is naturally challenging for individuals with different theoretical paradigms to collaborate with each other; however, each discipline evolves from reflective feedback that colleagues from other disciplines can provide. The product of interdisciplinary collaboration can advance knowledge for each discipline and for collective knowledge in an area of interest.

CHALLENGES ASSOCIATED WITH DEVELOPING EVIDENCE FOR PRACTICE

The following are several different challenges in developing evidence for practice:
- Producing generalizable evidence
- Disseminating evidence in an accessible and relevant format
- Implementing evidence into practice

First, evidence needs to be generalizable to the professional's current practice environment. Consideration should be given to contextual factors including policy guidelines and the client's circumstances (Glasgow, Magid, Beck, Ritzwoller, & Estabrooks, 2005; Nananda, 2005). Second, disseminating evidence to maximize uptake by professionals requires that the evidence be accessible and relevant. Remaining current with EBP research requires professionals to be vigilant in seeking out evidence (Stegink-Jansen, 2002). Barriers to accessing evidence may include lack of time, lack of access to resources, or a lack of desire to enhance current knowledge and skills (Hannes et al., 2005). Therefore, evidence should be presented in a format that is efficient for the professional to digest and applicable to current practice.

Third, implementing evidence into current practice or "closing the gap between what is known and what is practiced" (Weaver, Warren, & Delaney, 2005) is a challenge faced across health care disciplines. This challenge exists within the larger context of the practice environment and includes the health care profession, the organization or institution, and the interdisciplinary team. Implementing evidence into practice requires the support of the practice environment (Hannes et al., 2005; Ketefian, 2001; Reimer et al., 2005) to seek out information and a willingness to change current practice if evidence supports this change. Rogers (1995) proposed that professionals need to identify the key players that are both early adopters of innovation and are well respected by the constituent groups to get groups to adopt new ideas. This means that professionals need to identify key leadership that can influence both administrative and staff in order to adopt new ideas.

An Example Illustrating the Contribution of Research and Evidence to Developing Evidence-Based Knowledge for Practice and Knowledge Development

All of the ideas presented in this chapter and throughout this book are platitudes if there is no evidence that knowledge development and evolution actually occur in these ways. Those of us who are further along on our professional journey have a sense of knowledge development from our own lived experiences, but it is inefficient for a discipline to rely on "living it" to see the power of knowledge development. As disciplines mature, we must be willing to conduct formal analyses of knowledge development; this not only includes the facts and data from studies but also the evolution of insights at each new point in the knowledge development process. Without scholars willing to wonder, muse, and hypothesize about the meaning of information, all of the data in the world would not advance knowledge. Additionally, we need practitioners who are open to new ideas and who question current practice so that hypotheses can be tested and refined.

We will highlight these principles using a powerful example from the occupational therapy (and related disciplines') literature: the development of knowledge about sensory integration. This area of knowledge development illustrates all levels of evolution: individual scholars moving from novice to expert, the discipline increasingly incorporating advanced knowledge into the collective thinking, the impact of occupational therapy's work on other disciplines' knowledge development, and the opportunity for occupational therapy to embrace alternative constructs as interdisciplinary knowledge and demands evolve.

Early Developments and Insights

Occupational and physical therapy have a long history of relying on neuroscience literature to guide thinking about assessment and intervention. Many early theorists have discussed the importance of nervous system operations for the production of adaptive human behaviors (Ayres, 1955; Blashy & Fuchs, 1959; Bobath & Bobath, 1955; Cruickshank, Bice, & Wallen, 1957; Fay, 1948; Rood, 1952). These scholars were peers in the 1950s so much of their work was interdependent. For this discussion, we shall focus specifically on the evolution of sensory integration knowledge, which has been primarily attributed to Dr. A. Jean Ayres.

Dr. Ayres was an occupational therapist and licensed clinical psychologist whose early thinking arose from her study of neuroscience during her doctoral and postdoctoral work (Sieg, 1988). She had experience working with children and adults with various central nervous system conditions (Cruickshank, 1974). Therefore, from an individual perspective, we would say that Dr. Ayres was in her experienced professional period (see Table 2-1). As you recall from earlier in the chapter, this means that she would have created a personal database for decision making and would be sharing her perspectives with others. She was also seeking formal doctoral and postdoctoral education at this time, foreshadowing her intent to enter the expert professional period.

Dr. Ayres was fascinated by what she observed in children with cerebral palsy and learning disabilities. She began to hypothesize about the nature of these children's performance difficulties based on her studies and her professional experiences. She emphasized visual motor functions and perceptual and proprioceptive facilitation to improve upper extremity function (Henderson, Llorens, Gilfoyle, Myers, & Prevel, 1974). She wrote several articles to share her ideas with others (Ayres, 1954, 1958, 1960, 1963), as most do in the experienced professional period.

At the discipline level, Dr. Ayres was generating an impact in two ways. First, she was beginning to change the course of occupational therapy thinking. Second, those in related disciplines who also had an interest in children's perceptual motor skills considered Dr. Ayres a visionary scholar. Dr. William Cruickshank (1974), a noted scholar of education and psychology and one of Dr. Ayres' peers, stated in a review of Dr. Ayres early work, "... the writings of Jean Ayres ... have been instrumental in setting new directions for a total discipline, or at least have directed the profession of occupational therapy in two areas that are historically and functionally different ... prior to 1955" (p. viii).

Testing Hypotheses to Gain New Perspectives

After publishing her ideas and insights on children's perceptual motor skills and completing her postdoctoral education, Dr. Ayres began to test her theoretical ideas with larger samples and sound measurement methods. These actions represent the expert professional period of her individual career path. She was quite prolific in writing during this period, reporting on her findings, interpreting the results in light of her own and the work of other scholars, and making more refined hypotheses for subsequent research.

In order to test some of the theoretical constructs, Dr. Ayres identified available methods and constructed some of her own methods of measuring children's sensory, perceptual, motor, and praxis abilities. In her 1965 article, "Patterns of Perceptual Motor Dysfunction in Children," she reported on the first of several factor analytic studies, a creative and insightful work for the time. Using data from 100 children with perceptual deficits and 50 typically developing children, Dr. Ayres hypothesized that there were five syndromes representing dysfunction: apraxia, tactile and visual perception, tactile defensiveness, bilateral integration, and poor figure–ground perception.

With this study and subsequent work to refine these patterns, Dr. Ayres began to validate theoretical constructs that would provide a specific focus for occupational therapy research for the next 5 decades and beyond. Simultaneously, this contribution has influenced work in related disciplines by informing them of occupational therapy's significant and unique contributions and advancing knowledge to their work as well.

Dr. Ayres continued to elucidate perceptual motor and sensory integrative constructs in a series of factor analytic studies (Ayres, 1965, 1966a, 1966b, 1969a, 1969b, 1971, 1972a, 1972b). She and colleagues standardized the Southern California Sensory Integrative Tests, which enabled professionals to identify specific types of sensory integrative performance problems (Ayres, 1989).

By 1972, Dr. Ayres had identified the following five types of sensory integrative dysfunction:

1. Visual/tactile/kinesthetic form and space perception
2. Motor planning and tactile perception
3. Tactile perception, hyperactivity, distractibility, and tactile defensiveness
4. Postural and ocular muscle control
5. Auditory language functions

She increasingly refined her measures in her studies so that she could illustrate these categories of performance problems with more clarity. Because she had demonstrated the presence of several of these factors across study populations, she spoke with more confidence about their integrity and applicability to assessment and intervention planning in practice situations. Dr. Ayres also conducted other studies to examine the effectiveness of interventions based on her hypotheses (Ayres, 1972a, 1976). These intervention studies informed therapists as to how they might apply her ideas in their practice.

The Second Generation Develops Insights

As Dr. Ayres traversed through her expert professional period, she was influencing many younger therapists with her ideas. The knowledge that Dr. Ayres developed and validated through her research moved into occupational therapy curricula as core knowledge, and sensory integration theory and practice became inherent in service planning for children. From this, we can see that the novice professional begins his or her journey with knowledge that an expert professional provided for the field. As these second-generation colleagues moved from their novice periods into their experienced professional periods, they began making and testing hypotheses of their own.

Armed with the tools that Dr. Ayres provided (i.e., the data, the tests, new knowledge, expert insights), occupational therapists serving children began to emphasize sensory integration factors when evaluating and designing intervention programs. Occupational therapy graduate students and scholars who were studying Dr. Ayres's work began to design and implement intervention studies to evaluate the effectiveness of a sensory integrative approach in therapy. (Note: Because our purpose here is to examine the knowledge development process and not provide a comprehensive review of this literature, please review Bundy, Lane, Fisher, and Murray [2002] for an in-depth reporting of the work during this period.)

As this next generation of professionals was moving from experienced professionals into their expert professional period, there was a prolific period for testing hypotheses and generating insights about the role of sensory integration in persons' performance. Dr. Ayres had provided such a rich foundation of ideas that what began as a few musings and insights had now become a whole body of ideas to consider. Because Dr. Ayres was so vigilant at disseminating her ideas in writing and in presentations (due to the fact that she was mentoring others), the possibility of advancing knowledge multiplied geometrically with this new cohort of novices emerging to experienced professionals. For example, Ottenbacher (1982) found 49 articles reporting on research about sensory integrative interventions. His meta-analysis revealed a positive effect for sensory integrative interventions, but only 8 of the articles met his criteria for inclusion in the review process. Other studies reported more equivocal results (Feagans, 1983; Ferry, 1981; Ottenbacher & Short-DeGraff, 1985), suggesting that further work still needed to be done to demonstrate the appropriate application of sensory integrative constructs for EBP.

Another important event in knowledge development at the discipline level occurred during this time. Because there was more information available about the constructs and application (both effective and ineffective) of sensory integration, scholars from other disciplines began to consume this knowledge with mixed results. For example, Arendt, MacLean, and Baumeister (1988) published a critique of sensory integration therapy as it might be applied to persons with mental retardation and reported that it would be inappropriate to apply these methods based on the available evidence. The editor recognized the provocative nature of this topic and invited five scholars in occupational therapy to respond to this article. The entire series of articles is published in one volume, providing an excellent example of scholarly discourse. From a knowledge development perspective, critiques such as these are not possible until knowledge has developed to the point that others can study it and consider their own perspective on the idea.

It was also during this period that scholars conducted clinical trials of sensory integration interventions (Humphries, Snider, & McDougall, 1993; Humphries, Wright, McDougall, & Vertes, 1990; Humphries, Wright, Snider, & McDougall, 1992; Kaplan, Polatajko, Wilson, & Faris, 1993; Polatajko, Kaplan, & Wilson, 1992; Polatajko, Law, Miller, Schaffer, & Macnab, 1991; Wilson & Kaplan, 1994; Wilson, Kaplan, Fellowes, Gruchy, & Faris, 1992). These research teams reported similar results (i.e., that sensory integration therapy was equally effective as other interventions [e.g., perceptual motor, tutoring, traditional interventions], not more effective at affecting sensorimotor outcomes, and that results on the impact of sensory integration on academic performance were equivocal).

These studies reflect the maturation of therapists' thinking about sensory integration and its increasing visibility in the larger professional arenas. There was more interest and pressure to demonstrate the usefulness of these new ideas. Those outside the "web of belief" were appropriately asking questions about the claims of effectiveness. It was time for researchers to study the nature and scope of sensory integration practices and for those in practice to understand when sensory integration interventions would be the appropriate or inappropriate choice to make. This process of refinement had an important impact on knowledge generation in that it illuminated the possible limitations of this knowledge for particular intervention practices. It is critical that both effective and ineffective methods become clear in the research; this establishes the parameters for proper use of knowledge and invites scholars to reconceptualize the nature and meaning of their constructs for use in practice and in subsequent research.

The "Renaissance Period"

So here we are more than 2 decades after all of this activity. We have another cohort of occupational therapy professionals who are in their experienced and expert professional periods, only this time they have been able to study not only the knowledge that Dr. Ayres provided but also all of the knowledge that the first cohort provided (who are now in their expert professional periods). This breadth of information and distance from the original seeds of knowledge provide a new vantage point for considering the ideas. Additionally, the culture of scholarly endeavors has matured, affording new tools and strategies for testing the fidelity of knowledge and the effectiveness of its application in practice.

Great things happened, as they do when knowledge has the time to settle in, and scholars can take a fresh look with new tools. Occupational therapy scholars who have been studying neuroscience and sensory integration knowledge added clarity to some of Dr. Ayres's original ideas, as well as proposed new ideas for consideration. As an indication of the available accumulating knowledge, L. Miller and Lane (2000) produced a three-part series of articles that provided a taxonomy of definitions related to sensory integration and sensory processing, inviting scholars to use consistent terms for this burgeoning body of knowledge.

As one example of knowledge being reformulated, Dr. Ayres discussed tactile defensiveness and gravitational insecurity as conditions in which the person was unable to tolerate touch and movement input, respectively (Ayres, 1972b). Researchers revisited one's inability to process sensory input as part of modulating the amount and type of information that a person might need for creating adaptive responses. They used the knowledge developed until then and applied contemporary methods of research to characterize sensory modulation as a range of responses to sensory events (Baranek, Foster, & Berkson, 1997; Dunn, 2000), thus broadening the original ideas and observations of this topic. We have also broadened ideas about the domain of study.

In the early years, sensory integration concepts and treatment methods were the focus of the research but, in more recent years, scholars have identified constructs that are more properly classified in the larger context of sensory processing. Though sensory integration is a component of sensory processing (i.e., the nervous system's capacity to process sensory input; L. Miller & Lane, 2000), the term *sensory processing* encompasses the application of broader neuroscience constructs to the human experience (i.e., the way in which the nervous system receives, modulates, integrates, and organizes incoming sensory information; L. Miller & Lane, 2000). Studies of children with poor coping skills (Williamson & Szczepanski, 1999), poor regulatory abilities (DeGangi, 2000), autism (Baranek et al., 1997; Kientz & Dunn, 1997), and fragile X syndrome (Belser & Sudhalter, 1995) provided evidence that a broader consideration was appropriate. Additionally, studies of intervention in natural settings (Case-Smith & Bryan, 1999; Kemmis & Dunn, 1996) have suggested that some of the findings of ineffectiveness of sensory integration interventions may be related to a too-narrow perspective.

With a broader perspective, it becomes imperative for scholars to conduct studies with scholars from other disciplines. Furthermore, scholars from other disciplines are finding sensory processing knowledge from the literature themselves and using knowledge from occupational therapy to inform their research programs.

For example, DeGangi, Sickel, Wiener, and Kaplan (1996) studied fussy babies by combining occupational therapy methods and psychophysiological methods and found that there are distinct patterns of performance, indicating hyperresponsivity to stimuli. Baranek et al. (1997) conducted a factor analysis of behaviors of children and adults with developmental disabilities and found two factors that both supported the idea of sensitivities to sensory input. L. Miller and colleagues (MacIntosh, Miller, Shyu, & Hagerman, 1999; L. Miller et al., 1998) have reported behavioral and psychophysiological data indicating poor sensory modulation in children with fragile X syndrome and identified a distinct pattern of performance they call *sensory modulation disorder*. Dunn and colleagues (Dunn, 1994; Dunn & Brown, 1997; Dunn & Westman, 1997; Ermer & Dunn, 1998; Kientz & Dunn, 1997) reported on distinct patterns of children's responses to sensory events in daily life based on disabilities such as autism and attention deficit–hyperactivity disorder (ADHD). Belser and Sudhalter (1995) found distinct arousal difficulties in children with fragile X syndrome when compared to children with autism and ADHD, and they hypothesized about their ability to modulate input for responding.

During the early part of the 21st century, other disciplines have taken a strong interest in sensory processing as an important factor in children's and adults' lives. Knowledge development about sensory processing has taken two paths. First, researchers have reported about more vulnerable populations, suggesting that sensory processing is a factor in the manifestation of the conditions and should be a consideration for both assessment and intervention planning. For example, researchers have reported about distinct patterns of sensory processing in adults with post-traumatic stress, bipolar disorder, schizophrenia, obsessive–compulsive disorder, and autism (Brown, Cromwell, Filion, Dunn, & Tollefson, 2002; Crane, Goddard, & Pring, 2009; Reike & Anderson, 2009). Researchers studying children have reported specific sensory processing patterns for those with feeding needs, autism spectrum, and atopic dermatitis (Ben-Sasson et al., 2009; Engel-Yeger et al., 2007; Nadon et al., 2011).

Second, sensory processing has entered into public knowledge. There is a growing awareness that sensory processing ideas, which began with studies about vulnerable populations, are actually applicable to everyone. For example, Engel-Yeger (2008) found a relationship between activity choices and sensory processing patterns in typical children. Engel-Yeger and Dunn (2011) found that levels of pain catastrophizing, and affect, are positively related to particular sensory processing patterns in typical adults. Others reported relationships between sensory patterns and core features of children who are gifted (Dunn, 2009a; Gere et al., 2009). Additionally, magazines such as *Newsweek*, *Time*, and *Cosmopolitan*; newspapers such as the *London Times*; and radio stations have carried articles about sensory patterns on people's behaviors (e.g., Ali, 2007; Heitman, 2008; Rix, 2007; Wallis, 2007). Summarizing knowledge for public consumption, books are available for the public as well (e.g., Dunn, 2007). Dr. Ayres would be so proud of this evolution of knowledge from her humble yet astute initial observations.

Contemporary Developments Illustrating Expert Interprofessional Discourse

In the last 10 years within occupational therapy, ideas of sensory integration and sensory processing have been diverging (Dunn, 2009b). Expert colleagues with a sensory integration focus emphasize person factors as the source of difficulties; intervention methods focus on highly specified therapy approaches to resolve the sensory integration difficulties. Some also advocate for a new diagnosis to identify people with sensory processing disorders. Expert colleagues have reviewed the intervention research on sensory integration and found it to be equivocal (Baranek, 2002; Pollock, 2009).

Experts from other disciplines are also weighing in on sensory integration. For example, Zimmer and Desch (2012) published a policy statement for the American Academy of Pediatrics about sensory integration therapies. They indicated that there is not a universally accepted framework for diagnosing sensory processing disorders and so recommended that their colleagues refrain from using this diagnosis. They went on to say that parents need to be informed about the limited and inconclusive research concerning the effectiveness of sensory integration therapy.

Expert colleagues with a sensory processing focus emphasize knowing how a person's sensory patterns interact with environmental or activity features to affect participation. Intervention methods emphasize making adjustments to environments and activities based on the person's sensory patterns to support the person's participation in daily life. This difference in emphasis reflects the belief that sensory processing concepts are a reflection of persons within their authentic lives; therefore, solutions to challenging situations are not focused on the person as disordered but rather on finding the best match between person and context. Experts with this focus embrace interdisciplinary research that indicates adjustments in authentic contexts and routines are effective methods for supporting functional outcomes (e.g., Dunst, Bruder, Trivette, & Hamby, 2006; King et al., 2003). By adding sensory processing knowledge to this evidence, professionals have more knowledge to inform intervention planning.

So we see that across more than 6 decades, the story evolves as the professionals evolve. Novices begin their journey on paths that have been forged by the experts that came before them. A young professional studying sensory information today begins in a very different place than Dr. Ayres did and so has new challenges to face. Dr. Ayres did not have the benefit of the last 60 years of discussion to inform her thinking. She was a pioneer, so it is likely that she would be coming up with pioneering ideas for this decade if she were doing her work now. Many more professionals are discussing these ideas because of her. With open minds and novices to forge ahead, who knows where these ideas will take us?

Personal Reflection—by Winnie Dunn

My professional development occurred during the periods I have briefly described. As a novice in 1972, I had the advantage of Dr. Ayres's work from the onset of my studies to be an occupational therapist. Looking back, I certainly had no idea that I, as a novice, was part of this new direction (as Dr. Cruickshank called it). I just thought of sensory integration as part of occupational therapy knowledge. At that time, the role of researcher was a distant and disconnected one from practice. I certainly began to realize the power of this knowledge evolution as I attended workshops and studied. If someone had told me then that I would be contributing to this body of knowledge, I would have laughed and dismissed the comment. That is the way of novices—we do not have insight about the impact we have on others and ourselves; nevertheless, the impact occurs.

For me, it was the plague of a practice dilemma for which I could not find an answer in my books and references that pressed me toward insight. I was completely focused on solving my dilemma without any awareness that this was the beginning of my research career. It was many years later that I was able to identify the beginning of my "researcher self."

In the last few years, as I have studied sensory processing and developed sensory profile tools for research and practice, I came upon some of my work pages from my novice period. I found a diagram I had been trying to formulate that contained the same constructs that I reported in an article in 1997 (Dunn, 1997). What strikes me is that it took me more than 20 years to achieve clarity about these ideas; yet, it also strikes me that I had these ideas more than 20 years ago!

It is also exciting to see the interprofessional discourse that is taking place today. We used to be obscure as a discipline, but now people from many disciplines refer to our literature, use our tools and ideas to inform their work, and have new perspectives for us to consider. The journey from novice to expert, from an obscure discipline to one that is in the limelight, is part of this process we have been discussing in this chapter. Remaining open to the journey is the perennial test of whether an individual professional and a collective discipline will thrive.

I relay this experience because novices can get discouraged, feeling that they will never learn and know what their mentors do. I invite you to be aware of the raw material ideas you produce during your novice period; perhaps we need to plant those seeds early so that we can release them to the public at a later date. Pay attention to your own development and how it affects you, the persons you serve, and your profession. Yes, you affect knowledge development with every action you take. Experts are sometimes encumbered by their own history, making it difficult to see knowledge in a new way; in the role of the novice entering the world of knowledge development, you serve as the reminder that the process is unfolding as it should.

CONCLUSION

In this chapter, we considered how knowledge develops. There are simultaneous activities occurring that enable knowledge to emerge and evolve. Professionals develop along their respective career paths, profiting from the work that has come before them and gathering their own information and insights along the way. As individuals in a profession gather and discuss their ideas, collective insights form as hypotheses that can be formulated and tested. As data become available, professionals reformulate their hypotheses and gain new insights. Interdisciplinary discourse also advances knowledge by adding perspectives to evolving ideas. These are the processes that occur to produce evidence for practice.

There is still much to discover about the nature of rehabilitation interventions and their appropriate application in practice. With the wealth of colleagues attending to this body of knowledge, there is no doubt that this journey will continue and be a fruitful source of knowledge development. It is through the persistent processes of professionals moving from novice to expert and disciplines evolving that this will occur.

TAKE-HOME MESSAGES

✓ Knowledge develops at many different levels—simultaneously within a discipline and in collaboration with other disciplines.

✓ The tension between practice and knowledge development is inevitable and acts in a positive way as the source for the advancement of knowledge.

✓ The role of the individual professional within a discipline area passes through four distinct stages: preservice experience, novice professional period, experienced professional period, and expert professional period. Knowledge, skill, and professional reasoning evolve through these stages.

✓ An understanding of how knowledge develops must include recognition of the three different vantage points for knowledge (individual professional, professional within a discipline, and professionals across disciplines).

✓ Novices can enact a positive influence on knowledge development by becoming aware of their research selves, choosing a methodical and critical approach to finding and implementing new knowledge, and encouraging new ideas.

✓ There are different responsibilities for the practitioner in each of the three different vantage points for the development of knowledge:

Individual Professional

• Remaining aware of the influence of one's own personal beliefs/biases.

• Evaluating effectiveness through questioning current information and seeking answers.

• Willingness to use this information to abandon ineffective practices.

Professional Within a Discipline

- Challenging current beliefs and sharing information with colleagues.
- Introducing new ideas and formally testing hypotheses.

Professionals Across Disciplines

- Conducting research collaboratively and being open to other points of view.
- Remaining aware of how decisions are being made by a variety of disciplines, because this may impact families/clients.
- Facilitating awareness of various approaches to problem solving between disciplines.
- Recognizing that there are several challenges in developing evidence in rehabilitation: producing generalizable evidence, evidence dissemination, and the implementation of evidence into practice.

LEARNING AND EXPLORATION ACTIVITIES

The purpose of this chapter is to introduce the different vantage points at which knowledge develops and to demonstrate how these levels interact in practice.

1. Select one of the following topics of rehabilitation practice that interests you:

    a. Treatment of acute low back pain

    b. Outcomes of medical versus stroke units for person experiencing a stroke

    c. Home-based treatment for persons with arthritis

    d. School-based treatment for children with cerebral palsy

    e. Community reintegration for persons with schizophrenia

2. Complete the following activities for the topic you have selected:

    a. Using your current knowledge and a literature search, construct a preliminary professional reasoning strategy to guide treatment and practice for this topic area. Focus on what you know as a student and the elements of practice that should be put into place based on the evidence that you find.

    b. Interview a practitioner in the same topic area. Ask him or her to tell you about his or her professional reasoning strategy to guide practice.

    c. Compare the results of what you found and what you discussed with the practitioner. Are the two approaches congruent? If not, what are the differences? Why might these differences occur, and how do they relate to the development of knowledge in rehabilitation practice?

3. Three arms of knowledge development within professions contribute to EBP: the individual professional's path, intradisciplinary development, and interdisciplinary development. Think of an example in current practice. How will each of these arms address the issue in order to contribute to EBP?

4. Think of a population with which you have already worked or a population that you are interested in working with in the future (e.g., children with cerebral palsy, older adults with dementia, teenagers with eating disorders). List any assumptions or personal beliefs that you carry about that population. How will these beliefs affect your use of the evidence surrounding this population? How may they affect intradisciplinary development? Interdisciplinary development?

REFERENCES

Ali, L. (2007). You and your quirky kid. *Newsweek* (Pacific Edition). Published 9/24/2007; 150(13):38.

Antiila, H., Suoranta, J., Malmivaara, A., Makela, M., & Autti-Ramo, I. (2008). Effectiveness of physiotherapy and conductive education interventions in children with cerebral palsy: A focused review. *American Journal of Physical Medicine & Rehabilitation, 87*(6), 478–501.

Arendt, R., MacLean, W., & Baumeister, A. (1988). Critique of sensory integration therapy and its application in mental retardation. *American Journal on Mental Retardation, 92*, 401–411.

Ayres, A. J. (1954). Ontogenetic principles in the development of arm and hand functions. *American Journal of Occupational Therapy, 8*(3), 95–99, 121.

Ayres, A. J. (1955). Proprioceptive facilitation elicited through the upper extremities: Part 3: Special applications to occupational therapy. *American Journal of Occupational Therapy, 9*(3), 121–126.

Ayres, A. J. (1958). The visual motor function. *American Journal of Occupational Therapy, 12*(3), 130–138.

Ayres, A. J. (1960). Occupational therapy for motor disorders resulting from impairment of the central nervous system. *Rehabilitation Literature, 21*, 302–310.

Ayres, A. J. (1963). The development of perceptual motor abilities: A theoretical basis for treatment of dysfunction. *American Journal of Occupational Therapy, 17*(6), 221–225.

Ayres, A. J. (1965). Patterns of perceptual motor dysfunction in children. *Perception and Motor Skills, 20*, 335–368.

Ayres, A. J. (1966a). Interrelations among perceptual motor abilities in a group of normal children. *American Journal of Occupational Therapy, 20*(6), 288–292.

Ayres, A. J. (1966b). Interrelationships among perceptual motor functions in children. *American Journal of Occupational Therapy, 20*(2), 68–71.

Ayres, A. J. (1969a). Deficits in sensory integration in educationally handicapped children. *Journal of Learning Disabilities, 2*, 160–168.

Ayres, A. J. (1969b). Relation between Gesell development quotients and later perceptual motor performance. *American Journal of Occupational Therapy, 23*(1), 11–17.

Ayres, A. J. (1971). Characteristics of types of sensory integrative dysfunction. *American Journal of Occupational Therapy, 25*(7), 329–334.

Ayres, A. J. (1972a). Improving academic scores through sensory integration. *Journal of Learning Disabilities, 5*, 338–343.

Ayres, A. J. (1972b). Types of sensory integrative dysfunction among disabled learners. *American Journal of Occupational Therapy, 26*(1), 13–18.

Ayres, A. J. (1976). *The effect of sensory integrative therapy on learning disabled children: The final report of a research project*. Los Angeles, CA: University of Southern California.

Ayres, A. J. (1989). Sensory Integration and Praxis Tests. Los Angeles: Western Psychological Services.

Bairstow, P., Cochrane, R., & Rusk, I. (1991). Selection of children with cerebral palsy for conductive education and the characteristics of children judged suitable and unsuitable. *Developmental Medicine & Child Neurology, 33*(11), 941–942.

Baranek, G. T. (2002) Efficacy of sensory and motor interventions for children with autism. *Journal of Autism and Developmental Disorders, 32*(5):397-422.

Baranek, G., Foster, L., & Berkson, G. (1997). Sensory defensiveness in persons with developmental disabilities. *Occupational Therapy Journal of Research, 17*(3), 173–185.

Barbour, R. S., & Barbour, M. (2003). Evaluating and synthesizing qualitative research: The need to develop a distinctive approach. *Journal of Evaluation in Clinical Practice, 9*(2), 179–186.

Belser, R., & Sudhalter, V. (1995). Arousal difficulties in males with fragile X syndrome: A preliminary report. *Developmental Brain Dysfunction, 8*, 270–279.

Ben-Sasson, A., L. Hen, L, Fluss, R., Cermak, S. Engel-Yeger, B, & Gal, E. (2009). A meta-analysis of sensory modulation symptoms in individuals with autism spectrum disorders. *Journal of Autism and Developmental Disorders, 39*(1), 1–11.

Blashy, M., & Fuchs, R. (1959). Orthokinetics: A new receptor facilitation method. American *Journal of Occupational Therapy, 13*(5), 226–234.

Bobath, K., & Bobath, B. (1955). Tonic reflexes and righting reflexes in the diagnosis and assessment of cerebral palsy. *Cerebral Palsy Review, 16*(5), 4–10.

Bochner, S., Center, Y., Chapparo, C., & Donelly, M. (1999). How effective are programs based on conductive education? A report of two studies. *Journal of Intellectual and Developmental Disability, 24*(3), 227–242.

Brown, T., Cromwell, R., Filion, D., Dunn, W., & Tollefson, N. (2002). Sensory processing in schizophrenia: Missing and avoiding information. *Schizophrenia Research, 55*(1–2), 187–195.

Bundy, A., Lane, S., Fisher, A., & Murray, E. (2002). *Sensory integration theory and practice*. Philadelphia, PA: F.A. Davis Company.

Case-Smith, J., & Bryan, T. (1999). The effects of occupational therapy with sensory integration emphasis on preschool-age children with autism. *American Journal of Occupational Therapy, 53*(5), 489–497.

Chinn, C., & Brewer, W. (1993). The role of anomalous data in knowledge acquisition: A theoretical framework and implications for science instruction. *Review of Educational Research, 63*(1), 1–49.

Clark, P. G. (2004). Institutionalizing interdisciplinary health professions programs in higher education: The implications of one story and two laws. *Journal of Interprofessional Care, 18*(3), 251–261.

Cooper, B. A., Cohen, U., & Hasselkus, B. R. (1991). Barrier-free design: A review and critique of the occupational therapy perspective. *American Journal of Occupational Therapy, 45*(4), 344–350.

Crane, L., Goddard, L., & Pring, L. (2009). Sensory processing in adults with autism spectrum disorders. *Autism, 13*(215), 215–228.

Cruickshank, W. (1974). Foreword. In A. Henderson, L. Llorens, E. Gilfoyle, C. Myers, & S. Prevel (Eds.), *The development of sensory integrative theory and practice: A collection of the works of A. Jean Ayres*. Dubuque, IA: Kendall/Hunt Publishing.

Cruickshank, W., Bice, H., & Wallen, N. (1957). *Perception and cerebral palsy*. Syracuse, NY: Syracuse University Press.

Darrah, J., Watkins, B., Chen, L., & Bonin, C. (2004). Conductive education intervention for children with cerebral palsy: An AACPDM evidence report. *Developmental Medicine and Child Neurology, 46*(3), 187–203.

DeGangi, G. (2000). *Pediatric disorders of regulation in affect and behavior: A therapist's guide to assessment and treatment*. San Diego, CA: Academic Press.

DeGangi, G., Sickel, R., Wiener, A., & Kaplan, E. (1996). Fussy babies: To treat or not to treat? *British Journal of Occupational Therapy, 59*(10), 457–464.

Dunn, W. (1994). Performance of typical children on the sensory profile: An item analysis. *American Journal of Occupational Therapy, 48*(11), 967–974.

Dunn, W. (1997). A conceptual model for considering the impact of sensory processing abilities on the daily lives of young children and their families. *Infants and Young Children, 9*(4), 23–35.

Dunn, W. (2000). The sensations of everyday life: Empirical, theoretical, and pragmatic considerations. *American Journal of Occupational Therapy, 55*(6), 608–620.

Dunn, W. (2007). *Living sensationally: Understanding your senses*. London, England: Jessica Kingsley Publications.

Dunn, W. (2009a). Invited commentary on sensory sensitivities in gifted children. *American Journal of Occupational Therapy, 63*(3), 296–300.

Dunn, W. (2009b). *Sensory processing concepts and applications in practice*. Continuing Education on CD series. Bethesda, MD: American Occupational Therapy Association.

Dunn, W., & Brown, C. (1997). Factor analysis on the sensory profile from a national sample of children without disabilities. *American Journal of Occupational Therapy, 51*, 490–495.

Dunn, W., & Westman, K. (1997). The sensory profile: The performance of a national sample of children without disabilities. *American Journal of Occupational Therapy, 51*, 25–34.

Dunst, C. J. (2002). Family-centered practices: Birth through high school. *Journal of Special Education, 36*(3), 139–147.

Dunst, C. J., Deal, A. G., & Trivette, C. M. (1996). *Supporting & strengthening families: Methods, strategies and practices* (Vol. 1). Cambridge, MA: Brookline Books.

Dunst, C. J., Bruder, M. B., Trivette, C. M., & Hamby, D. W. (2006). Everyday activity settings, natural learning environments, and early intervention practices. *Journal of Policy and Practice in Intellectual Disabilities, 3*, 3–10.

Engel-Yeger, B. (2008). Sensory processing patterns and daily activity preferences of Israeli children. *Canadian Journal of Occupational Therapy, 75*(4), 220–229.

Engel-Yeger, B., & Dunn, W. (2011). Relationship between pain catastrophizing level and sensory processing patterns in typical adults. *American Journal of Occupational Therapy, 65*, 1–10.

Engel-Yeger, B., Habib-Mazawi, S., Parush, S., Rozenman, D., Kessel, A., & Shani-Adir, A. (2007). The sensory profile of children with atopic dermatitis as determined by the sensory profile questionnaire. *Journal of the American Academy of Dermatology, 57*(4), 610–615.

Ermer, J., & Dunn, W. (1998). The sensory profile: A discriminant analysis of children with and without disabilities. *American Journal of Occupational Therapy, 52*(4), 283–290.

Fay, T. (1948). The neurophysical aspects of therapy in cerebral palsy. *Archives of Physical Medicine, 29*(6), 327–334.

Feagans, L. (1983). A current view of learning disabilities. *Journal of Pediatrics, 102*(4), 487–493.

Ferry, P. C. (1981). On growing new neurons: Are early intervention programs effective? *Pediatrics, 67*(1), 38–41.

Fertman, C. I., Dotson, S., Mazzocco, G. O., & Reitz, S. M. (2005). Challenges of preparing allied health professionals for interdisciplinary practice in rural areas. *Journal of Allied Health, 34*(3), 163–168.

Feyerbend, P. (1993). *Against method* (3rd ed.). London, England: Verso.

Gere, D., Capps, S., et al. (2009). Sensory sensitivities of gifted children. *American Journal of Occupational Therapy, 63*(3), 288–295.

Glasgow, R. E., Magid, D. J., Beck, A., Ritzwoller, D., & Estabrooks, P. A. (2005). Practical clinical trials for translating research to practice: Design and measurement recommendations. *Medical Care, 43*(6), 551–557.

Gross, A. R., Kay, T. M, Kennedy, C., Gasner, D., Hurley, L., Yardley, K., et al. (2002). Clinical Practice guidelines on the use of manipulation or mobilization in the treatment of adults with mechanical neck disorders. *Manual Therapy, 7*(4), 193–205.

Hannes, K., Leys, M., Vermeire, E., Aertgeerts, B., Buntinx, F., & Depoorter, A. M. (2005). Implementing evidence-based medicine in general practice: A focus group based study. *BMC Family Practice, 9*, 6–37.

Heitman, B. (2009). Max out your postsex bliss. *Cosmopolitan*. December 2009. Available at: www.cosmo.ph/sex/mattress-moves/11-ways-to-max-out-your-postsex-bliss. Accessed October 7, 2013.

Henderson, A., Llorens, L., Gilfoyle, E., Myers, C., & Prevel, S. (1974). *The development of sensory integrative theory and practice: A collection of the works of A. Jean Ayres.* Dubuque, IA: Kendall/Hunt Publishing.

Humphries, T., Snider, L., & McDougall, B. (1993). Clinical evaluation of the effectiveness of sensory integrative and perceptual motor therapy in improving sensory integrative function in children with learning disabilities. *Occupational Therapy Journal of Research, 13*(3), 163–182.

Humphries, T., Wright, M., McDougall, B., & Vertes, J. (1990). The efficacy of sensory integration therapy for children with learning disability. *Physical and Occupational Therapy in Pediatrics, 10*(3), 1–17.

Humphries, T., Wright, M., Snider, L., & McDougall, B. (1992). A comparison of the effectiveness of sensory integrative therapy and perceptual-motor training in treating children with learning disabilities. *Journal of Developmental Behavior and Pediatrics, 13*(1), 31–40.

Kaplan, B. J., Polatajko, H. J., Wilson, B. N., & Faris, P. D. (1993). Reexamination of sensory integration treatment: A combination of two efficacy studies. *Journal of Learning Disabilities, 26*(5), 342–347.

Kemmis, B., & Dunn, W. (1996). Collaborative consultation: The efficacy of remedial and compensatory interventions in school contexts. *American Journal of Occupational Therapy, 50*(9), 709–717.

Ketefian, S. (2001). Issues in the application of research to practice. *Revista Latino-Americana de Enfermagem, 9*(5), 7–12.

Kientz, M., & Dunn, W. (1997). A comparison of the performance of children with and without autism on the sensory profile. *American Journal of Occupational Therapy, 51*(7), 530–537.

King, G., Law, M., King, S., Rosenbaum, P., Kertoy, M., & Young, N. (2003). A conceptual model of factors affecting the recreation and leisure participation of children with disabilities. *Physical & Occupational Therapy in Pediatrics, 23*(1), 63–90.

Kuhn, T. (1996). *The structure of scientific revolutions* (3rd ed.). Chicago, IL: University of Chicago Press.

Lonton, A. P., & Russell, A. (1989). Conductive education—Magic or myth? *Zeitschrift für Kinderchirurgie, 44*(Suppl. 1), 21–23.

MacIntosh, D., Miller, L., Shyu, V., & Hagerman, R. (1999). Sensory modulation disruption, electrodermal responses, and functional behaviors. *Developmental Medicine & Child Neurology, 41*, 608–615.

Miller, L., & Lane, S. (2000). Toward a consensus in terminology in sensory integration theory and practice, part 1: Taxonomy of neurophysiological processes. *Sensory Integration Special Interest Section Quarterly, 23*(1), 1–4.

Miller, L., McIntosh, D., McGrath, J., Shyu, V., Lampe, M., Taylor, A., et al. (1998). Electrodermal responses to sensory stimuli in individuals with fragile X syndrome: A preliminary report. *American Journal of Medical Genetics, 83*, 268–279.

Miller, P. A., Solomon, P., Giacomini, M., & Abelson, J. (2005). Experiences of novice physiotherapists adapting to their role in acute hospitals. *Physiotherapie Canada, 57*(2), 145–153.

Moore, M. E., Vaughan, K. T. L., Hayes, B. E., & McLendon, W. (2005). Developing an interdisciplinary collaboration center in an academic health sciences library. *Medical References Services Quarterly, 24*(4), 99–107.

Nadon, G., Feldman, D.E., Dunn W., & Gisel E. (2011). Mealtime problems in children with autism spectrum disorder and their typically developing siblings: A comparison study. *Autism. 15*(1), 98-113.

Nananda, F. (2005). Challenges in translating research into practice. *Journal of Women's Health, 14*(1), 87–95.

Ottenbacher, K. (1982). Sensory integration therapy: Affect or effect? *American Journal of Occupational Therapy, 36*, 571–578.

Ottenbacher, K., & Short-DeGraff, M. (1985). *Vestibular processing dysfunction in children.* Binghamton, NY: Haworth Press.

Polatajko, H., Kaplan, B., & Wilson, B. (1992). Sensory integration treatment for children with learning disabilities: Its status 20 years later. *Occupational Therapy Journal of Research, 12*(6), 323–341.

Polatajko, H., Law, M., Miller, J., Schaffer, R., & Macnab, J. (1991). The effect of a sensory integration program on academic achievement, motor performance, and self-esteem in children identified as learning disabled: Results of a clinical trial. *Occupational Therapy Journal of Research, 11*(3), 155–174.

Pollock, N. (2009). Sensory integration: A review of the current state of the evidence. Occupational Therapy Now, 11(5), 6-10.

Quine, W., & Ullian, J. (1978). *The web of belief* (2nd ed., pp. 9–34). New York, NY: McGraw-Hill.

Rappolt, S., & Tassone, M. (2002). How rehabilitation therapists gather, evaluate, and implement new knowledge. *The Journal of Continuing Education in the Health Professions, 22*, 170–180.

Reddihough, D. S., King, J., Coleman, G., & Catanese, T. (1998). Efficacy of programmes based on conductive education for young children with cerebral palsy. *Developmental Medicine & Child Neurology, 40*(11), 763–770.

Reike, E., & Anderson, D. (2009). Adolescent/adult sensory profile and obsessive–compulsive disorder. *American Journal of Occupational Therapy, 63*(2), 138–145.

Reimer, B., Sawka, E., & James, D. (2005). Improving research in the addictions field: A perspective from Canada. *Substance Use & Misuse, 40*, 1707–1720.

Rix, J. (2007, October 20). Are you a sensory junkie or a nervous wreck? *London Times.*

Rodehorst, T. K., Wilhelm, S. L., & Jensen, L. (2005). Use of interdisciplinary simulation to understand perceptions of team members' roles. *Journal of Professional Nursing, 21*(3), 159–166.

Rogers, E. (1995). *Diffusion of innovations* (4th ed.). New York, NY: The Free Press.

Rood, M. (1952). Neurophysiological mechanisms utilized in the treatment of neuromuscular dysfunction. *American Journal of Occupational Therapy, 10*(4), 220–225.

Rosenbaum, P., King, S., Law, M., King, G., & Evans, J. (1998). Family-centred service: A conceptual framework and research review. *Physical and Occupational Therapy in Pediatrics, 18*(1), 1–20.

Schachter, K. A., & Cohen, S. J. (2005). From research to practice: Challenges to implementing national diabetes guidelines with five community health centers on the U.S.–Mexico border. *Preventing Chronic Disease, 2*(1), 1–6.

Schell, B. (1998). Clinical reasoning: The basis of practice. In M. Neistadt & E. Crepeau (Eds.), *Willard and Spackman's occupational therapy* (9th ed.). Philadelphia, PA: Lippincott, Williams & Wilkins.

Schell, B., & Schell, J. (2007). *Clinical and professional reasoning in occupational therapy.* Philadelphia, PA: Lippincott, Williams & Wilkins.

Sieg, K. (1988). A. Jean Ayres. In B. Miller, K. Sieg, F. Ludwig, S. Shortridge, & J. Van Deusen (Eds.), *Six perspectives on theory for practice of occupational therapy* (pp. 95–142). Rockville, MD: Aspen Publishers.

Solomon, P., & Miller, P. A. (2005). Qualitative study of novice physical therapists' experiences in private practice. *Physiotherapie Canada, 57*(3), 190–198.

Stegink-Jansen, C. W. (2002). Outcomes, treatment effectiveness, efficacy, and evidence-based practice: Examples from the world of splinting. *Journal of Hand Therapy, 15*(2), 136–143.

Steinfeld, E., & Shea, S. (1993). Enabling home environments. Identifying barriers to independence. *Technology and Disability, 2*(4), 69–79.

Wallis, C. (2007, December 10) Making sense of your senses. *Time.*

Weaver, C. A., Warren, J. J., & Delaney, C. (2005). Bedside, classroom and bench: Collaborative strategies to generate evidence-based knowledge for nursing practice. *International Journal of Medical Informatics, 74*, 989–999.

Wilkins, S., Jung, B., Wishart, L., Edwards, M., & Gamble-Norton, S. (2003). The effectiveness of community-based occupational therapy education and functional training programs for older adults: A critical literature review. *Canadian Journal of Occupational Therapy, 4*(70), 214–225.

Williamson, G., & Szczepanski, M. (1999). Coping frame of reference. In P. Kramer & J. Hinojosa (Eds.), *Frames of reference for pediatric occupational therapy* (pp. 431–468). Philadelphia, PA: Lippincott, Williams & Wilkins.

Wilson, B. N., & Kaplan, B. J. (1994). Follow-up assessment of children receiving sensory integration treatment. *Occupational Therapy Journal of Research, 14*(4), 244–266.

Wilson, B. N., Kaplan, B. J., Fellowes, S., Gruchy, C., & Faris, P. (1992). The efficacy of sensory integration treatment compared to tutoring. *Physical and Occupational Therapy in Pediatrics, 12*(1), 1–36.

Zimmer, M., & Desch, L. (2012). Sensory integration therapies for children with developmental & behavioral disorders. Retrieved from http://pediatrics.aappublications.org/content/early/2012/05/23/peds.2012-0876

SUGGESTED READINGS

Center for Universal Design, North Carolina State University. Retrieved from http://www.ncsu.edu/project/design-projects/udi/

Chen, Y. H., Rodhers, J., & McConachie, H. (2009). Restricted & repetitive behaviours, sensory processing and cognitive style in children with ASD. *Journal of Autism and Developmental Disorders, 39*, 635–642.

Fisher, A. G., Murray, E. A., & Bundy, A. C. (1991). *Sensory integration theory and practice.* Philadelphia, PA: F. A. Davis Company.

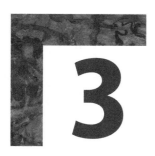

3

BECOMING AN EVIDENCE-BASED PRACTITIONER

Aliki Thomas, PhD, OT(c), Erg and Annie McCluskey, PhD, MA, DipCOT

LEARNING OBJECTIVES

After reading this chapter, the student/practitioner will be able to:
- Name the steps in the process of evidence-based practice.
- Describe the evidence-based practice competencies required by health practitioners.
- Describe the effectiveness of educational interventions to improve evidence-based practice (EBP) competencies.
- Recognize his or her own practice style traits and how personal traits can impact on practice.

INTRODUCTION

The process of becoming an evidence-based practitioner appears relatively simple at first glance. In our experience, learning to write focused questions and search more effectively are the easier skills to learn, although both require practice. Learning to critically appraise research is more challenging, as we will discuss in this chapter, partly because of a need to interpret statistics and understand a range of research designs. Then there is the matter of using these skills to inform practice—more difficult than it first appears. Finally, changing practice in line with new evidence is one of the most challenging aspects of becoming an evidence-based practitioner.

The focus of this chapter is on becoming an evidence-based practitioner. In this chapter we present EBP as a developmental journey that begins during entry-level education programs and continues throughout professional practice. Although evidence-based practitioners are expected to demonstrate the requisite competencies upon graduation, these competencies will be further refined through years of practice. In our experience as researchers and educators, evidence-based practitioners need to continuously evaluate their practice and reflect upon the benefits and outcomes of using evidence to support clinical decision making.

This chapter describes how you can become an evidence-based practitioner. The chapter has been informed by research on teaching and learning EBP across the health professions. First, we

Law M., & MacDermid, J. C.
*Evidence-Based Rehabilitation: A Guide
to Practice, Third Edition* (pp 37–63).
© 2014 SLACK Incorporated.

present the steps of the EBP process. Second, we describe EBP competencies required by health care practitioners. Third, we summarize current evidence on the effectiveness of educational interventions to improve EBP competencies and suggest methods for teaching EBP that are grounded in educational theory. We conclude the chapter with a description of methods for measuring change and improvements in EBP competencies and the benefits of knowing your own practice style traits.

Evidence-Based Practice as a Developmental Journey

Successful integration of research evidence in clinical practice is highly dependent upon an individual's experience and expertise in a domain (Craik & Rappolt, 2006; Strauss, Ball, Balcombe, Sheldon, & McAlister, 2005). It is unrealistic to expect new graduates and novice practitioners to demonstrate expert-like competencies in EBP at the end of their entry-level education. However, it is realistic to expect that academic programs, through gradual development, will lay the foundation of EBP and—during the course of the program—move students along a trajectory of learning and progressive development of EBP competencies.

The concept of a developmental trajectory toward superior performance and expertise is part of a new chapter in expertise research that supports a developmental pattern rather than the dichotomous expert–novice orientation of earlier research. In the past, researchers studied "exceptional people" (Chi, 2006, p. 21) to understand how they performed in their domain and how they differed from the general population. Contemporary studies of expertise have been oriented toward studying the developmental and multidimensional nature of expertise in order to identify developmental markers that can shift individuals from novice to expert (Ackerman, 1996, 2000, 2003; Alexander, 2003; Lajoie, 2003).

Researchers in the health sciences are now interested in identifying these developmental markers of superior performance in order to help learners and entry-level practitioners move toward expert-like performance in various domains of practice. A recent study by Thomas, Saroyan, and Snider (2011) sought to identify such a trajectory by examining the differences in EBP behaviors among occupational therapy (OT) students and experienced clinicians and identifying the extent to which these behaviors corresponded to the decisions represented in an EBP reference model (Thomas, Saroyan, & Lajoie, 2011). Students from three different academic levels (n = 53) and expert clinicians (n = 9) were asked to respond to five questions that reflected the steps of the EBP process. Qualitative and quantitative data analyses of group differences showed that students had greater breadth of knowledge of the aspects of EBP that are formally taught in the OT program (posing a clinical question, searching the literature, and appraising the literature) but that their knowledge was not as well organized as the knowledge represented in a reference model based on information gleaned from expert clinicians. Experienced clinicians' practice behaviors were most consistent with the decisions illustrated in the model in the final two steps of the EBP process (decision making and reevaluation), which may be a result of their extensive clinical experience. Therefore, a shift in the trajectory of EBP competency development may occur, from *instruction dependent* to *experience dependent*. Performance of the first three steps of the EBP process may be dependent upon formal education and explicit instruction, whereas competence in integrating scientific evidence and evaluating EBP outcomes may occur more gradually, with sustained practice and feedback.

The notion of incremental development of EBP competencies suggests that once foundational knowledge is present, development toward different levels of expertise must be scaffolded along the way (Collins, Brown, & Newman, 1989). Students and novice clinicians can move toward superior levels of skills and performance in various aspects of EBP through sustained exposure and practice with clients in a given area.

Steps in the Process of Evidence-Based Practice

Although different authors have proposed variations in the steps of the EBP process, there is general consensus about the following five steps:

1. Posing a clinical question

2. Searching for the evidence

3. Appraising the literature

4. Making a decision

5. Assessing the effectiveness of the intervention (or test/assessment) and one's proficiency with the EBP process

Step 1: Posing a Clinical Question

The first step of the process involves formulating a clear and answerable question derived from a client's problem or need. Although a practitioner may be confident that he or she has identified a clinical problem, it is important that the question be directly relevant to the problem at hand, phrased to facilitate searching for a precise answer, focused, and well-articulated.

The clinical question is referred to as "P.I.C.O." question and captures four components: (P) the target population, (I) the intervention (assuming that the question is about a therapy or intervention of some sort), (C) the comparison to another group or another intervention, and (O) the desired outcome of the intervention. The "P"—target population—can be about a primary problem (e.g., quality of life, people with decreased hand function), a client's main concern or complaint (e.g., pain, loss of sensation, decreased vision), or a disease or health status (e.g., depression, arthritis, stroke). The intervention—"I"—refers to the treatment that is being considered for the person. The intervention may be a treatment approach, an adjunctive therapy, a medication, or recommendation to use a product or procedure. Intervention can also be replaced by a test or assessment (e.g., whether one test is better than another for screening or measuring a domain). The "C"—comparison—refers to an alternative treatment (or test). A comparison is optional in the P.I.C.O. question because often practitioners do not wish to compare treatments. The fourth component is the outcome of interest, or "O." The outcome specifies what result(s) the practitioner (or client) expects to accomplish, improve, or affect. The outcome should be measurable. Specific outcomes will yield better search results and allow the practitioner to find studies of interest. When defining the outcome, terms such as *more effective* are inadequate. Instead, it is preferable to state "more effective in preventing contractures" or in "decreasing edema." Examples of outcomes include reductions in pain, improvements in hand function or rates of return to work, and decreased hospital lengths of stay. Consider the following example for which we may need to formulate a clinical P.I.C.O. question:

> Mr. V. is a 75-year-old man who lives alone in a two-storey home. His past medical history includes high blood pressure, bilateral cataracts, and osteoarthritis in the knees. Mr. V. fell while getting out of bed one night to go the bathroom. He was taken to the emergency department where an x-ray revealed a right hip fracture. He then had a hemiarthroplasty. The surgery was successful and 3 days later he was transferred to a rehabilitation hospital. His rehabilitation is progressing well. It is 2 weeks prior to his discharge and the team is considering the recommendation that Mr. V. take part in the hospital's outpatient multicomponent falls prevention program. Mr. V. and his son have been informed that he may be invited to attend the falls prevention program. They ask you if participating in the program will be of added benefit given that he has received rehabilitation and whether the likelihood of future falls will be reduced if he attends the fall prevention program.

The P.I.C.O. question for this scenario might be: *In the older population living in the community (P), does a fall prevention program (I) reduce the risk of future falls (O) compared to traditional rehabilitation (C)?*

Notice how in this P.I.C.O. question, we translated "Mr. V. is a 75-year-old man who lives alone in a two-storey home" into "older population living in the community" in order to clearly state the population. Hence, when you consider the concepts and terms to use in your P.I.C.O. question, you need to be specific enough to ensure that your search yields relevant results but not so specific that you come away empty-handed.

Although the P.I.C.O. question generally includes four components, the composition of the P.I.C.O. question depends on the type of question being asked. P.I.C.O. questions can be about a therapy/treatment intervention, diagnosis, etiology, prognosis, or appropriate/accurate assessment. Consider the following example of a P.I.C.O. question with three components:

> Mr. P. is a 54-year-old engineer who was diagnosed with rheumatoid arthritis 6 months ago. His doctor sent him to occupational therapy for evaluation and treatment for the arthritis. As his therapist, you will recommend that he participate in a joint protection education program to minimize the pain and joint stiffness. You want to know whether there is evidence to support joint protection education for people with rheumatoid arthritis.

The P.I.C.O. question for this scenario could be: *For adults with rheumatoid arthritis (P), does joint protection education (I) improve function and reduce stiffness (O)?*

In Chapter 5, P.I.C.O. questions as the basis for literature searching are discussed again in detail.

Step 2: Searching for the Evidence

This step of the process requires a search for the best available research to help answer the clinical (P.I.C.O.) question. Before starting a search we recommend that you prepare by checking your P.I.C.O. question and identifying the key concepts in your question, relevant synonyms, and alternate terms or spelling as well as relevant databases to search. Although many practitioners report a lack of confidence and skill in searching for scientific evidence, this is a skill that can be acquired and one that can be supported by a librarian or colleague with experience in searching scholarly databases. When you are ready to search it is important that you aim to find clinical research evidence. Studies that report clinical data will likely be more relevant for your client. You should also aim to find papers using the best methods for a particular type of clinical question. Although randomized controlled trials (RCTs) are considered the gold standard for research about therapy effectiveness, these studies will not be useful if you are looking for research about clients' experiences following a major burn or play patterns of preschool children with autism. You may need to keep searching until the best available evidence is located.

There are two common search challenges. First, there are many available sources of information, including many scholarly databases. If you are a novice at searching for research papers, you may find it difficult to sift through the numerous databases and you may find it equally challenging to decide which ones are more credible or likely to yield the type of research you are looking for. As most sophisticated searchers would tell you, do not despair! There are several traditional databases, such as PubMed, Embase, CINAHL, and PsychINFO, that catalogue much of the published rehabilitation research. Alternatively, you can use specialist databases, journals, and Web sites of preappraised research such as the Cochrane Library, OTseeker, and the Physiotherapy Evidence Database (PEDro) that contain peer-reviewed appraisals on a specific topic. You can also find critically appraised papers at http://www.otcats.com or in journals such as the *Australian Occupational Therapy Journal* and the *American Journal of Occupational Therapy* (Evidence Brief Series). Chapter 5 details specific search strategies and tips for ensuring your searches are comprehensive and well-targeted.

A second challenge when searching for evidence is determining what is legitimate evidence (Maynard, 1994). This question has been central to an ongoing debate about EBP (Mowinski-Jennings & Loan, 2001). Skeptics have often criticized the process of EBP for use of evidence hierarchies and the narrow and overly prescriptive nature of systematic reviews (Marks, 2002). The RCT has also been under attack because such trials sometimes produce findings that are inapplicable to specific clients (Rolfe, 1998; Welsh & Lyons, 2001). Another criticism has been about the apparent lack of regard for qualitative research. Because EBP has been primarily grounded in quantitative approaches and experimental designs, findings from qualitative studies have seldom been considered as legitimate sources of evidence. Consequently, critics argue that qualitative research has not taken its rightful place within EBP (and is rarely included in clinical practice guidelines), despite the popularity of qualitative research and its potential to capture the complex relationships of clients and their illness experiences (Forbes & Griffiths, 2002; Hammel, 2001; Herbert, Sherrington, Maher, & Mosely, 2001; Miles, Grey, Polychronis, Price, & Melchiorri, 2004). Within the OT profession, Reagon, Bellin, and Boniface (2008) proposed a framework that includes a broader view of evidence and sources of evidence other than empirical research and RCTs. Textbooks, research, colleagues, clinical experience, clients and their families, outcome measurement, and observation also constitute valid sources of evidence (Bennett & Bennett, 2000; Egan, Dubouloz, von Zweck, & Vallerand, 1998; Hammell, 2001).

To benefit clients and improve clinical outcomes, practitioners can become consumers of research and weigh the advantages and disadvantages of various sources of evidence to determine how these sources should inform practice.

Step 3: Appraising the Literature

Not all available evidence is of good quality, nor is all available evidence useful. It takes skill, experience, and practice to decide which evidence to select to answer your question. The third step of the EBP process allows us to decide on quality and relevance of the literature. Critical appraisal is about assessing the trustworthiness, value, and relevance of the literature for a particular patient and context.

Critical appraisal is one of the most challenging steps of the EBP process for many practitioners. Several studies have consistently shown that a lack of skill in critical appraisal—particularly in interpreting statistics and understanding various research designs—is one of the major obstacles to using evidence to inform practice (Dubouloz, Egan, Vallernad, & von Zweck, 1999; Salbach, Jaglal, Korner-Bitensky, Rappolt, & Davis, 2007; Teasell et al., 2008; Welch & Dawson, 2006). Critical appraisal is a skill that is being taught in most entry-level health sciences programs, including OT and physical therapy programs. The hope is that this skill will help graduates become better research consumers. As will be discussed later in this book, knowledge translation researchers are designing and assessing the effectiveness of various strategies for assisting practitioners in developing and using critical appraisal skills and implementing evidence into practice.

When critically appraising research, you are addressing three broad questions: What are the results? Are the results valid? How will these results help me work with my client? The answers to these questions will help you assess the research you have found and assist you in making a decision as to whether you can use the findings for your client.

Critical appraisal of published research can be conducted in one of two ways. The first method involves using a critical appraisal form or checklist. There are many available critical appraisal tools that provide useful frameworks for evaluating studies using different research designs. One of the most widely used and easiest scales to use when appraising RCTs is the PEDro scale (Maher, Sherrington, Herbert, Moseley, & Elkins, 2003). This scale is used by systematic reviewers and practitioners to rate the methodological quality of a study and potential biases during client recruitment to a trial, measurement, and data analysis. That scale is used to rate trials on the PEDro and

OTseeker Web sites and is taught in many health science programs. The PEDro scale and guidelines for use can be downloaded free from both of these Web sites (www.pedro.org.au and www.otseeker.com). You can find other appraisal checklists for systematic reviews, studies comparing one test or measure with another, and qualitative studies on the Web site of the Oxford-Based Center for Evidence-Based Medicine (www.cebm.net/index.aspx?o=1157) or at the McMaster University site of the Canadian Occupational Therapy Evidence-Based Practice Research Group (www.srs-mcmaster.ca/Default.aspx?tabid=630).

In a 2004 systematic review of the content of critical appraisal tools, Katrak, Bialocerkowski, Massy-Westropp, Saravana Kumar, and Grimeer summarized the content, intent, construction, and psychometric properties of published critical appraisal tools to identify common elements and their relevance to allied health research. The authors found that of the 121 published critical appraisal tools, 87% were specific to a research design and most tools were developed for use with experimental studies. Guidelines on how to administer the tools were provided in 43% of cases. According to Katrak and colleagues (2004), there is variability in intent, components, construction, and psychometric properties of published critical appraisal tools. There is no "gold standard critical appraisal tool for any study design, nor is there any widely accepted generic tool that can be applied equally well across study types." No tool was specific to allied health research requirements. Hence, interpretation of critical appraisal of research needs to be considered in light of the properties and intent of the critical appraisal tool chosen for the task. Chapter 6 also provides extensive information on critical appraisal and the tools to use in this process.

Another method for evaluating the quality of research is to refer to critically appraised topics (or CATs) or critically appraised papers (CAPs). A CAT is a synopsis of evidence on a specific topic of interest and is typically focused around a clinical question. When professionals summarize a single study, the outcome is a CAP. Usually more than one study is included in a CAT. CATs are one way for busy practitioners to collate and share their appraisals. Although a CAT is like a shorter and less rigorous version of a systematic review that summarizes the best available research evidence on a topic, some CATs have not been formally peer reviewed. The lack of peer review presents an important limitation in that the reader cannot be assured that a complete search of the literature has been conducted or that an accurate interpretation of the methods, results, and statistics has been made. This limitation needs to be considered when using CATs or CAPs to guide your practice. Many universities are now using CATs as assignments designed to evaluate learners' skills and knowledge. There are a small number of free Web sites containing CATs or CAPs, such as the University of Michigan Department of Paediatrics (www.med.umich.edu/pediatrics/ebm/Cat.htm) and the OT-CATS site (www.otcats.com). CATs are also discussed in detail in Chapter 10.

Step 4: Making a Decision

In the fourth step of the EBP process, the practitioner engages in collaborative decision making with the client to decide whether and how the information gleaned from the literature can be applied to the client's problem and context. Appropriate decision making integrates the context, values, and preferences of the client as well as the available resources which include the available research evidence and the practitioner's expertise. Several researchers have asserted that success in decision making comes with experience and expertise in an area of practice, after encountering a range of client problems (Craik & Rappolt, 2006; Davidoff, 1999; Haynes, 2002; Rappolt, 2003; Rolfe, 1998; Straus, Richardson, Glasziou, & Haynes, 2005). Hence, although graduates from health sciences programs are expected to use evidence to inform their practice, the ease and sophistication with which they are able to do so will increase with experience.

To assist you in deciding whether and how you can apply the evidence, ask yourself the following questions:
- Were the study participants similar to my clients?
- Is the intervention realistic in my setting?
- Does the comparison treatment reflect my current practice?
- Were the outcomes in line with our treatment goals?
- How big was the benefit in relation to the risk of an adverse event due to treatment or to the costs?
- Are there social or cultural factors that might affect suitability or acceptance?
- What are the wishes of the client and family?
- Does the strength of the evidence warrant clinical use?

Step 5: Assessing the Effectiveness of the Intervention (or Test/Assessment) and One's Proficiency With the Evidence-Based Practice Process

The final step of the EBP process involves two parts: Evaluating the outcome of the intervention you implemented and evaluating your skill in navigating the different steps of the process. In evaluating the outcome of the decision you made to implement a specific intervention you may want to ask yourself the following questions:
- Were you able to implement the evidence, and did you do so routinely with clients, if that was your intention?
- Did the intervention result in positive outcomes?
- Did the benefits outweigh the harm?
- Did the benefits outweigh the costs?
- Were clients satisfied with the intervention and was it what they expected?
- Was the intervention feasible, and did you implement it with fidelity (i.e., as closely as possible to that delivered in the original study/studies, with the same dosage and intensity)?
- Were the outcomes from this intervention superior to usual care or no intervention?
- Were you satisfied with your delivery of the intervention?

In answering the questions you can reflect upon the reasons why the intervention may not have been successful or what factors influenced your client's satisfaction with the program. This final assessment will allow you to modify any actions or decisions you make in the future if a similar problem arises.

It is also good practice to engage in a self-assessment of your ability to undertake the EBP process and determine areas where there may be shortcomings in your skills. This self-assessment may, for example, highlight that you need to hone your critical appraisal skills, that you need to learn how to overcome common barriers to implementation, or that you could consult more experienced practitioners to discuss the specifics about implementing a given treatment intervention. The following are some questions that can help guide your personal assessment:
- How did I do progressing through the steps of EBP?
- Which steps were easy/difficult for me (e.g., searching or critical appraisal or implementation)?
- How did I respond to limited evidence, poor quality evidence, or inconclusive evidence?
- Did I respond to my clients' concerns?
- Did I take into consideration the constraints in the environment?

- Do I need to acquire any new skills?
- Did I consult with peers and more experienced colleagues in addition to consulting with my client and published research?

Practitioners and supervisors may also wish to use a standardized tool such as the PERFECT (Professional Evaluation and Reflection on Change Tool) as part of an annual self-assessment (Menon et al., 2010). The PERFECT tool has four sections and 33 questions to promote reflection about practice change, including barriers and enablers to change. The tool is freely available on the Strokengine Assess Web site (http://strokengine.ca/).

EVIDENCE-BASED PRACTICE COMPETENCIES REQUIRED BY GRADUATE HEALTH PRACTITIONERS

Practitioners frequently make decisions on how to proceed with their clients (Mattingly & Fleming, 1994). Clinical decision making (or evidence-based decision making) is the end point in a process requiring clinical reasoning, problem solving, and awareness of the client and his or her context (Clark, Scott, & Krupa, 1993; Dubouloz et al., 1999). The interaction of research evidence with clinical expertise and client values (Bennett & Bennett, 2000; Haynes, Deveraux, & Guyatt, 2002; Rappolt, 2003; Sackett, Rosenberg, Richardson, & Haynes, 1997) is believed to help with evidence-based decision making.

There is limited research to explain how practitioners develop EBP skills such as writing clinical questions and searching for and appraising evidence. Rappolt (2003) explored the role of expertise in evidence-based OT and found that therapist competence in moving through the five steps of the EBP process was a function of their research skills, knowledge, and experience. She suggested that in order for therapists to be evidence-based practitioners they need to acquire the following skills: the ability to identify clinical issues, reflection and reasoning skills to help with problem identification, the ability to gather and appraise evidence, problem-solving skills, the ability to evaluate the entire process, and sufficient knowledge and experience to draw from in order to make clinical decisions. Lloyd-Smith (1997) discussed the actions of searching, retrieving, and critically appraising literature (Step 2) but did not address the skills that may be involved in the other stages. Rosenberg and Donald (1995) argued that success in EBP is contingent upon some level of expertise that can only be achieved with time and practice. They also claimed that critical appraisal is a required skill for EBP. Profetto-McGrath (2005) proposed that critical thinking requires specific knowledge, skills, and processes that support the decision making needed in EBP. The authors found that nurse practitioners use judgment to plan and provide care. Questioning, critical appraisal, evaluation, and application were requisite skills influenced by, and necessary for, critical thinking. Miles and colleagues (2004) also suggested that judgment is a necessary skill for EBP, particularly when deciding whether statistical results are applicable for specific patient problems. Because research facts "never really speak for themselves," therapists need to interpret and make sense of data. Craik and Rappolt (2003) examined the self-reported use of research in practice of expert therapists in order to identify the processes involved in translating research into practice. They found that clinical decision making by occupational therapists involved a reflective and evaluative component. Clinical experience and structured reflection, which is considered "a necessary component for building knowledge and applying research findings to clinical care," were both necessary for decision making. Using a grounded theory approach, Craik and Rappolt (2006) examined the self-reported research utilization behaviors of 11 occupational therapists working in stroke rehabilitation. They found that clinicians' experiences, active engagement in continuing education, involvement in research, and mentoring of students contributed to their capacity to translate research evidence into practice.

The researchers identified clinical, research, teaching, and reflective practice skills as four key skill sets that were important contributors to successful application of research evidence in OT practice.

McCluskey, Home, and Thomson (2008) described the development of EBP competencies in an earlier edition of this book. Their study involved 106 occupational therapists who attended a 2-day EBP workshop. After 18 months, the researchers interviewed a subgroup ($n = 10$) of the most active participants, based on frequency of searching and appraisal activities from self-report diaries. Within this subgroup of practitioners, the level of knowledge and engagement with EBP varied. Novices rarely engaged in search and appraisal activities and possessed basic skills, limited knowledge, and a negative attitude toward EBP; they spoke at length about barriers such as lack of time. At the other end of the continuum, competent non-experts engaged in search and appraisal activities regularly, had achieved competency with these skills, and demonstrated extensive knowledge and a very positive attitude to EBP; they rarely complained about barriers such as lack of time, they just "did" EBP. Apprentices were somewhere in between. Three key strategies were used to advance EBP competencies: (1) finding time for and prioritizing EBP above other activities; (2) actively developing their skills and knowledge by teaching others and seeking help, particularly with appraisal; and (3) staying focused, being persistent when barriers were encountered, and maintaining EBP work habits. Conditions or factors that helped participants develop their EBP competencies included (a) readiness for change; (b) personal and organizational expectations; (c) the presence of deadlines; and (d) the availability of support at work, particularly from managers. Further research is now needed to confirm whether this typology, theory of change, and attitudinal differences are similar or different across health practitioners and settings.

Collectively, this literature suggests that being an evidence-based practitioner involves drawing on clinical experience, acquiring teaching and reflective practice skills, as well as critical thinking and problem-solving skills, in order to identify a clinical problem. Then, through the appropriate use of various sources of evidence, practitioners need to be able to formulate a plan to address the client's problem within their social context. The studies suggest that in order to apply research findings in clinical decision making, clinicians must be able to pose a good clinical question and have a skill set that facilitates the searching and appraisal of the literature.

EDUCATIONAL INTERVENTIONS AND STRATEGIES TO IMPROVE EVIDENCE-BASED PRACTICE COMPETENCIES

The Sicily statement describes a recommended curriculum and minimum requirements for training health professionals to practice in an evidence-based manner (Dawes et al., 2005). Curricula to deliver EBP competencies should be grounded in the five-step process of EBP. Instruments that are freely available and measure competence at each stage of the process, as well as changes in skill, knowledge, and behavior, should be used with students and graduates. In this section we summarize existing research on the effectiveness of educational interventions to improve EBP knowledge, skills, and behaviors. We then offer suggestions for teaching EBP in universities and further promoting EBP competencies in practice. In the final section of this chapter we discuss instruments for measuring change.

Effectiveness of Evidence-Based Practice Educational Interventions

Student Learners

Teaching activities described in the health sciences literature are designed to address one or more of the required EBP skills and are typically aligned with the five EBP steps. Few teaching approaches address all five EBP steps and fewer have demonstrable success in teaching all of the skills needed to adequately and consistently integrate EBP into practice.

Five systematic reviews, conducted between 1998 and 2007, examined the effectiveness of teaching interventions on knowledge of critical appraisal, attitudes, skills, and EBP behavior in health sciences students. Flores-Mateo and Argimon (2007) studied the effect sizes for different instructional interventions aimed at improving EBP knowledge, attitudes, skills, and behaviors in postgraduate health care education (medicine, nursing, and allied health professions). They found small improvements for all four outcomes when these were measured alone but rather large improvements (effect size > .79) in knowledge and skill in EBP when these were measured together in a total score. These findings notwithstanding, the authors were critical of many of the studies in the review because of poor study quality and lack of validated outcome measures. Norman and Shannon (1998) showed that instruction in critical appraisal resulted in positive gains on medical students' knowledge of critical appraisal, without providing evidence of gains sustained over time or translated into practice.

Coomarasamy, Taylor, and Khan's (2003) systematic review of the teaching of critical appraisal revealed improvements in knowledge of critical appraisal but not in EBP attitudes, skills, or behaviors. Coomarasamy and Khan (2004) reviewed the effect of standalone versus integrated courses (teaching of EBP integrated within clinical practice) on critical appraisal knowledge, skills, attitudes, and behaviors. They found that the former improved knowledge only, whereas the integrated approach showed improvement in all four outcomes (knowledge of critical appraisal, skills, attitudes, and behaviors), supporting the use of authentic teaching situations and the situated aspect of learning (Lave & Wenger, 1991). A later systematic review by Hyde, Deeks, and Milne (2006) examined the teaching of critical appraisal and the impact of this teaching on client care, client outcomes, and knowledge of critical appraisal. The review, which included only one RCT, indicated that teaching improved knowledge of critical appraisal by 25%; however, there were no data reported on client outcomes.

As a whole these reviews suggest that teaching interventions, particularly skills-based workshops, have a greater impact on knowledge and skill than they do on sustainable EBP behaviors. Improvements in EBP knowledge seem to vary according to the level of the learner, whether undergraduate or postgraduate. EBP instruction may have a greater impact on learning and acquisition of EBP-related knowledge, skills, and attitudes if integrated into real-life contexts using authentic situations such as those provided during fieldwork and clerkships, which support the value of situated learning and the use of authentic teaching situations (Lave & Wenger, 1991). According to Hatala and Guyatt (2002) and Gruppen (2007), the findings from these reviews must be interpreted with caution due to a number of limitations including infrequent use of randomization in experimental designs, a heavy reliance on quantitative methods for measuring and explaining the complex forms of EBP competencies, the short duration of interventions in university environments where there is a rapid student turnover and limited time for longitudinal studies, and repeated use of self-reports of knowledge and skill instead of objective measures of performance and behavior.

Practitioners

A recent Cochrane review evaluated whether educational interventions improve the frequency and quality of questions asked and written by health care practitioners (Horsley et al., 2010). The authors found only four studies examining interventions to improve question formulation and none focusing on the frequency of questions formulated. Risk of methodological bias was generally high. Three of the four studies showed improvements in question formulation in physicians, resident medical officers, or mixed allied health populations in the short- to moderate-term follow-up. Only one study examined sustainability of effects after 1 year, by which time skills had deteriorated. The review showed some small improvements in the quality of questions written by health practitioners following training (and in some cases the use of written pamphlets), but improvements do not appear to be sustained over time.

A FRAMEWORK FOR PROMOTING EVIDENCE-BASED PRACTICE IN EDUCATION AND PRACTICE

In the Educational Environment

Education that primarily targets content knowledge or discrete skills ignores the need for the kind of deeper learning that enables students to link classroom learning to real-life practice (Bransford & Schwartz, 1999). University programs should provide students with opportunities to acquire strategies that help them to learn on their own. Such a process helps to develop prolific, self-regulated learners. The main purpose of instruction and design of effective learning environments is learning by doing and learning in context (Lajoie & Azevedo, 2006). Constructivist and situated learning paradigms are useful for the design of learning environments that foster the cognitive and metacognitive skills needed for EBP. Two major assumptions of these theories are that learning in context facilitates meaningful learning and, with the help of peers and teachers, students can draw upon existing knowledge and experiences to construct new knowledge and develop problem-solving skills, clinical reasoning abilities, and self-monitoring behaviors. For example, when working with simulated case vignettes, students can draw from their existing knowledge of sciences such as anatomy, physiology, or psychology to form a new understanding of the impact of an evidence-based treatment intervention on a specific problem or impairment. Clinicians can draw from experiential knowledge to judge whether a recommended intervention could be applied to a new client. Accumulated experiences and knowledge can be useful stepping stones toward acquisition of a different and more advanced set of skills.

Proceeding through the five steps of EBP requires a balance of skills in each step (Dawes et al., 2005). Curricula designed to promote knowledge, skills, and attitudes toward EBP grounded in the five-step process and in different clinical situations can help students see the EBP process as a continuum. Teaching methods that help learners acquire and integrate cognitive and self-monitoring strategies and discover, use, and manage knowledge (Collins et al., 1989) can support the move along the trajectory of developing expertise in EBP (Lajoie, 2003).

We propose that instructional design that targets EBP competencies in the health professions be based on five salient constructivist characteristics about learners and the learning context. Instructors should do the following:

- Consider the learner's existing knowledge, beliefs, and attitudes regarding EBP.
- Understand the salient role of social negotiation and collaboration with peers in order to incorporate evidence in clinical decision making.
- Acknowledge that learning situations, content, and learning activities are meant to foster self-analysis, problem solving, higher-order thinking, and deep understanding; as such, they must be relevant and authentic and represent the natural complexities of the world.
- Support collaborative learning that exposes students to alternative viewpoints and affords them the opportunity to pursue apprenticeship learning.
- Scaffold learners from what is presently known to what is to be known, thereby facilitating the learner's ability to perform just beyond the limits of current ability (Ernest, 1995; Honebein, 1996; Jonassen, 1991, 1994; von Glasersfeld, 1995; Vygotsky, 1978; Wilson & Cole, 1991).

Accordingly, EBP can be taught in a socially constructed environment in the classroom and in authentic learning contexts such as those afforded by fieldwork. In these contexts, students should be encouraged to engage in discussion, debate, reflection, and problem solving with peers and experts and ultimately solve problems that reflect the broad scope of scenarios they are likely to encounter in the future. The content and context of learning can be structured and guided by the teacher in collaboration with the learner. The teacher could model the EBP process and its underlying skills, scaffold students through practice, and progressively fade the support, allowing students to engage in EBP autonomously.

The use of collaborative learning methods, case-based methods, and cognitive apprenticeship offers much promise for promoting the development of EBP competencies. Table 3-1 (Thomas, Saroyan, & Dauphinee, 2011) shows these three approaches and highlights the main objectives, processes, instructor roles, and desired outcomes of each approach.

Collaborative learning (CL) requires learners to work in small groups. During the process of cooperatively solving problems, learners generate self-explanations and construct inferences about a specific problem, which ultimately helps them integrate and solidify new understanding and solve problems (Slavin, 1991). Engaging in discussions, problem solving, and questioning (Johnson & Johnson, 1993) allows students to test each other's understanding and build knowledge. The types of constructive activities involved in CL also trigger metacognitive activities. In attempting to solve problems, learners monitor their understanding and become aware of errors and misunderstandings. Group problem solving improves awareness of misunderstandings, which in turn triggers help-seeking behaviors and explanations, promoting better understanding and problem resolution (Johnson & Johnson, 1993). CL contexts afford many opportunities for working on EBP cases where learners can discuss client scenarios and integrate the EBP steps in a group setting.

Cases are frequently used in traditional and problem-based learning health sciences curricula (Evenson & Hmelo, 2000; Hmelo-Silver, 2004). The objective of case-based instruction is "learning through problem solving" (Hmelo-Silver, 2004, p. 239). While working with cases, students learn content, strategies, and self-directed learning by solving problems (Hmelo-Silver, Duncan, & Chinn, 2007) and actively construct knowledge in a collaborative manner with peers. The instructor's role is to guide the process through open-ended questioning that facilitates problem solving, reasoning, and the application of existing and prior knowledge. In problem-based learning environments, the case (or problem) is typically a multifaceted but realistic problem used to facilitate learning and reasoning (Barrows, 2000; Evenson & Hmelo, 2000). In health sciences curricula, clinical cases are designed to promote knowledge acquisition, problem solving, and working through the decision-making process. Cases can range from simple scenarios targeting surface-type issues (identification of the client's occupational performance issues) to more complex vignettes designed to promote analysis, synthesis, and application of knowledge. Cases contain explicit detail and appropriate cues, allowing the clinical image to emerge. By selecting the important information among the less pertinent information in a case (McKeachie, 1986), either with support from peers or instructors, students can begin to identify the more relevant assessments and treatments. Focusing on the significant aspects of the case facilitates understanding of the nature of the problem (Rogers & Holm, 1991). Neistadt, Wight, and Mulligan (1997) found that the use of cases in OT education led to improved intervention plans and understanding of clinical reasoning concepts. The authors proposed that improvements were due to instructors explicitly modeling their expert problem-solving and clinical reasoning skills before students attempted to solve a similar case. Using case studies, Reed (1996) developed and evaluated a 12-week course designed to help foster problem-solving skills in OT students. Students in that program were not only more confident in their selection of assessment and treatment interventions but they could apply effective problem-solving skills to determine solutions to complex pediatric patient problems. Case-based methods can have great potential for evoking both the knowledge and skills required for evidence-based decision making.

The cognitive apprenticeship framework as a social constructivist approach to the teaching of EBP offers much promise. It can promote the required EBP skills and competencies by exposing students to authentic practices through activity and social interaction. Cognitive apprenticeship embeds learning in activities that make deliberate use of the social context. Social interaction and collaboration with peers and with the teacher promote conceptual understanding and the development of problem-solving skills (Collins et al., 1989). In cognitive apprenticeship, students are given ill-defined tasks and real-world problems representing authentic situations. The tasks start by being slightly more difficult than students can manage independently, requiring the support of peers and instructors to succeed.

The techniques in cognitive apprenticeship include modeling, scaffolding, coaching, articulation, reflection, and observation. Modeling, scaffolding, and coaching are designed to assist students in integrating a set of cognitive and metacognitive skills through processes of observation and guided practice. Modeling provides students with a concrete reference to expert performance. It provides a glimpse into the expert's internal cognitive processes and helps students understand the thinking involved in solving problems. The process requires that the expert's (in this case the instructor's) knowledge be made explicit if it is to contribute to the developing knowledge and practice of novices (in this case the students; Bereiter & Scardamelia, 1993; Ethell & McMeniman, 2000; Mayer, 1987). In *coaching*, instructors observe learners while they carry out a task. During the observations, the instructor offer hints, cues, feedback, and reminders as needed and suggests new tasks that will help bring the learner's performance closer to expert performance. Learners begin to assume a greater role in the activity by carrying out and integrating skills through highly interactive feedback and suggestions. *Articulation* involves learners talking out loud about their knowledge, reasoning, or problem-solving processes. This helps students not only consolidate their knowledge, but it also helps them to compare and contrast their understanding with peers and the expert (instructor). Ultimately, the instructor has a basis for refining and expanding the student's understanding. In *scaffolding*, the teacher provides support to help learners carry out a task. This is done by carrying out parts of the overall task the learner cannot yet manage by providing physical supports or by providing suggestions and help along the way and as needed. The *fading* stage occurs when the student is capable of independent exploration of learning (Collins et al., 1989). Exploration pushes students to try out hypotheses, methods, and strategies similar to those that experts use to solve problems (Collins, 1991); encourages learner autonomy in defining and solving problems; and enhances discovery of new knowledge and acquisition of general problem-solving skills (Shunk, 2000).

Classrooms and clinical milieus that incorporate cognitive apprenticeship principles place teaching and learning practices within rich and varied contexts that are meaningful and authentic to students. In the classroom, clinical cases, collaborative learning groups, and clinical experiences can be woven though the curriculum, providing authentic learning opportunities for students to enter into cognitive apprenticeship with practicing clinicians and instructors. The didactic portion of the curriculum also offers opportunities for cognitive apprenticeship. Instructors can model their thought processes and verbalize their problem-solving processes while working on cases (Graham, 1996; Maudsley & Strivens, 2000). In fieldwork, preceptors can demonstrate and model the EBP skills and behaviors that students are expected to learn. Gradually, preceptors can reduce their direct assistance and shift from modeling to guiding or facilitating learning with the objective of engaging the student in the EBP process independently (Sullivan & Bossers, 1998).

Interventions That Change Practice

Considerable research has been published about the self-reported barriers to EBP (e.g., McCluskey, 2003; Salbach et al., 2007), such as lack of time, skills, and the ability to search for, appraise, and understand statistical analyses. In addition, considerable research exists about what practitioners think might help them to be more evidence based, such as more education and

Table 3-1

Suggestions for Teaching Evidence-Based Practice in Occupational Therapy Education

	COLLABORATIVE LEARNING	CASE-BASED METHOD	COGNITIVE APPRENTICESHIP
Objectives	• Improve understanding and problem resolution • Foster metacognitive awareness and metacognitive skills • Improve awareness of misunderstandings • Trigger help-seeking behaviors	• Learning content and strategies • Learning through problem solving • Improve self-directed learning • Actively construct knowledge in a collaborative manner with peers	• Embed learning in activities that make deliberate use of the social context • Promote conceptual understanding and development of problem-solving skills • Integrate a set of cognitive and metacognitive skills
Process	• Work in small groups to solve problems (integrate and solidify new understanding) • Construct inferences about a specific problem-solving situation • Test each other's understanding and knowledge-building through discussion, problem solving, and questioning	• Work with cases ranging in difficulty and level of detail • Select the important information among less pertinent information in a case with support from peers and instructors	• Work with ill-defined tasks and real-world problems representing authentic situations • Five-step process: modeling, scaffolding, coaching, articulation, exploration *Modeling* • Expert makes knowledge explicit, providing students with a concrete reference of expert/teacher performance • Helps learners understand the thinking involved in problem solving *Scaffolding* • Expert/teacher provides support to help learners carry out a task (carrying out parts of the overall task the learner cannot yet manage by providing physical supports or by providing suggestions and help along the way and as needed) *Coaching* • Expert/teacher observes learners while they carry out a task and offers hints, cues, feedback, reminders (as needed), and new tasks to bring the learner's performance closer to expert performance

(continued)

Table 3-1 (continued)

Suggestions for Teaching Evidence-Based Practice in Occupational Therapy Education

	COLLABORATIVE LEARNING	CASE-BASED METHOD	COGNITIVE APPRENTICESHIP
			Articulation • Learners talking out loud about their knowledge, reasoning, or problem-solving processes *Exploration* • Learners try out hypotheses, methods, and strategies similar to those that experts use to solve problems on their own • Compare their results to expert's/teacher's
Role of instructor	• Facilitate problem solving, reasoning, and the application of existing and prior knowledge	• Guide the learning process through open-ended questioning • Facilitate problem solving, reasoning, and the application of existing and prior knowledge	• Provide support and cueing in the initial stages of learning • Model and demonstrate expert-like decisions, knowledge, strategies • Progressively scaffold and remove support to facilitate learner autonomy
Outcomes	• Acquisition of content knowledge and problem-solving strategies • Generation of self-explanations • Improved self-monitoring skills	• Acquisition of content knowledge, strategies, and self-directed learning • Active construction of knowledge	• Greater role in learning • Independent performance of tasks • Integration of cognitive and metacognitive skills

From "Evidence-Based Practice: A Review of Theoretical Assumptions and Effectiveness of Teaching and Assessment Interventions in Health Professions," by A. Thomas, 2011, *Advances in Health Sciences Education: Theory and Practice, 16*(2). With kind permission from Springer Science and Business Media.

easy-to-read evidence summaries (e.g., Salbach, Veinot, Jaglal, Bayley, & Rolf, 2011). However, closing evidence-practice gaps depends on actual change in practice, not pondering what might change practice and not only improving search and appraisal skills. We have already reported that progressive evidence-based practitioners do not seem to worry about or discuss barriers much (McCluskey et al., 2008); they just "get on and do it." Therefore, a brief summary of effective interventions targeted at changing practitioner behavior is now presented, with a more detailed review in later chapters.

A series of Cochrane and non-Cochrane reviews have shown that small changes of up to 10% can be achieved using the following interventions: (a) printed educational materials such as clinical guidelines and guideline summaries; (b) educational meetings including workshops, conferences, and inservice sessions to address knowledge or clinical skills (e.g., cognitive behavioral therapy; Kramer & Burns, 2008); (c) reminders that prompt a practitioner to perform or avoid performing a test or intervention; (d) audit of client records followed by written or oral feedback about performance to create urgency and drive change; and (e) client-mediated information, where clients take evidence to their treating practitioner to help drive change. For a detailed review, see McCluskey (2010). Updates on these interventions can be found on the Web site of the Cochrane review group for Effective Practice and Organisation of Change (www.epoc.cochrane.org/en/index.html) and the free Canadian Web site "Treatment for Change" (www.cadth.ca/en/resources/rx-for-change/database/browse).

MEASURING CHANGE IN EVIDENCE-BASED PRACTICE COMPETENCIES

Review of the Evidence

Until about 1998, published assessment instruments focused mostly on the evaluation of critical appraisal, essentially ignoring the other EBP steps. Furthermore, the majority of instruments measured EBP knowledge and skills but did not objectively assess behaviors in actual practice. Most important, few had established validity and reliability (Shaneyfelt et al., 2006). In the last decade, several instruments have been developed to address the shortage of measures with strong psychometric properties that incorporate all steps of EBP. Green (1999) conducted a systematic review of evaluation instruments in graduate medical education training in the areas of clinical epidemiology, critical appraisal, and evidence-based medicine. The main objective of the studies included in Green's (1999) review was to improve critical appraisal skills (other EBP steps were excluded) in resident-directed small-group seminar teaching using scores on multiple-choice examination as the outcome measure. Only 4 of the 18 studies met minimum methodological standards for controlled trials and of the 7 studies that evaluated the effectiveness of teaching critical appraisal skills, the effect sizes ranged from no effect to a 23% net absolute increase in test scores. Green (1999), however, reported problems with the studies, including incomplete description of curriculum development, absence of behavioral objectives and clearly defined educational strategies, and inadequate evaluations of the curricula that introduced limitations to the systematic review process.

A 2006 systematic review by Shaneyfelt and colleagues identified 115 articles on assessment of EBP, representing 104 unique instruments administered primarily to medical students and postgraduate medical trainees. Although the majority of available valid instruments were self-report measures of skills in searching for and appraising the literature, the authors highlighted two instruments with strong psychometric properties that evaluated most of the EBP steps: (1) the Fresno Test (Ramos, Schafer, & Tracz, 2003), which uses two clinical vignettes and asks students to formulate a clinical question, acquire the evidence, appraise it, and then apply the evidence for the client depicted in the vignette; and (2) the Berlin Questionnaire (Fritsche, Greehalgh, Falck-Ytter,

Neumayer, & Kunz, 2002), which measures EBP knowledge and skills using a 15-item multiple choice test. Although the Berlin Questionnaire is easier to score than the Fresno Test, the Berlin Questionnaire does not evaluate all of the EBP steps (Agrawal, Szatmari, & Hanson, 2008).

Other instruments reviewed by Shaneyfelt and colleagues (2006) targeted fewer EBP steps and were specific to certain types of EBP curricula. In a 2007 review, Flores-Mateo and Argimon compiled 22 distinct assessment methods for evaluating the EBP skills, knowledge, behaviors, and attitudes of postgraduate health care workers. The authors described several problems with studies in their review including poorly reported feasibility of implementation, underreporting of time needed to administer and score the instruments, and lack of instrument validation. Only 45% ($n = 10$) of the instruments were validated with at least two or more types of evidence of validity or reliability. In addition, most instruments had limited applicability to different teaching modalities or to different curricula in the health professions.

CONSIDERATIONS FOR ASSESSMENT OF EVIDENCE-BASED PRACTICE COMPETENCIES

In the Classroom

To be compatible with and support a constructivist model of teaching and learning, assessment should be targeting both the process and the product of learning. We propose that the design of EBP assessment methods be grounded in the five-step process where competence is evaluated using different assessment tools that target the different skills involved in each step. Table 3-2 (Thomas, Saroyan, & Dauphinee, 2011) illustrates the key assumptions and features of assessment design and provides examples for application in EBP assessment.

Assessment of learning and competence in EBP requires careful planning. Instructors can design valid, reliable, and authentic assessments that take place in authentic environments similar to those in which the learner is expected to apply the newly acquired knowledge (Boston, 2003). Dynamic assessment evaluates learners' understanding and performance in EBP during a term of instruction. It also provides useful and immediate feedback to both the student and the instructors (Brown, Campione, Webber, & McGilly, 1992; Lajoie & Azevedo, 2006; Palinscar, 1998). This feedback reinforces students' metacognitive abilities and helps instructors to better scaffold student learning (Vygotsky, 1978), to modify the content and process of instruction, and to make recommendations to students for areas of improvement (Palinscar, 1998).

Assessment methods must clearly capture and be aligned with the learning objectives (Fenwick & Parsons, 2000; Frederiksen & Collins, 1990; Kelson, 2000). Both the methods and the manner in which they are used must converge with the specific expectations as previously stated in learning outcomes. Assessments should contain explicit criteria regarding what is expected from the student. Because the EBP process contains various steps and associated skills, the notion of transparency allows learners to know exactly what aspects are being evaluated and how (Bass & Glaser, 2004; Frederiksen & Collins, 1990; Frederiksen & White, 1997; Pellegrino, Chudowsky, & Glaser, 2001; Shepard, 2000, 2001; Wolf & Reardon, 1996). Access to evaluation criteria satisfies a basic fairness criterion and helps students develop their understanding of standards in a domain (Shepard, 2001).

When possible, instructors should use a broad range of formative and summative assessments (Pellegrino et al., 2001). No one single test score can capture the complexity of EBP and its five related steps. A wide range of assessments allows instructors to address the diversity of learner needs and develop a holistic understanding of what EBP knowledge and skills have been acquired (Fenwick & Parsons, 2000) and enhances validity and fairness of inferences by giving students various ways to show their competence in EBP (Pellegrino et al., 2001). Assessments should

Table 3-2

Assumptions and Features of Assessment Design and Examples of Application in Assessment of Evidence-Based Practice

ASSUMPTION	FEATURES	APPLICATION TO ASSESSMENT OF EVIDENCE-BASED PRACTICE
Planning and authenticity	• Planning of valid, reliable, and authentic assessments • Assessment takes place in authentic environments • Assessment tasks resemble the challenges learners will encounter in the course of ordinary living	• Teacher ask questions such as: "How should students demonstrate knowledge and competence in EBP?" "At what level should students be able to resolve problems at the end of an instructional episode?" "What important aspects of a student's performance do we want to draw inferences from when measuring student achievement in EBP?" "What situations and tasks should we observe to make the appropriate inferences?" • Assessments using simulated clients, real clients during fieldwork, and cases histories
Dynamic assessment	• Evaluates progress in knowledge and performance during the problem-solving process • Evaluates learners throughout a term of instruction to capture the degree of development in learning • Offers immediate feedback to both the learners and the teacher who use this information to scaffold the next steps of instruction, modify content and process of instruction, and make recommendations to learners for areas of improvement • Makes it possible to use assessment as a learning vehicle in a formative, rather than in a summative, way	• Assessment of EBP competencies throughout a term of instruction and in each of the academic years • Integration of EBP concepts across assignments • Regular feedback on EBP knowledge, skills, and behaviors
Alignment of assessment with learning outcomes	• Assessment methods converge with specific expectations stated in the learning outcomes	• If novice learners are expected to know the definition and purpose of EBP, assessment should target surface-type knowledge • If desired outcome is synthesis of research findings and integration of findings in clinical decision making, assessment should target these higher level skills in addition to surface knowledge regarding critical appraisal

(continued)

Table 3-2 (continued)

Assumptions and Features of Assessment Design and Examples of Application in Assessment of Evidence-Based Practice

ASSUMPTION	FEATURES	APPLICATION TO ASSESSMENT OF EVIDENCE-BASED PRACTICE
Transparency	• Presents learners with explicit evaluation criteria • Satisfies a basic fairness criterion • Helps learners develop their understanding of standards in a domain	• Assessment of critical appraisal skills; provide a detailed checklist with explicit criteria for the different areas of critical appraisal
Using a range of formative and summative assessments	• One way of meeting the diversity of learner needs • Helps to gain a holistic understanding of what knowledge and skills have been acquired • Enhances validity and fairness of inferences by giving learners various ways of showing competence • Formative assessment removes high-stakes element of assessment and informs learning	• Utilize different assessment methods that target the different skills involved in the five EBP steps for various clinical scenarios (e.g., essay questions, oral presentations, and client simulations) • Feedback on assignment that are not graded (e.g., searching for literature with a librarian, practice of critical appraisal using different checklists, etc.)
Group performance	• Assessment that targets group performance and contributions of individuals to that performance • Reflects many real-life situations involving interactions with others and contributions from many people	• Assessment of the contribution of various group members in working on a case depicting an EBP scenario
Focus on thinking and cognitive processes	• Assessment that targets the thinking and the cognitive processes involved in a domain, as opposed to emphasizing acquisition of content knowledge only	• May involve problem solving and decision making in the face of varying or conflicting scientific evidence regarding a treatment

From "Evidence-Based Practice: A Review of Theoretical Assumptions and Effectiveness of Teaching and Assessment Interventions in Health Professions," by A. Thomas, 2011, *Advances in Health Sciences Education: Theory and Practice, 16*(2). With kind permission from Springer Science and Business Media.

be designed to target group performance and group contributions to complex EBP situations because many real-life situations will require interactions with others. Assessment should focus on the thinking and the cognitive processes involved in EBP (decision making, problem solving) as opposed to emphasizing acquisition of content knowledge only (Pellegrino et al., 2001; Royer, Cisero, & Carlo, 1993; Shepard, 2000).

Lastly, authentic and performance-based assessments represent the complex thinking and problem-solving skills that are necessary for successful EBP in the world today. They are useful for assessing the process and product of learning (Bransford & Schwartz, 1999; Lajoie, 2003; Lajoie & Azevedo, 2006; Linn, Baker, & Dunbar, 1991; Pellegrino et al., 2001) and can be developed to reflect the types of competencies needed in most occupations and professions (Graue, 1993; Schuwirth & van der Vleuten, 2006; Shepard, 1989).

In Practice

The Fresno Test mentioned previously in this section was recently shortened and adapted for use with occupational therapists (the Adapted Fresno Test of Competence in EBP; McCluskey & Bishop, 2009) and physical therapists (Tilson, 2010). The test involves a practitioner reading a short clinical scenario and then writing a focused question to guide searching, describing search strategies, and answering questions about study design and interpretation. Each answer is scored, and the total score reflects competence in EBP. The Adapted Fresno Test was used to measure change in the EBP competence of over 100 occupational therapists following a 2-day workshop (McCluskey & Lovarini, 2005). The instrument is sensitive to change in novice practitioners but less discriminating with practitioners who already have some competence in EBP (McCluskey & Bishop, 2009).

A new test, the Knowledge of Research Evidence Competencies (K-REC) Test, is based on the Adapted Fresno Test and is sensitive to change in the skills and knowledge of entry-level physical therapy students (Long et al., 2011). The K-REC has also been validated for use with other entry-level health science students (human movement) and recent graduates (Lewis, Williams, & Olds, 2011). This tool is the only one validated for use with entry-level students in the allied health professions (Lewis et al., 2011).

HOW PRACTICE STYLE TRAITS MAY INFLUENCE PRACTICE

What individual practitioners consider to be credible sources of evidence varies, as does the weighting assigned to workload and waiting lists and willingness to diverge from peer norms. These three factors, referred to as *practice style traits*, may help to differentiate those who do and those who do not become evidence-based practitioners (Wyszewianski & Green, 2000). Understanding our own practice style traits and those of our peers (and students) can be helpful when trying to close evidence-practice gaps and select implementation strategies (Korner-Bitensy, Menon-Nair, Thomas, Boutin, & Arafah, 2007). Active seekers of evidence may become the opinion leaders of tomorrow.

A framework for classifying the practice style traits of practitioners was proposed by Wyszewianski and Green (2000) and is being used increasingly to classify practitioners using the Practice Style Questionnaire. The four traits proposed are seeker, receptive, traditionalist, and pragmatist. *Seekers* guide their practice using published research more than personal experience or expert advice. *Receptives* are more likely to defer to respected experts for advice but have some inclination toward using published evidence and changing practice. *Traditionalists* view clinical experience and respected experts as the most reliable sources of information. *Pragmatists* focus on practical matters, are easily influenced, and will change their practice based on workload demands and patient flow rather than published evidence. In a sample of 243 Canadian occupational therapists and physical therapists working in stroke rehabilitation (Korner-Bitensky et al., 2008) the most prevalent trait was pragmatist (56% for occupational therapists, 54% physical therapists) and the least prevalent was seeker (2% for occupational therapists, 11% for physical therapists). When the study was repeated with student occupational therapists and physical therapists ($n = 178$) the results were essentially the same, with < 1% of seekers. What these findings suggest is that very few students and practitioners who attend lectures and workshops on EBP may be adopters or opinion leaders. Educators need to cater more to the pragmatists, rather than the seekers. Furthermore, helping practitioners identify their own practice style and attitudes to practice change may help when implementing evidence.

CONCLUSION

In this chapter, we presented the steps of the EBP process and the key actions required to successfully go through each step. We also presented findings from recent research on the most effective educational strategies that can be used to support students and practitioners in their use of evidence in practice. Available and validated measures of EBP can be used to monitor one's skills. Becoming an evidence-based practitioner rests upon a balance of knowledge, skills, and attitudes that begin to develop during formal education and are further refined with clinical practice.

TAKE-HOME MESSAGES

✓ Competencies that an evidence-based practitioner will need to acquire include skills and knowledge to help write focused questions, the ability to search for and appraise evidence, and translate evidence into practice.

✓ EBP competencies begin during formal training and are further developed and refined with clinical practice.

✓ Effective EBP educational interventions for students and practitioners should be grounded in learning theories and be informed by current research in knowledge translation.

✓ There are available validated measures of EBP competence for students and practitioners.

WEB LINKS

Occupational Therapy Systematic Evaluation of Evidence

www.otseeker.com

This free database contains records of over 7,500 systematic reviews and preappraised randomized trials relevant to OT practice.

Physiotherapy Evidence Database

www.pedro.org.au

This free Web site contains records of over 20,000 clinical practice guidelines, systematic reviews, and preappraised randomized trials relevant to physical therapy practice.

Canadian Agency for Drugs and Technology in Health: Treatment for Change

www.cadth.ca/en/resources/rx-for-change/database/browse

This Canadian site provides updates of interventions aimed at changing professional practice such as audit and feedback, educational meetings, and clinical practice guidelines. The level of evidence is shown and summaries are updated every one to two years.

Cochrane Review Group: Effective Practice and Organisation Change

www.epoc.cochrane.org/en/index.html

This free Web site contains systematic reviews of interventions aimed at changing practitioner skills, knowledge, attitudes, and behaviors, as well as changing systems and organizations.

EVIDENCE-BASED PRACTICE LEARNING RESOURCES

The Adapted Fresno Test of Evidence-Based Practice Competence

This test measures change in EBP skills and knowledge, such as the ability to search for and critically appraise research papers. The test is intended for use with rehabilitation practitioners and has been validated to date with occupational therapists. The test contains two clinical scenarios followed by seven questions and asks respondents to write a focused clinical question, describe search strategies, and identify suitable study designs related to the scenario.

The Adapted Fresno Test is most useful for demonstrating change in novice learners of EBP, with the test content aimed at this population. Novice learners demonstrated a mean change of 26.8 points on the 156-point Adapted Fresno Test scale immediately after a 2-day training workshop on EBP. The test takes 20 minutes to complete and 20 minutes to score and is currently being used by rehabilitation practitioners to measure change in EBP competence following workplace-based training. A description and sample are provided in the paper published by McCluskey and Bishop (2009). A full copy can be provided free of charge from the first author by e-mail. A different version of the Fresno test had been developed and adapted for use with physical therapists (Tilson, 2010) and is also available from the author.

The Knowledge of Research Evidence Competencies Test

Developed and validated for use with physical therapy students, graduates, and, more recently, with human movement science students (Lewis et al., 2011; Long et al., 2011). Based on the Fresno test, the Knowledge of Research Evidence Competencies (K-REC) contains one clinical scenario and nine questions. Available from the authors upon request.

REFERENCES

Ackerman, P. L. (1996). A theory of adult intellectual development: Process, personality, interest and knowledge. *Intelligence, 22*, 229–259.

Ackerman, P. L. (2000). Domain-specific knowledge as the "dark-matter" of adult intelligence: Gf/Gc, personality and interest correlates. *Journal of Gerontology: Psychological Sciences, 55*(2), 69–84.

Ackerman, P. L. (2003). Aptitude complexes and trait complexes. *Educational Psychologist, 38*, 85–93.

Agrawal, S., Szatmari, P., & Hanson, M. (2008). Teaching evidence-based psychiatry: Integrating and aligning the formal and hidden curricula. *Academic Psychiatry, 32*(6), 470–474.

Alexander, P. A. (2003). The development of expertise: The journey form acclimation to proficiency. *Educational Researcher, 32*, 10–14.

Barrows, H. S. (2000). *Problem-based learning applied to medical education.* Springfield, IL: Southern Illinois University School of Medicine.

Bass, M. K., & Glaser, R. (2004). *Developing assessments to inform teaching and learning.* Los Angeles, CA: Graduate School of Education, University of California, Los Angeles.

Bennett, S., & Bennett, J. W. (2000). The process of evidence-based practice in occupational therapy: Informing clinical decisions. *Australian Occupational Therapy Journal, 47*, 171–180.

Bereiter, C., & Scardamalia, M. (1993). *Surpassing ourselves: An inquiry into the nature and implications of expertise.* La Salle, IL: Open Court.

Boston, C. (2003). *Cognitive science and assessment.* Retrieved from ERIC database.

Bransford, J. D., & Schwartz, L. D. (1999). Rethinking transfer. A simple proposal with multiple implications. *Review of Research in Education, 24*, 61–100.

Brown, A. L., Campione, J. C., Webber, L. S., & McGilly, K. (1992). Interactive learning environments: A new look at assessment and instruction. In B. R. Gifford, & M. C. O'Connor (Eds.), *Changing assessments: Alternative views of aptitude, achievement and instruction* (pp. 121–212). Boston, MA: Kluwer.

Chi, M. T. H. (2006). Two approaches to the study of experts' characteristics. In N. Charness, P. Feltovich, & R. Hoffman (Eds.), *Cambridge handbook of expertise and expert performance*. Cambridge: Cambridge University Press.

Clark, C., Scott, E., & Krupa, T. (1993). Involving clients in program evaluation and research: A new methodology for occupational therapy. *Canadian Journal of Occupational Therapy, 60*, 192–199.

Collins, A., Brown, J. S., & Newman, S. E. (1989). Cognitive apprenticeship: Teaching the craft of reading, writing and mathematics. In L. B. Resnick (Ed.), *Knowing, learning, and instruction: Essays in honor of Robert Glaser* (pp. 453–494). Hillsdale, NJ: Lawrence Erlbaum Associates.

Coomarasamy, A., & Khan, S. K. (2004). What is the evidence that postgraduate teaching in evidence-based medicine changes anything? A systematic review. *British Medical Journal, 329*, 1–5.

Coomarasamy, A., Taylor, R., & Khan, S. K. (2003). A systematic review of postgraduate teaching in evidence-based medicine and critical appraisal. *Medical Teacher, 25*, 77–81.

Craik, J., & Rappolt, S. (2003). Theory of research utilization enhancement: A model of occupational therapy. *Canadian Journal of Occupational Therapy, 70*(5), 266–275.

Craik, J., & Rappolt, S. (2006). Enhancing research utilization capacity through multifaceted professional development. The *American Journal of Occupational Therapy, 60*, 155–164.

Davidoff, F. (1999). In the teeth of the evidence. The curious case of evidence-based medicine. *The Mount Sinai Journal of Medicine, 66*, 75–83.

Dawes, M., Summerskill, W., Glasziou, P., Cartabellotta, A., Martin, J., Hopayian, K., …, Osborne, J. (2005). Sicily statement on evidence-based practice. *BMC Medical Education, 5*, 1.

Dubouloz, C. J., Egan, M., Vallerand, J., & von Zweck, C. (1999). Occupational therapists' perceptions of evidence-based practice. *American Journal of Occupational Therapy, 53*, 445–453.

Egan, M., Dubouloz, C. J., von Zweck, C., & Vallerand, J. (1998). The client-centered evidence-based practice of occupational therapy. *Canadian Journal of Occupational Therapy, 65*, 136–143.

Ernest, P. (1995). The one and the many. In L. Steffe & J. Gale (Eds.). *Constructivism in education* (pp. 459–486). NJ: Lawrence Erlbaum Associates.

Ethell, G. R., & McMeniman, M. M. (2000). Unlocking the knowledge in action of an expert practitioner. *Journal of Teacher Education, 51*, 87–101.

Evenson, D., & Hmelo, C. (2000). *Problem based learning: A research perspective on learning interactions*. Mahwah, NJ: Erlbaum.

Fenwick, T., & Parsons, J. (2000). *The art of evaluation. A handbook for educators and trainees*. Toronto, ON: Thompson Educational Publishing.

Flores-Mateo, G., & Argimon, J. (2007). Evidence based practice in postgraduate healthcare education: A systematic review. *BMC Health Services Research, 7*, 119–119.

Forbes, A., & Griffiths, P. (2002). Methodological strategies for the identification and synthesis of "evidence" to support decision-making in relation to complex health care systems and practices. *Nursing Inquiry, 9*, 141–155.

Frederiksen, J. R., & Collins, A. (1990). A systems approach to educational testing. *Educational Researcher, 18*, 27–32.

Frederiksen, J. R., & White, B. Y. (1997). *Reflective assessment of student's research within an inquiry-based middle school science curriculum*. Paper presented at the annual meeting of the American Educational Research Association, Chicago, IL.

Fritsche, L., Greenhalgh, T., Falck-Ytter, Y., Neumayer, H. H., & Kunz, R. (2002). Do short courses in evidence based medicine improve knowledge and skills? Validation of Berlin questionnaire and before and after study of courses in evidence based medicine. *British Medical Journal, 325*(7376), 1338.

Graham, C. L. (1996). Conceptual learning processes in physical therapy students. *Physical Therapy, 76*, 856–865.

Graue, M. E. (1993). Integrating theory and practice through instructional assessment. *Educational Assessment, 1*, 283–309.

Green, M. L. (1999). Graduate medical education training in clinical epidemiology, critical appraisal, and evidence-based medicine: A critical review of curricula. *Academic Medicine, 74*(6), 686.

Green, L., Gorenflo, D. W., & Wyszewianski, L. (2002). Validating an instrument for selecting interventions to change physician practice patterns: a Michigan Consortium for Family Practice Research study. *Journal of Family Practice,* 51(11):938-42.

Gruppen, L. D. (2007). Improving medical education research. *Teaching and Learning in Medicine, 19*(4), 331–335.

Hammell, K. W. (2001). Using qualitative research to inform the client-centered evidence-based practice of occupational therapy. *British Journal of Occupational Therapy, 64*, 228–234.

Hatala, R., & Guyatt, G. (2002). Evaluating the teaching of evidence-based medicine. *Journal of the American Medical Association, 288*(9), 1110–1112.

Haynes, R. B. (2002). What kind of evidence is it that evidence-based medicine advocates want health care providers and consumers to pay attention to? *British Medical Council Health Services Research, 2,* 3.

Haynes, R. B., Devereaux, P. J., & Guyatt, G. H. (2002). Clinical expertise in the era of evidence-based medicine and patient choice. *American College of Physicians Journal Club, 136,* A11–A14.

Herbert, D. R., Sherrington, C., Maher, C., & Mosely, M. A. (2001). Evidence-based practice—Imperfect but necessary. *Physiotherapy Theory and Practice, 17,* 210–211.

Hmelo-Silver, C. E. (2004). Problem-based learning: What and how do students learn? *Educational Psychology Review, 16*(3), 235–266.

Hmelo-Silver, C. E., Duncan, R. G., & Chinn, C. A. (2007). Scaffolding and achievement in problem-based and inquiry learning: A response to Kirschner, Sweller, and Clark (2006). *Educational Psychologist, 42*(2), 99–107.

Honebein, P. (1996). Seven goals for the design of Constructivist learning environments. In B. Wilson (Ed.), *Constructivist learning environments* (pp. 17–24). NJ: Educational Technology Publications.

Horsley, T., O'Neill, J., McGowan, J., Perrier, L., Kane, G., & Campbell, C. (2010). Interventions to improve question formulation in professional practice and self-directed learning. *Cochrane Database of Systematic Reviews, 5,* CD007335. doi:10.1002/14651858.CD007335.pub2

Hyde, J. P., Deeks, J., & Milne, J. (2006). *Teaching critical appraisal skills in health care settings. Review.* John Wiley & Sons.

Johnson, R. T., & Johnson, D. W. (1993). Implementing cooperative learning. *Education Digest, 58,* 62–66.

Jonassen, D. (1991). Evaluating constructivist learning. *Educational Technology, 36,* 28–33.

Jonassen, D. (1994). Thinking technology. *Educational Technology, 34,* 34–37.

Katrak, P., Bialocerkowski, E. A., Massy-Westropp, N., Saravana Kumar, V. S., & Grimeer, A. K. (2004). A systematic review of the content of critical appraisal tools. *BMC Medical Research Methodolology, 4,* 22.

Kelson, C. A. (2000). Epilogue. Assessment of students for proactive lifelong learning. In D. H. Evenson & C. E. Hmelo (Eds.), *Problem-based learning. A research perspective on learning interactions* (pp. 315–344). Mahwah, NJ: Lawrence Erlbaum.

Korner-Bitensky, N., Menon-Nair, A., Thomas, A., Boutin, E., Arafah, A.M. (2007). Practice style traits: do they help explain practice behaviours of stroke rehabilitation professionals? *Journal of Rehabilitation Medicine.* 39(9):685-692.

Kramer, T., & Burns, B. (2008). Implementing cognitive behavioural therapy in the real world: A case study of two mental health centres. *Implementation Science, 3,* 14.

Lajoie, S. P. (2003). Transitions and trajectories for studies of expertise. *Educational Researcher, 32,* 21–25.

Lajoie, S. P., & Azevedo, R. (2006). Teaching and learning in technology-rich environments. In P. A. Alexander & P. Winne (Eds.), *Handbook of Educational Psychology* (2nd ed., pp. 803–821). Mahwah, NJ: Erlbaum.

Lave, J., & Wenger, E. (1991). *Situated learning: Legitimate peripheral participation.* Cambridge, MA: Cambridge University Press.

Lewis, L. K., Williams, M. T., & Olds, T. S. (2011). Development and psychometric testing of an instrument to evaluate cognitive skills of EBP in the health professional disciplines. *BMC Medical Education. 11,* 77.

Linn, R., Baker, E., & Dunbar, S. (1991). Complex performance-based assessment: Expectations and validation criteria. *Educational Researcher, 20*, 15–21.

Lloyd-Smith, W. (1997). Evidence-based practice and occupational therapy. *The British Journal of Occupational Therapy, 60*, 474–478.

Long, K., McEvoy M., Lewis, L. K., Wiles, L., Williams, M., & Olds, T. (2011). Entry level training in evidence-based practice: Does it change knowledge and attitudes? *Internet Journal of Allied Health.*

Maher, C. G., Sherrington, C., Herbert, R. D., Moseley, A. M., & Elkins, M. (2003). Reliability of the PEDro scale for rating quality of randomized controlled trials. *Physical Therapy, 83*(8), 713–721.

Marks, D. F. (2002). *Perspectives on evidence-based practice.* Retrieved from www.nice.org.uk/niceMedia/pdf/persp_evid_marks.pdf

Mattingly, C., & Fleming, M. (1994). *Clinical reasoning: Forms of inquiry in a therapeutic practice.* Philadelphia, PA: F. A. Davis.

Maudsley, G., & Strivens, J. (2000). Promoting professional knowledge, experiential learning and critical thinking for medical students. *Medical Education, 34*, 535–544.

Mayer, R. E. (1987). *Educational psychology. A cognitive approach.* New York, NY: Harper Collins.

Maynard, A. (1994). Evidence-based medicine: An incomplete method for informing treatment choices. *Lancet, 349*(9045), 126.

McCluskey, A. (2003). Occupational therapists report a low level of knowledge, skill and involvement in evidence-based practice. *Australian Occupational Therapy Journal, 50*, 3–12.

McCluskey, A. (2010). Implementing evidence into practice. In T. Hoffmann, S. Bennett, & C. Del Mar (Eds.), *Evidence-based practice across the health professions* (pp. 318–339). Sydney, Australia: Churchill Livingstone.

McCluskey, A., & Bishop, B. (2009). The Adapted Fresno Test of Competence in Evidence-Based Practice. *Journal of Continuing Education in the Health Professions, 29*(2), 1–8.

McCluskey, A., Home, S., & Thompson, L. (2008). Becoming an evidence-based practitioner. In M. Law & J. MacDermid (Eds.), *Evidence-based rehabilitation: A guide to practice* (pp. 35–60). Thorofare, NJ: SLACK Incorporated.

McCluskey, A., & Lovarini, M. (2005). Providing education on evidence-based practice improved knowledge but did not change behaviour: A before and after study. *BMC Medical Education, 5*, 40.

McKeachie, J. W. (1986). Teaching psychology: Research and experience. In V. P. Makosley (Ed.), *The G. Stanley Hall lecture series* (Vol. 6). Washington, DC: American Psychological Association.

Menon, A., Cafaro, T., Loncaric, D., Moore, J., Vivona, A., Wynands, E., & Korner-Bitensky, N. (2010). Creation and validation of the PERFECT: A critical incident tool for evaluating change in the practices of health professionals. *Journal of Evaluation in Clinical Practice, 16*, 1170–1175.

Miles, A., Grey, J. E., Polychronis, A., Price, N., & Melchiorri, C. (2004). Developments in the evidence-based practice debate. *Journal of Evaluation in Clinical Practice, 10*, 129–142.

Mowinski-Jennings, B. M., & Loan, L. A. (2001). Misconceptions among nurses about evidence-based practice. *Journal of Nursing Scholarship, 33*(2), 121.

Neistadt, E. M., Wight, J., & Mulligan, E. S. (1997). Clinical reasoning case studies as teaching tools. *The American Journal of Occupational Therapy, 52*, 125–132.

Norman, G. R., & Shannon, I. S. (1998). Effectiveness of instruction in critical appraisal (evidence-based medicine) skills: A critical appraisal. *Canadian Medical Association Journal, 158*, 177–181.

Palinscar, A. M. (1998). Social constructivist perspectives on teaching and learning. *Annual Review of Psychology, 49*, 345–375.

Pellegrino, J. W., Chudowsky, N., & Glaser, R. (2001). *Knowing what students know: the science and design of educational assessment.* Washington, DC: National Academy Press.

Profetto-McGrath, J. (2005). Critical thinking and evidence-based practice. *Journal of Professional Nursing, 21*, 364–371.

Ramos, K. D., Schafer, S., & Tracz, S. M. (2003). Validation of the Fresno test of competence in evidence based medicine. *BMJ (International Ed.), 326*(7384), 319.

Rappolt, S. (2003). Evidence-based practice forum. The role of professional expertise in evidence-based occupational therapy. *American Journal of Occupational Therapy, 57*, 589–593.

Reagon, C., Bellin, W., & Boniface, G. (2008). Reconfiguring evidence-based practice for occupational therapists. *International Journal of Therapy and Rehabilitation, 15*(10), 428–436.

Reed, C. (1996). Improving the ability of master's level occupational therapy students to strategically problem solve when providing services to children and youth. *Dissertation Abstracts International.*

Rogers, J. C., & Holm, M. B. (1991). Occupational therapy diagnostic reasoning: A component of clinical reasoning. *American Journal of Occupational Therapy, 45*, 1045–1053.

Rolfe, G. (1998). *Expanding nursing knowledge: Understanding and researching your own practice.* Oxford, England: Butterworth Heinemann.

Rosenberg, W., & Donald, A. (1995). Evidence-based medicine: An approach to clinical problem solving. *British Medical Journal, 310*, 1122–1125.

Royer, M. J., Cisero, A. C., & Carlo, S. M. (1993). Techniques and procedures for assessing cognitive skills. *Review of Educational Research, 63*, 201–243.

Sackett, D. L., Rosenberg, W. M., Richardson, W. S., & Haynes, R. B. (1997). *Evidence-based medicine: How to practice and teach EBM.* Edinburgh, Scotland: Churchill, Livingston.

Salbach, N. M., Jaglal, S. B., Korner-Bitensky, N., Rappolt, S., & Davis, D. (2007). Practitioner and organizational barriers to evidence-based practice of physical therapists for people with stroke. *Physical Therapy, 87*(10), 1284–1303.

Salbach, N. M., Veinot, P., Jaglal, S. B., Bayley, M., & Rolfe, D. (2011). From continuing education to personal digital assistants: What do physical therapists need to support evidence-based practice in stroke rehabilitation? *Journal of Evaluation in Clinical Practice, 17*, 786–793.

Schuwirth, L. W. T., & van der Vlauten, C. P. M. (2006). Challenges for educationalists. *British Medical Journal, 333*(7567), 544–546.

Shaneyfelt, T., Baum, K. D., Bell, D., Feldstein, D., Houston, T. K., Kaatz, S., …, Green, M. (2006). Instruments for evaluating education in evidence-based practice: A systematic review. *Journal of the American Medical Association, 296*(9), 1116–1127.

Shepard, L. A. (1989). Why we need better assessment. *Educational Leadership, 46*, 5–9.

Shepard, L. A. (2000). The role of assessment in a learning culture. *Educational Researcher, 29*, 4–14.

Shepard, L. A. (2001). The role of classroom assessment in teaching and learning. In V. Richardson (Ed.), *Handbook of research on teaching* (pp. 1066–1101). Washington, DC: American Educational Research Association.

Shunk, D. H. (2000). Learning theories: An educational perspective (3rd ed). Upper Saddle River, NJ: Prentice Hall.

Slavin, R. E. (1991). Synthesis of research of cooperative learning. *Educational Leadership, 48*, 71–82.

Straus, S. E., Ball, C., Balcombe, N., Sheldon, J., & McAlister, F. A. (2005). Teaching evidence-based medicine skills can change practice in a community hospital. *Journal of General Internal Medicine, 20*, 340–343.

Straus, S. E., Richardson, W. S., Glasziou, P., & Haynes, R. B. (2005). *Evidence-based medicine. How to practice and teach EBM* (3rd ed.). Edinburgh, Scotland: Churchill Livingstone.

Sullivan, T. M., & Bossers, A. (1998). Occupational therapy fieldwork levels. *National Newsletter of the Canadian Association of Occupational Therapists, 15*, 8–9.

Teasell, R. W., Foley, N. C., Salter, K., Bhogal, S. K., Jutai, J., & Speechley, M. R. (2008). *Evidence-based review of stroke rehabilitation* (11th ed.). Canadian Stroke Network.

Thomas, A., Saroyan, A., & Dauphinee, W. D. (2011). Evidence-based practice: A review of theoretical assumptions and effectiveness of teaching and assessment interventions in health professions. *Advances in Health Sciences Education: Theory and Practice, 16*(2), 253–276.

Thomas, A., Saroyan, A., & Lajoie, S. P. (2011). Creation of an evidence-based practice reference model in falls prevention: Findings from occupational therapy. *Disability and Rehabilitation.*

Thomas, A., Saroyan, A., Snider, M. L. (2011). Evidence-based practice behaviors: A comparison amongst occupational therapy students and clinicians. *Canadian Journal of Occupational Therapy.*

Tilson, J. K. (2010). Validation of the modified Fresno test: Assessing physical therapists' evidence-based practice knowledge and skills. *BMC Medical Education, 10*, 38.

von Glasersfeld, E. (1995). A constructivist approach to teaching. In L. P. Steffe & J. E. Gale (Eds.), *Constructivism in education* (pp. 3–15). Hillsdale, NJ: Lawrence Erlbaum.

Vygotsky, L. (1978). *Mind in society: The development of higher psychological processes.* Cambridge, MA: Harvard University Press.

Welch, A., & Dawson, P. (2006). Closing the gap: collaborative learning as a strategy to embed evidence within occupational therapy practice. *Journal of Evaluation in Clinical Practice, 12*(2), 227.

Welsh, I., & Lyons, C. M. (2001). Evidence-based care and the case for intuition and tacit knowledge in clinical assessment and decision making in mental health nursing practice: An empirical contribution to the debate. *Journal of Psychiatric and Mental Health Nursing, 8*, 299–305.

Wilson, B., & Cole, P. (1991). A review of cognitive teaching models. *Educational Technology Research and Development, 39*, 47–64.

Wolf, D. P., & Reardon, S. F. (1996). Access to excellence through new forms of student assessment. In J. B. Baron & D. P. Wolf (Eds.), *Performance-based student assessment: Challenges and possibilities* (pp. 1–31). Chicago, IL: University of Chicago Press.

Wyszewianski, L., Green, L.A. (2000). Strategies for changing clinicians' practice patterns. A new perspective. *The Journal of Family Practice.* 49(5):461-464.

SUGGESTED READINGS

Bransford, J. D., Brown, A., & Cocking, R. (2000). *How people learn: Brain, mind, experience, and school.* Washington, DC: National Academy Press.

Miller, L., Bossers, A., Polatajko, H. J., & Hartley, M. (2001). Competency based fieldwork evaluation for health sciences students. *Occupational Therapy International, 8*, 244–262.

Philibert, D. B., Snyder, P., Judd, D., & Windsor, M. M. (2003). Practitioners' reading patters, attitudes and use of research reported in occupational therapy journals. *The American Journal of Occupational Therapy, 57*, 450–458.

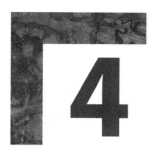

OUTCOME MEASUREMENT IN EVIDENCE-BASED REHABILITATION

Joy C. MacDermid, PhD, PT Reg (Ont), FCAHS;
Mary Law, PhD, OT Reg (Ont), FCAHS; and Susan L. Michlovitz, PT, PhD, CHT

LEARNING OBJECTIVES

After reading this chapter, the practitioner will be able to:

- Describe an outcome measure and how these measures fit into evidence-based practice (EBP).
- Relate outcome measurement to the *International Classification, Functioning, Disability and Health* (ICF).
- Differentiate between different types of outcome measures for rehabilitation practice.
- Develop skills to find and select appropriate outcome measures.
- Use a standardized process to appraise the quality of individual studies of outcome measures.
- Use standardized criteria to evaluate the relative merits of an outcome measure.
- Design an outcome measure strategy for use with individual patients.
- Use outcome measures scores to make decisions about current status and set goals for individual patients.
- Use outcome measures to make decisions about changes resulting from rehabilitation interventions.
- Identify barriers to implementing outcome measures in practice and recognize potential solutions and opportunities to overcome the barriers.

The purposes of this chapter are to (a) provide the practitioner with the foundations for finding, selecting, and applying evidence-based outcome measures to patient-centered care and (b) incorporate these measures in an evaluation process that determines the impact of evidence-based clinical decisions.

Law M., & MacDermid, J. C.
Evidence-Based Rehabilitation: A Guide
to Practice, Third Edition (pp 65–104).
© 2014 SLACK Incorporated.

Outcome Measures Are Integral to Evidence-Based Practice

First you ask the clinical question, find the evidence, evaluate it, and make a decision. Then you must complete the fifth step in the EBP process by evaluating the outcomes of your evidence-based decisions. Evaluation of the impact of an evidence-based choice is critical to the ongoing individualization of rehabilitation programs to optimize outcomes for individual patients. The process of routine outcome administration in practice is critical to the development of expertise as an evidence-based practitioner. Outcome measures selected for patient evaluation and decisions should be valid and reliable and able to measure the impacts of the rehabilitation interventions provided to patients. The following are desirable qualities of these measures:

- Be easy for the practitioner to access/apply and provide minimal inconvenience or discomfort for the patient.
- Be relevant and applicable across different contexts (clinical conditions/severity, language/literacy, cultures, environments).
- Have clearly defined standardized procedures to allow consistent application and interpretation.
- Have the ability to assist with diagnosis/classification, goal setting, prognosis, and/or measurement of treatment effectiveness for individual patients.
- Reflect domains of patients' health that may be affected by rehabilitation.
- Provide a consistent numeric metric that can accurately quantify treatment effects associated with different interventions.
- Have sufficient comparative data to norms and others with similar conditions.
- Have strong consistent measurement properties across different patient populations and contexts.

Any single outcome measure is unlikely to fulfill all measurement purposes because the measurement properties that optimize different measurement purposes can be competing. Fortunately, a spectrum of outcome measures is available to evaluate relevant aspects of rehabilitation practice. Though the evidence is incomplete on most measures with respect to all of the criteria previously listed, rehabilitation has a strong tradition of evaluating clinical measurement as one of its foundational scientific principles. Thus, there is a substantial—but imperfect—body of evidence to inform how we evaluate the outcomes of our interventions. Clinicians should be able to understand the properties of different outcome measures and apply an evidence-based approach to selecting and interpreting the scores obtained from an outcome evaluation process. When evaluating the impact of a clinical decision, it is important to match the evaluation indicator to the type of decision that was made and to the focus of rehabilitation.

Basic Purposes of Clinical Measurement

Clinical measurement can serve three different purposes:

1. Evaluate change over time (treatment effectiveness, maturation, and decline in status)
2. Discriminate between or among different groups (diagnosis, classification)
3. Predict future status (diagnosis or outcome)

A measure is labeled an outcome measure if it is used to evaluate change following interventions (treatment effectiveness). This type of use for a measure is the most common clinical purpose of measurement. Outcome measures can help us determine whether a change occurs in an aspect of functioning and/or health following rehabilitative intervention. Evaluation over time may also be used to measure maturation effects (as is sometimes required in pediatrics) or decline, which can be measured as an indication of the functional implications of aging or disease. The form of validity that is most relevant to this function is *responsiveness*—the ability of a measure to detect change over time.

The second most common purpose for using a measure of patient status is to discriminate between subgroups. Discrimination can result in classification into clinically meaningful diagnostic or classification subgroups. Diagnostic measures typically include clinical diagnostic tests performed by the therapist but can also include patient-report measures designed for diagnosis. For example, when diagnosing carpal tunnel syndrome, we can use a hand diagram (Katz & Stirrat, 1990) or a diagnostic questionnaire (Kamath & Stothard, 2003). Classification can also separate different clinical subgroups to establish their treatment needs or functional capability. For example, it has been shown that a classification system is useful to divide patients with low back pain into different clinical subgroups that require different treatment approaches (Fritz, Delitto, & Erhard, 2003). Others have developed a staging system for functional independence across the activities of daily living (ADL), sphincter management, mobility, and executive function domains (ASME) using the Functional Independence Measure (FIM) in a manner consistent with the ICF model as a method for "assessment and goal setting in terms that are meaningful to patients and their caregivers" (Stineman, Ross, Fiedler, Granger, & Maislin, 2003). Discriminative (known groups) validity is the most related measurement property for this type of clinical tool application.

Lastly, measures are sometimes used to predict a patient's future status. For example, the Movement Assessment of Infants, a neuromotor assessment tool, has been used to predict which infants will be diagnosed with cerebral palsy at a future follow-up (Harris et al., 1984). The FIM has been used to predict discharge status for stroke patients, correctly predicting outcomes in 70% of cases (Mauthe, Haaf, Hayn, & Krall, 1996). Others have shown that the Quebec Task Force Classification is discriminative at intake, whereas the pain pattern classification procedures—including centralization and non-centralization—help predict return to work 1 year after rehabilitation. Thus, these measures have different types of validity—the Quebec Task Force Classification is discriminative but not predictive, whereas centralization is predictive (Werneke & Hart, 2004). Predictive validity is the most relatable measurement property for this type of clinical tool application.

Reasons to Measure Outcomes in Practice

Measuring outcomes in practice can benefit the individual patient–therapist interaction by focusing the interaction to achieve relevant goals and outcomes. The potential to improve recognition of the role of rehabilitation in the health care system can be reinforced if appropriate measures are selected and reported. Finally, routine outcome measurement can support the scientific foundations of the profession.

Practice that is evidence based is by definition reflective, because it incorporates formal evaluation of the impact of decision making as the fifth step of the process. Using standardized measures to make decisions about individual patients has the potential to improve decision making. For example, routine administration of the Canadian Occupational Performance Measure (COPM) has been associated with improvements in practice parameters such as knowledge of the patient's perspective on outcome and clinical decision making (Colquhoun, Letts, Law, MacDermid, & Edwards, 2012). Unfortunately, there is often limited and inconclusive evidence about the effects of routine administration of standardized outcome evaluation on the outcomes achieved (Colquhoun, Letts, Law, MacDermid, & Edwards, 2010).

There are potential benefits to incorporating routine outcome measurement in practice beyond the immediate patient encounter. Standardized outcome processes allow rehabilitation professionals to provide data on the benefits of rehabilitation to referral sources and payers, thereby strengthening the role of rehabilitation in the health care system. Routine outcome evaluation is becoming an increased expectation within the health care system. The increased burden of an aging population, expansion of the use of technology, and global economic challenges all place pressure on the sustainability of the health care system. The ever increasing need to demonstrate to payers and administrators that health care dollars are being allocated to worthy services makes it imperative that rehabilitation providers capture the impacts of their interventions. Practitioners who have an integrated evidence-based approach that includes outcome evaluation into their clinical practice will be prepared to justify their services.

Outcome Measures Are Not Just for Research

Evaluation of outcomes is distinct from clinical research. In fact, it is important that clinicians know measuring outcomes is not performed for research purposes. Standardized measures should be used for decision making regarding individual patients. However, practice-based evidence can be an important driver of EBP. Evidence derived from practice can identify priority areas for research where outcomes are suboptimal or identify practice variations that suggest that optimization of care might be improved. Further, with the increasing acknowledgment of the importance of effectiveness research, the importance of observational research documenting the clinical outcomes achieved in practice is increasingly being valued (Jette & Keysor, 2002).

FRAMEWORKS AND DEFINITIONS FOR UNDERSTANDING HEALTH OUTCOMES

The biomedical model defines *health* as the absence of disease. This model assumes that diseases or injuries lead to dysfunction that can result in reduced health. Historically, the biomedical model has significantly influenced rehabilitation and its approach to outcome measurement. Though there was inherent value in this model as a contributor to the development of rehabilitation, it falls short from embracing the essence of rehabilitation because it implies that accurate diagnosis and identification of the biological defects can directly lead to selection of interventions that will maximize health outcomes. Measurement in a biomedical framework focuses on structural or system integrity to evaluate the success of an intervention. The influence of this model on rehabilitation practice is seen in areas that continue to emphasize measures of impairment as treatment outcomes.

The biomedical model has played a critical role in the development and recognition of rehabilitation. Advancements in recognizing pathology, defining physical and mental impairments, and designing interventions to mitigate these impairments have been achieved using this model. Typically, rehabilitation practice focuses on maximizing functional movement, activity, and communication as a means of restoring meaningful participation. Many rehabilitation practitioners continue to rely on the medical model when it comes to evaluating outcomes by focusing on impairment measures to evaluate their treatment programs (Abrams et al., 2006; MacDermid, Wojkowski, Kargus, Marley, & Stevenson, 2010). The benefits of rehabilitation can be underestimated when outcome assessment focuses on impairments because the benefits of rehabilitation practice are achieved by implementing interventions that allow people to become more functional and assume valued life roles—sometimes in the absence of any change of impairment. Furthermore, as the burden of chronic disease and episodic illnesses increases, this underestimation will become increasingly problematic because the relative importance of impairment reduction versus adaptation/self-management will increasingly shift toward the latter.

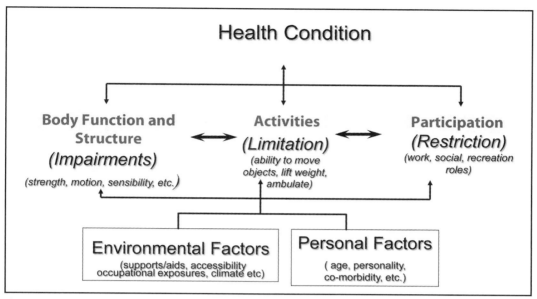

Figure 4-1. Interaction of concepts. (From The *International Classification of Functioning, Disability and Health,* by the World Health Organization, 2001, Geneva, Switzerland. Adapted with permission.)

The International Classification of Functioning, Disability, and Health

Measuring health outcomes requires a conceptual framework for understanding health. The most internationally accepted standard is a classification system for understanding functioning and disability that was introduced in 2001 by the World Health Organization (WHO): the *International Classification of Functioning, Disability and Health* (Finger, Cieza, Stoll, Stucki, & Huber, 2006; Rimmer, 2006; Steiner et al., 2002; Stucki et al., 2002; Stucki, Cieza, & Melvin, 2007; Stucki, Ewert, & Cieza, 2002, 2003; Stucki, Maksimovic, Davidovic, & Jorga, 2007; Figure 4-1). The ICF, is a classification of health and health-related domains. As a conceptual model it is a biopsychosocial model that acknowledges the interaction between different aspects of health, individual attributes, and their environment. As a language, it allows us to classify the domains of health from body, individual, and societal perspectives by means of two lists: a list of body functions and structure and a list of domains of activity and participation. Because an individual's functioning and disability occur in a context, the ICF also includes a list of environmental factors. Although personal factors also impact on health, they are not specifically coded within the ICF.

The ICF has become the most internationally accepted model of health and is used by a variety of health care providers. Its biopsychosocial view of health is well aligned with the approach taken to rehabilitation by most rehabilitative disciplines. This model portrays an interactive relationship among impairments, activities, and participation, mediated by environmental context and personal factors. Rehabilitation therapists are familiar with the interactive nature of the components of the ICF because it is part of our assessment of the etiological factors that contribute to disability; it is also used in intervention planning. Rehabilitation measures often focus on measuring disability. The ICF attempts to mainstream disability by highlighting that all individuals experience health decrements or limitations.

The ICF has core values of universality, parity, neutrality, and environmental awareness. *Universality* means that the ICF should apply to all persons, regardless of their health condition. The *parity* principle suggests that disability should not be differentiated by etiology/type of health condition. For example, mental and physical conditions that affect functioning and disability should not be differentiated as more vital components of disability. The *neutrality* principle focuses on the need to use neutral language in classification so that both positive and negative aspects of functioning and disability can be reflected. The fourth ICF principle is the necessity to include the environment because the ICF embraces the social model of disability. Environmental factors considered in the ICF include physical factors such as climate, terrain, and the built environment; social/cultural attitudes; laws/policies/institutions; and other aspects of environment.

The ICF has developed terms to define different aspects of health (Grimby & Smedby, 2001; Steiner et al., 2002; Stucki et al., 2002; www.who.int/classifications/icf/en). *Body functions* are physiological or psychological functions of body systems (WHO, 1980). *Body structures* are anatomical parts of the body such as organs, limbs, and their components. *Impairment* is the loss or abnormality of psychological, physiological, or anatomical structure or function. Examples of impairments that rehabilitation therapists measure include mobility of joints, control of movement, and sensation (Table 4-1).

Activity is the execution of a task or action by an individual. *Participation* is involvement in a life situation. Inability in these areas can be termed *activity limitations* or *participation restrictions*, respectively. Activity limitations can be measured in a variety of ways. For example, patients may perform standardized tests in a clinical setting by recording the time to complete the test (e.g., time to up-and-go) or may evaluate performance in a qualitative way. Conversely, clinicians may administer questionnaires where patients can self-report difficulties in performing tasks. Many self-report functional scales contain both activity- and participation-type items. Recently, there has been a greater interest in the development of measures of participation that focus on a person's functioning within everyday environments in their home and community.

Contextual factors are an integral component of ICF and consist of environmental factors (the physical, social, and attitudinal environment in which people live and conduct their lives) and personal factors. The ICF model is increasingly being used as a conceptual framework for rehabilitation practice and clinical research. However, the ICF is much more than a framework to explain health. It is also a hierarchical classification, a common language that allows for uniform indication across disciplines and about disability.

International Classification of Functioning, Disability, and Health *Qualifiers*

The ICF uses qualifiers to record the presence and severity of a problem on a 5-point scale (*no impairment*, *mild*, *moderate*, *severe*, and *complete*). At present, there is no consistent metric for defining the qualifiers, although standardized outcome measures linked to ICF codes may form a bridge between existing health measures and ICF. The clinical measurement literature is increasingly reporting studies where items on health or disability scales are being linked to ICF codes (Cieza et al., 2005; Weigl et al., 2003). This process involves identifying which ICF code(s) best represent the content of items on self-report questionnaires (Cieza et al., 2005).

For activity and participation domains, ICF uses two qualifiers: performance and capacity. It is important to note that these words are used in a different way than in some other rehabilitation contexts. In the ICF, a performance qualifier describes what an individual does in his or her current environment, and capacity describes an individual's ability to execute a task or an action. Conversely, in other rehabilitation contexts we often think about performance being a test that is performance based and capacity to be a specific type of test that focuses on establishing someone's maximum capacity in some aspect of physical function. For example, it is common to use performance-based tests that assess dexterity, balance, gait, memory, etc. Capacity tests such as functional capacity assessment or functional residual capacity (cardiorespiratory) tests focus on establishing what a

Table 4-1

Definitions of the Dimensions Considered in the Context of a Health Condition

DIMENSIONS	DEFINITIONS	LIMITATIONS	EXAMPLES OF TARGET OUTCOMES

Body functions and structure	Body functions are the physiological and psychological functions of the body systems. Body structures are the anatomical parts of the body such as organs, limbs, and their components	Impairments are problems in body function or structure such as a significant deviation or loss	• Range of motion
			• Balance
			• Strength
			• Sensibility
			• Muscle tone
			• Wound size
			• Visual tracking
			• Praxis
			• Tidal volume
			• Heart rate
			  ○ Nerve conduction
			  ○ Imaging results

Activity	The performance of a task or action by an individual	Activity limitations are difficulties an individual may have in the performance of activities	• Walking • Lifting a glass • Dexterity • Functional capacity • Overhead lift • Transfer • Eating • Dressing • Toileting • Throwing a ball • Making a bed
Participation	An individual's involvement in life situations in relation to health conditions, body functions and structures, activities, and *contextual factors	Participation restrictions are problems an individual may have in the manner or extent of involvement in life situations	Ability to participate in: • Work • Community • Family life • Advocacy • Lived experiences • Usual social roles

*Contextual factors: An integral component of the classification, consisting of environmental factors (the physical, social, and attitudinal environment in which people live and conduct their lives) and personal factors.

(continued)

Table 4-1 (continued)

Definitions of the Dimensions Considered in the Context of a Health Condition

DEFINITIONS IN *INTERNATIONAL CLASSIFICATION OF FUNCTIONING, DISABILITY, AND HEALTH*
Body functions are physiological functions of body systems (including psychological functions).
Body structures are anatomical parts of the body such as organs, limbs, and their components.
Impairments are problems in body function or structure such as a significant deviation or loss.
Activity is the execution of a task or action by an individual.
Participation is involvement in a life situation.
Activity limitations are difficulties an individual may have in executing activities.
Participation restrictions are problems an individual may experience in involvement in life situations.
Environmental factors make up the physical, social, and attitudinal environment in which people live and conduct their lives.

From The *International Classification of Functioning, Disability and Health*, by the World Health Organization, 2001, Geneva, Switzerland. Reprinted with permission.

person is capable of doing and hence are consistent with the ICF definition. Athletic therapists think about performance in relation to athletic performance. As therapists we are aware that patients do not always perform what they are capable of performing, and this may be an important consideration in our rehabilitation planning. Questions that ask patients about "how often did you do this" versus "can you do this" may tap into those differences, but we know that it is much more complex than expecting our patients to differentiate these two concepts.

The ICF is a hierarchical classification system where one can specify the content by finding codes that provide the ICF standard terminology (codes). As one moves down the hierarchical structure, the level of detail becomes more precise and more exclusive. At the top, for chapter level, broad categories of health are specified. Table 4-2 is a list of the chapters covered by ICF. For example, if you wish to say that someone had problems with activities of daily life, at the ICF chapter level that might come under self-care. If you wish to be more detailed about what aspects of self-care had limitations, then you would drill down to the level of detail you wish to reach. This hierarchical structure allows people to describe things at the level of detail appropriate to their purpose.

The ICF Web site provides training materials for learning the ICF and its applications (www.who.int/classifications/icf/en). It also provides an online version of the ICF classification system (http://apps.who.int/classifications/icfbrowser). Using the online version, people can enter the limitation or function that they wish to describe and find the ICF codes and their definitions.

One of the challenges in using the ICF, particularly for clinicians, is the large number of codes and understanding of what level of detail to use them. In recognition of this difficulty, the ICF Research Branch has led the development of core sets. These are reduced sets of codes that go through a formal process to be recognized by an international consensus as most relevant for specific patient subgroups or areas of practice. Users are not restricted from using other codes, but it does provide a vehicle for focusing on the most relevant codes and potentially devising applications around the core sets. There are an increasing number of core sets available and these can be downloaded from the Web site (www.icf-research-branch.org/download/viewcategory/5.html). They

Table 4-2

Chapters in *International Classification of Functioning, Disability, and Health*

BODY FUNCTION
Mental functions
Sensory functions and pain
Voice and speech functions
Functions of the cardiovascular, hematological, immunological, and respiratory systems
Functions of the digestive, metabolic, and endocrine systems
Genitourinary and reproductive functions
Neuromusculoskeletal and movement-related functions
Functions of the skin and related structures

BODY STRUCTURE
Structure of the nervous system
The eye, ear, and related structures
Structures involved in voice and speech
Structure of the cardiovascular, immunological, and respiratory systems
Structures related to the digestive, metabolic, and endocrine systems
Structure related to genitourinary and reproductive systems
Structure related to movement
Skin and related structures

ACTIVITIES AND PARTICIPATION
Learning and applying knowledge
General tasks and demands
Communication
Mobility
Self-care
Domestic life
Interpersonal interactions and relationships
Major life areas
Community, social, and civic life

ENVIRONMENTAL FACTORS
Products and technology
Natural environment and human-made changes to environment
Support and relationships
Attitudes
Services, systems, and policies

From The *International Classification of Functioning, Disability and Health*, by the World Health Organization, 2001, Geneva, Switzerland. Reprinted with permission.

cross a spectrum of types of health disorders including cancer, musculoskeletal, neurological, mental health, and others. They are more closely linked to areas of practice and specific health disorders (e.g., hand conditions and vocational rehabilitation).

Core sets are developed by a structured process led by the ICF Research Branch, which provides consistency in process and ensures balanced, multidisciplinary, international evidence and expert-based consensus. The nature of each core set will vary to a certain extent by the consensus achieved.

The core set development process involves a rigorous review of the published health literature to define the concepts of health and disability that have been reported for given health conditions, qualitative work with the patient groups to define aspects of health and disability important to patients, and survey work with experts to obtain their perspectives on the health and disability issues for that health condition. This information is then presented to an international consensus panel that uses this information, their expertise, and discussion to arrive at a draft core set. The core sets then go on to additional validation performed by the ICF Research Branch. The finalized core sets are published by the ICF Research Branch in research publications and are openly available on their Web site. Each core set is actually composed of a comprehensive and a brief core set. The comprehensive core set is a set of codes that provides "everything that is needed, and nothing that is not" to describe the health and functioning of a person with that health disorder. Comprehensive core sets may be useful for multidisciplinary teams, clinical research, or other applications. The brief core set is a condensed set of codes that represents "the minimal set of codes that describe health and functioning" in that circumstance/condition. These are likely to be more relevant for an individual clinician because they provide a more manageable set of codes.

Applications of ICF in rehabilitation are rapidly emerging (Alviar, Olver, Brand, Hale, & Khan, 2011; Bilbao et al., 2003; Deathe et al., 2009; Geertzen, Rommers, & Dekker, 2011; Grill, Stucki, Boldt, Joisten, & Swoboda, 2005; Harty, Griesel, & van der Merwe, 2011; Hickson & Scarinci, 2007; Kuipers, Foster, Smith, & Fleming, 2009; Leyshon & Shaw, 2008; Lohmann, Decker, Muller, Strobl, & Grill, 2011; Maini, Nocentini, Prevedini, Giardini, & Muscolo, 2008; Oltman, Neises, Scheible, Mehrtens, & Gruneberg, 2008; Reed et al., 2009; Reinhardt, 2011; Rimmer, 2006; Soberg, Finset, Roise, & Bautz-Holter, 2008; Stucki et al., 2003, 2007; Tempest & McIntyre, 2006; Verhoef, Toussaint, Putter, Zwetsloot-Schonk, & Vliet Vlieland, 2008). The ICF has been used in rehabilitation for a wide variety of purposes including defining roles on multidisciplinary teams, framing multidisciplinary treatment and documentation, identifying the scope of measurement when adopting for measures for practice, and establishing rehabilitation needs. Many other potential applications are possible. As rehabilitation practitioners develop and share these applications, the ICF may become more fully realized and intuitively obvious.

FUNCTION, PARTICIPATION, HEALTH STATUS, AND QUALITY OF LIFE AS OVERARCHING REHABILITATION OUTCOMES

The WHO defines health as "a state of complete physical, mental, and social well-being and not merely the absence of disease and infirmity." This definition reflects domains often used to define health-related quality of life (HRQOL) that focus on physical, mental, and social domains (Jette, 1999). For example, the model of health adopted by the Patient-Reported Outcomes Measurement Information System (PROMIS), a large enterprise focused on the evaluation of outcomes (www.nihpromis.org), specifies these three domains as foundational in its conceptual model. The definition can apply to health promotion, recovery, and adaptation as processes that enhance health and hence is well-aligned with rehabilitation.

An overarching or global outcome that represents the ultimate goal for the patient can be useful to compare across different contexts. Potential concepts that fulfill this role for rehabilitation practice include function, participation, health status, quality of life (QOL), or HRQOL. Unfortunately, the terminology around many of these concepts is not used consistently in clinical or research applications. Further, different disciplines can adopt internal definitions and traditions that serve as barriers to external communication.

Generic outcome measures that represent broad aspects of health that are universally accepted include terms such as health, QOL, and HRQOL. These are often used interchangeably without considering differences in meaning among these terms. A systematic review (Post, de Witte, & Schrijvers, 1999) on QOL measurement noted that there are three types of constructs: health, well-being, or a superordinate construct that encompasses both. These authors found that the concept of QOL has been used to be synonymous with a variety of terms: "health status, physical functioning, perceived health status, subjective health, health perceptions, symptoms, need satisfaction, individual cognition, functional disability, psychiatric disturbance, well-being and often, several of these at the same time."

Rehabilitation practitioners usually do not view the terms listed previously as interchangeable. In some cases, there are discipline-specific preferred terms/definitions that represent overarching outcomes. For example, occupational therapists often view participation as an overarching outcome. However, they may not view participation in exactly the same terms as the ICF does (Hemmingsson & Jonsson, 2005). Athletic therapists may view participation as return to sport. Physical therapists often view function as a primary goal for the patient and thus have a tendency to see function as their overarching outcome. Speech language pathologists may see communication as their overarching goal. Rehabilitation therapists should examine what their core principles are with respect to these overarching goals and determine whether their evaluation processes capture these goals. There are positive and negative aspects of having discipline-specific overarching outcomes. These may be beneficial in that they are most directly linked to the identity or scope of practice of the discipline. However, broad outcomes that are not discipline specific and convey overall health may be more easily communicated outside of the profession.

Quality of Life

QOL generally has a broad context and is concerned with a person's overall satisfaction with respect to the aspects of his or her life that he or she considers to be important. HRQOL is concerned with QOL in the context of a given health status affecting that person. The National Institutes of Health (NIH) defines QOL as "the overall enjoyment of life." QOL may be affected by health, but the focus of QOL is generally broader and strongly emphasizes the individual's valuation of his or her overall circumstances in life. Hence, political, economic, cultural, and environmental factors might be considered to have a relatively larger impact on QOL than on health. The Constitution of the WHO defines QOL as "an individual's perception of their position in life in the context of the culture and value systems in which they live and in relation to their goals, expectations, standards and concerns" (WHO QOL, 1997; www.who.int/mental_health/evidence/who_qol_user_manual_98.pdf). The WHO considers QOL to be subjective experience that is not "simply equated with the terms 'health status,' 'life style,' 'life satisfaction,' 'mental state,' or 'well-being.' Rather, it is a multidimensional concept incorporating the individual's perception of these and other aspects of life."

There are two basic approaches to measuring QOL: multidimensional direct assessment and utility measures. Multidimensional measures try to tap into the important constructs that represent QOL, whereas utility measures focus directly on the evaluation process and try to calibrate someone's current QOL between defined anchors (e.g., death and perfect health). Because QOL by definition implies a valuation of the individual's perception of his or her satisfaction with life circumstances, one might expect questions that focus on the individual's satisfaction with his or her current status to be more representative of this concept. Health status measures also assess across domains of health but are more focused on establishing status rather than satisfaction with that health state. The most commonly used health status measure is the Short Form-36 (SF-36). A number of measures that are termed *disease-specific, quality-of-life measures* might more appropriately be framed as disease-specific health status measures, because they cross domains of health but do not directly assess whether people are satisfied with their current health state. The WHO has developed a QOL measure (WHOQoL-100) and a shorter version, the WHOQoL-BREF, that include the following domains: physical capacity, psychological, social relationships, environment, independence, and spirituality.

In summary, when selecting overarching outcomes, rehabilitation therapists need to consider the following:

- What conceptual framework underlies my practice?
- What aspects of overall health or QOL am I engaged in affecting?
- What measures are available that represent the dimensions of health and QOL that I am affecting?

Types of Outcome Measures—Considering Evaluator and Perspective

Outcome measures vary according to their structure, purpose, domain, and measurement methods and properties. Outcome scales require that measurements or ratings be performed. Measurements can be observer based (sometimes called *clinician-based outcomes*) or self-reported (sometimes called *patient-reported outcomes*). Patient-reported outcomes can actually be self-reported (using questionnaires) or based on interviews that use structured or semi-structured inquiries to obtain patient responses.

Traditionally in medicine and, subsequently, in rehabilitation, there has been a strong reliance on clinician-based outcomes ranging from physical impairment measures to composite observer-based scales where clinicians rate performance while observing patients perform a task. The assumption by many clinicians has been that these measures are more reliable than self-report measures. In fact, studies indicate the contrary. Well-constructed, self-reported measures generally demonstrate a higher level of reliability than physical impairment measures assessed at the same time (MacDermid, Ramos, Drosdowech, Faber, & Patterson, 2004; Marx, Bombardier, & Wright, 1999). Some impairment measurements are associated with a high degree of tester or occasion variability. For example, strength and endurance can vary substantially even within a single day in a medically stable person (Boadella, Sluiter, & Frings-Dresen, 2003; Coldwells, Atkinson, & Reilly, 1994).

Agreement between clinician-based outcomes (particularly at the impairment level) and self-reported measures of pain and disability has been shown to be only moderate across a wide spectrum of patient problems, suggesting that these provide distinct perspectives. In some subdisciplines, it is popular to use overall indices of outcome that combine clinician-based and patient-reported outcomes into a composite score. For example, the Mayo Elbow Performance Index (Morrey, An, & Chao, 1993) combines patient-based functional items with impairment-based measures of range of motion, strength, and stability to formulate a single score that ranges from 0 to 100. Different score ranges are provided with subjective ratings of either excellent, good, fair, or poor. Though combined scales are popular in some areas of practice, caution is advised for several reasons. Perhaps most important, combining impairment scores with self-reported function may limit a therapist's ability to differentiate what is driving disability. Think about a patient from your practice who, despite substantial physical impairment, was able to do many of tasks of his or her daily life—he or she would receive a moderate score. Now consider a patient who has very little physical impairment but reported more functional difficulties. He or she would also receive a moderate score. In these cases, a moderate score does little to show whether it is the impairment or the experience of disability that needs to be addressed. Unfortunately, many of these measures exacerbate their measurement problems by artificially assigning ratings of fair, excellent, and good to the scores. The weighting of different impairments is typically arbitrarily set and may not relate to the role of these specific impairments as contributors to function (Turchin, Beaton, & Richards, 1998). Therefore, we make the point that because self-rated and clinician-based impairment measures tap into different concepts, combining them in a composite score may be uninformative and is not recommended for monitoring individual patient status.

The fact that impairment measures and self-report measures of function tap into different constructs suggests that we should consider it necessary in many cases to measure both. Particularly in cases where therapists are implementing an intervention that is designed to change an impairment, it is important to measure whether that impairment changes. One cannot expect a treatment to work if we do not have proof that it, at a minimum, is causing the effects that we expected when deciding to implement it. However, because we are often interested in the greater good for patients, we cannot assume that changing impairments alone will necessarily result in changes in function, participation, or health. Therefore, we need to include more functionally relevant measures to determine whether the approach we take with our patients is useful.

Types of Outcome Measures Based on Underlying Theory

Two distinct theoretical approaches to assessment of outcomes have evolved over the years. Psychometric methods are most prevalent and rely on years of research in psychological measurement. These approaches are concerned with creating instruments where a specific domain of content is sampled and items are developed to represent this domain. Multivariate statistical methods, like factor analysis, are often used to determine the validity of these domain structures. Classical test theory is based on the concept that every score is composed of the true score and some error, and that clinical measurement can be defined and improved by understanding the nature of the measurement error.

Recently, other theories are emerging in clinical measurement research (e.g., item response or latent trait theory). Underlying this approach to clinical measurement is the assumption that we have a defined construct or latent trait that we are interested in representing through our clinical measurement process. Discrete item responses considered are observable manifestations of these traits, constructs, or attributes. Though the constructs may not be directly observable, they can be inferred from the manifest responses. The construct should be measurable on a scale and it should be possible to determine the difficulty of items along that scale. There is an assumption that item responses should reflect the difficulty along that scale and not be different for different classes of people (differential functioning). Item response theory or Rasch methods provide an alternative perspective on evaluating these attributes of measurement scales in rehabilitation.

Because QOL is a subjective evaluation, other methods have focused on decision theory as a basis for understanding how people value their life or health states. These methods are common in health economics where a one-dimensional measure of quality/utility is important to calculate the cost of interventions and associated changes in the health state. Utility scores range from 0 to 1, usually with 0 representing the worst-case scenario (death or worst possible health state) and 1 representing the best-case scenario (full health or best possible health). A variety of techniques such as standard gamble or time trade-off (Bakker, Rutten van Molken, van Doorslaer, Bennett, & van der Linden, 1993; Feeny et al., 2004; Sackett & Torrance, 1978; Smith & Dobson, 1993; Torrance, 1987) are used to establish a valuation for given health states. These techniques ask the person to make an inherently value-laden decision about the value he or she places on a given health state by using a series of decisions (choice options) to find a point of uncertainty or equivalence. For example, standard gamble patients might be asked whether they were willing to accept a specific probability of death or total disablement to attain a specific probability of optimal health. A similar approach is used in the time trade-off technique, by determining the amount of time people would be willing to trade off (loss of years of life) to achieve a better current QOL. Utility can also be measured using specific utility questionnaires (Torrance, 1987) or overall rating scales. In general, utility measures are not useful in clinical practice but are very helpful in clinical research—particularly if they include an economic analysis because they can be used to perform cost-effectiveness analysis. Quality-adjusted life years (QALY) are measures of life expectancy adjusted for QOL that can be determined once you have a utility measure. In economic studies, these types of outcome measures are used to evaluate how interventions affect the duration and quality of remaining life (Kaplan, Alcaraz, Anderson, & Weisman, 1996; Russell, Gold, Siegel, Daniels, & Weinstein, 1996). It is important for therapists to have a basic understanding of what a QALY is because it is important to read research about the cost/benefit of different treatment options and to communicate this to patients. It is unlikely that utility measures would be useful to assess individual patients in practice.

Types of Outcome Measures Based on Scope

Different types of outcome measures arise based on the domain structures. The most common types of instruments seen in rehabilitation include the following:

- Generic instruments such as quality of life, general health, utility, or participation.
- Disease- or symptom-specific measures that focus on the key aspects of a disease or symptom (e.g., stroke or pain).
- Regional or body part-specific measures that focus on a body area.
- Patient-specific measures such as the COPM or the Patient Specific Functional Scale where items are selected to be meaningful to a particular patient as opposed to being standardized across all respondents.

Structural Characteristics of Outcome Measures

Developers of outcome measures make fundamental decisions on the structure of scales/subscales, individual items, and response options when creating instruments. All of these decisions will have an impact on the clinical measurement properties, the clinical usefulness, and the acceptability and meaningfulness of the instrument to patients and clinicians.

Instructions for Administration and Completion

The structure of the instrument includes many different aspects of how tests are constructed from the instructions given to patients, the elements included in the test, and how they are scored and interpreted. The instructions provided to patients have a great influence on how they respond to the test or item. We know that standardization of methods is critical to obtaining reliable outcome measures. The literature has numerous examples showing that test instructions affect both impairment and self-report measures. For example, on a questionnaire, it matters whether we ask people to think about their current problem when responding to a question or if they are supposed to think about their overall status. Some instruments inquire about the person's difficulty performing a task without attribution to a specific health problem, whereas another scale might ask the same content but would frame the question by asking how the affected area or health problem contributed to their difficulty. For example, patients with upper extremity problems will report higher levels of disability when questions are attributed to their upper extremity than when responding to general questions (Marx et al., 2001). We observed that patients reported high levels of emotional impact on a disease-specific QOL instrument for rotator cuff but low impact on emotional health on the SF-36 where emotional health was placed in a more global context (MacDermid et al., 2004). It also matters whether we tell patients to think about a specific time interval. In acute conditions we may want to keep the interval fairly short ("right now" or a certain number of hours), whereas in more stable chronic conditions we might make the interval longer to achieve a more stable, average estimate.

Similarly, patients may respond differently depending on whether questions are framed in terms of capability or performance. Asking a person whether he or she *can* do something may elicit a different response that asking whether he or she *did* something. For example, a study comparing the relationship between capability and performance administered two versions of the Activities

Scale for Kids to 28 physically disabled children. The capability version asked children what they could do, whereas the performance version asked what they did do. Capability was found to exceed performance by approximately 18%, which the authors attributed to environmental context (Young, Williams, Yoshida, Bombardier, & Wright, 1996). This conclusion was supported in a separate study in children with cerebral palsy where children performed crawling or walking more often at home than in school or community environments (Tieman, Palisano, Gracely, & Rosenbaum, 2004).

Instructions provided to testers are also important and can be critical for impairment measures. In general, we know that standardization will enhance measurement properties like reliability and validity. It is important for therapists to measure things in the same way so that they can compare their data with reported clinical research or even other therapists' data. Unfortunately in some cases, test developers do not provide clear instructions or the detailed manuals often required to facilitate an appropriate level of standardization.

Outcome scales may be one-dimensional or have subscales that reflect different aspects of the health domain. For example, the SF-36 has eight different subscales that address different subdomains of health (Ware, 2003; Ware, Gandek, et al., 1998; Ware & Sherbourne, 1992). The physical and mental summary scores are intended to provide overall scores for two global and independent aspects of health. This can be important in rehabilitation because we often are interested in understanding the physical and psychosocial aspects of health problems. Factor analysis is a statistical process used to group items that behave similarly when a test is administered. This analysis is often used to determine whether items on a self-report measure follow the subscale's structure defined by the authors. In general, correlations between physical and mental summary scores on the SF-36 are quite low, suggesting that the questionnaire is able to measure two separate components of health (Ware, Kosinkski, et al., 1998).

Scoring of Instruments

Instruments will also vary on how individual questions and subscales are scored. Many patient-based outcomes are determined on the basis of questionnaires containing a range of scored items using Likert scaling or visual analog responses. Likert scaling of items provides a range of subjective options on an ordinal scale. Other instruments use a numeric 0 to 10 or visual analog response scale. In some cases, Likert and visual analog versions of the scale are available. In some pediatric scales, pictorial representations are used to represent different response options as a means of allowing young nonreaders to communicate their ratings.

Dealing With Missing Items

Instruments should provide instructions on how missing items are handled and other procedural elements. Regardless of the measurement approach, it is important for these instruments to contain sufficiently detailed instructions on how to score items, subscales, and total scores to ensure consistency across centers and clinical studies when instruments are applied in different situations.

Searching for Outcome Measures

One of the first steps in using outcome measures is selecting the appropriate measure. Methods for searching the research literature have been previously defined in Chapter 3 of this text. It is worth noting some special considerations that apply to outcome measures. First, many of the strategies that have been devised for refining search strategies do not apply very well to outcome measures. Second, finding studies of outcome measures does not necessarily lead to finding the measure itself. Many outcome measures may be mentioned in treatment studies or psychometric studies, but it is less common for the actual instruments themselves to be readily accessible.

Some textbooks and Web sites are designed for those who need to obtain the instruments, and a number of these resources are provided at the end of this chapter. The development of electronic repositories for databases that organize information about outcome measures can be a valuable way for clinicians to find outcome measures. A drawback of textbooks is that they can be out of date, so more recent information may be found on repositories if they are regularly updated. Readers are encouraged to explore some of these resources to understand the scope of measures available.

The overall process of selecting an outcome measure for practice is to do the following:

- Identify the conceptual framework and/or concepts that are important to measure (achieve alignment between your conceptual framework, your patient's issues, and your measurement purpose).

- Search scientific articles on outcome measures, articles addressing treatment effectiveness in a similar patient population, textbooks, and online outcome measure resources to identify a potential list of outcome measures/instruments.

- Remove any outcome measures that are not standardized, clearly not suited to your purpose or situation, or that have been shown to be unreliable or invalid for your purpose.

- Critically appraise your potential outcome scale(s) using a standardized process or instrument or evaluate fundamental measurement principles (see Appendix B).

- Determine whether the instrument can evaluate change, discriminate, or predict in the manner required for your population and purpose.

- Obtain the measures of interest and determine the scoring mechanism and any specific instructions on administration (including whether valid translations are available).

- Identify copyright, reimbursement issues, and ensure compliance.

- Devise and document a strategy as to what procedures will be followed in implementing outcome measures into practice (when they will be applied, who will provide them, how/when will they be scored, where the data will be retained, how the data will be used). Ensure that all parties involved participate in devising the implementation strategy and understand their roles.

- Pilot test either one or two instruments for a specified period and reevaluate the instrument's performance, feasibility, and implementation process.

- Finalize your choice and a set time frame to review outcomes data.

A number of practical issues must be considered when attempting to incorporate new measures into practice. Expect and prepare for a learning curve. Lack of adequate preparation will inevitably lead to frustration and an inability to use outcome measure scores in clinical decision making. Strategies for success include making the instruments readily available for use when needed, engaging clinicians throughout the process of adopting and implementing the measure, identifying the benefits to the clinic/clinician and patient for measurement, providing the measures to patients in a standardized way that fits with clinic flow, and having a strategy to ensure that forms are completed by all respondents. Certain payers or regulatory bodies may have predetermined outcome measures to be used within the context of care to their enrollees. If you choose to veer from that, document what is needed so that the person who will approve the rehabilitation plan has a clear understanding of your choice and rationale for a selected patient.

Developers of outcome measures have intellectual property rights with respect to their instruments, so it is important that these be respected. Many developers do not charge for the use of their instruments. In this case, it is advisable to contact the developer to request permission to use their instrument and inquire whether there is any documentation regarding proper administration or interpretation. In some cases, outcome measures and/or their supporting documentation must be purchased. Usually this is a one-time cost, but in some cases there can be ongoing charges for a license, for the measure forms, and/or for scoring. These practical issues may determine which measures are feasible in your practice. Some companies have developed platforms for administering, scoring, and providing interpretation of outcome measures in a computer-based format. Ongoing license fees for software and for reports are common in this case.

Examples of Outcome Measure Resources

"Physical Rehabilitation Outcome Measures: A Guide to Critical Appraisal" (Finch, Mayo, & Stratford, 2002) provides over 70 measures from a variety of areas within rehabilitation summarized on a standard format, including the following:

- Information on the developers
- Purpose
- A description of the measure
- Conceptual basis or construct measured
- Groups tests
- Translations available
- Typical reliability estimates
- Typical validity estimates
- Responsiveness and interpretability

In the occupational therapy field, Law, Baum, and Dunn (2005) have published a book that critically appraises measures of occupational performance. Reviews of measures in the areas of ADL, instrumental ADL, play, participation, work, and environment are included in this text.

We also highlight the following resources:

1. Rehabilitation Outcome Measures Database

   www.rehabmeasures.org/rehabweb/links.aspx

   Developing Web-based resources specific for rehabilitation that provides resources and links to other outcome measure databases

2. Canadian Interdisciplinary Network for CAM Research (IN-CAM)

   www.outcomesdatabase.org

   A database of outcome measures developed by complementary and alternative medicine

3. Patient-Reported Health Instruments (PHI)

   http://phi.uhce.ox.ac.uk/

   Compiled by the National Health Service and includes a searchable database of health instruments

4. Patient-Reported Outcome and Quality of Life Instruments Database (PROQOLID)

   www.proqolid.org

5. CAMHS Outcome Research Consortium (CORC)

   http://www.corc.uk.net/index.php?contentkey=81#HoN

   Outcome measures for children's mental health

6. StrokEngine Assess

   www.medicine.mcgill.ca/strokengine-assess

   Resources specific to stroke

7. The NIH Toolbox

   www.nihtoolbox.org/WebPart%20Pages/AboutUs.aspx

   Part of the NIH Neuroscience Blueprint initiative; seeks to develop brief yet comprehensive assessment tools measuring motor, cognitive, sensory, and emotional function. Upon completion, the toolbox will be available for use in longitudinal epidemiologic studies and prevention or intervention trials for people ages 3 to 85

8. Patient-Reported Outcomes Measurement Information System

   www.nihpromis.org

   PROMIS instruments use modern measurement theory to assess patient-reported health status for physical, mental, and social well-being to reliably and validly measure patient-reported outcomes for clinical research and practice. PROMIS instruments measure concepts such as pain, fatigue, physical function, depression, anxiety, and social function. PROMIS has constructed item banks and short standard (paper) forms. PROMIS instruments are available through the Assessment Center or by contacting the PROMIS Statistical Center at help@assessmentcenter.net

Evaluating Outcome Measures

Critical appraisal of outcome measures is more multidimensional than critical appraisal of individual effectiveness studies. The value of any given outcome measure is reflected across a spectrum of studies that must address initial development of the instrument and subsequent reliability and validity testing. Individual studies on psychometrics of measures will vary in quality and scope. Furthermore, it is important that reliability and validity be established in the clinical population for which the measure will be used. For example, an instrument designed to assess shoulder disability may be useful in most subgroups of patients but may be inappropriate to assess the high-level athlete or musician because of demand issues. Alternatively, it may be inappropriate in some subgroups of the target population if they have a unique impairment or disability issue. For example, although there are a number of measures that are made for people with shoulder problems, these may be less useful in patients with instability who are often young and healthy but have specific problems related to their instability.

Appraisal of outcome measure studies and outcome measures are two separate activities. Often when instruments are developed, researchers provide some preliminary data on the measurement properties of the tool. As the measure becomes more widely adopted, there will be an increasing volume of information describing the measurement properties of the tool in different populations and contexts. This is beneficial because we really need to understand how tools work under a variety of circumstances if we are to use them for our clinical practices, which tend to have diverse patients.

One form of critical appraisal focuses on evaluating the quality of individual articles. We have appended a scale to assist with evaluating individual clinical measurement articles. This scale has been used to summarize the quality of individual articles for a variety of rehabilitation or quality-of-life instruments (Forhan, Vrkljan, & MacDermid, 2009; MacDermid et al., 2009; Roy, Desmeules, & MacDermid, 2011; Roy, MacDermid, & Woodhouse, 2009, 2010). Critical appraisal of individual studies can be valuable to understand the measurement properties involved in using a tool. The MacDermid Critical Appraisal Tool consists of a 12-item checklist and the accompanying guide provides criteria for scoring the checklist. The items address the study question, methods, measurement process, analysis, and recommendations as indicated by the published study. It is available as an appendix in this book. The consistency of raters using the tool has been high.

An international group, the Consensus-Based Standards for the Selection of Health Status Measurement Instruments (COSMIN), has also developed an appraisal tool for appraising outcome instruments. The COSMIN checklist (Terwee et al., 2011) consists of 12 subscales (boxes) addressing different aspects of clinical measurement. Two boxes are used to evaluate general study requirements. Nine boxes are used to evaluate the quality of the assessment of the following measurement properties:

1. Internal consistency

2. Reliability

3. Measurement error

4. Content validity (including face validity)

5-7. Construct validity (subdivided into three boxes, about structural validity, hypotheses testing, and cross-cultural validity)

8. Criterion validity

9. Responsiveness

An additional box is used to evaluate the quality of a study on interpretability. The checklist has also been used to perform systematic reviews on measurement tools in rehabilitation (Hoang-Kim, Pegreffi, Moroni, & Ladd, 2011; Thorborg, Holmich, Christensen, Petersen, & Roos, 2011). The COSMIN checklist may be somewhat difficult to complete, as indicated by the complexity of the form/guide (www.cosmin.nl/images/upload/File/COSMIN%20checklist%20manual%20v6.pdf) and studies showing a moderate reliability (Mokkink et al., 2010).

There is a need for systematic reviews on rehabilitation tools because individual studies rarely provide sufficient information about a tool for the clinician to make a decision about whether it is optimal for use in practice. There is a wide scope of reliability and validity issues that need to be considered when adopting a tool. As such systematic reviews become more available in rehabilitation literature, it will be possible for clinicians to use these as a basis to make decisions about the selection of outcome measures.

When making overall selection decisions, particularly where no systematic review is available, we would recommend the outcome measures form and guidelines developed by Law et al. (Appendix B). This tool focuses on evaluating what is known about a specific outcome measure and deciding whether it is appropriate for your purpose.

There are many forms of reliability and validity, and the importance of each clinical measurement property varies with the purpose of using the outcome instrument. For example, when using instruments to evaluate change over time such as when following treatment, responsiveness—a component of validity—is particularly important. When using an instrument to determine to which group a patient belongs (determine a diagnosis or status such as "able to return to work"), discriminative validity is of importance. The ability to detect change and the ability to discriminate are two separate reasons we might want to use a measure that also requires different measurement properties. A measure can be very good at discriminating, but not at detecting change. Therefore, it is hard to say that a measure is high quality or low quality without stating about for what purpose. Psychometric properties may in fact compete with each other from a statistical point of view. There is no system of levels of evidence assigned to outcome measures as there would be for other areas of clinical practice such as prognosis and treatment effectiveness.

We will not review the basic concepts of reliability and validity as they apply to outcome measures. At the end of this chapter, there is a review of some the basic terminology as a quick reference. Understanding the basic premises of clinical measurement is important, however, and if the reader does not feel comfortable with these topics, the reader is advised to consult the resources listed at the end of this chapter.

Selecting Measures for Individual Patients

An emerging trend in some areas of practice is the development of consensus exercises to establish measures that could be used for routine administration and practice or as outcome measures for clinical research to provide more consistency in the reporting of health in disability outcomes in clinical research. These efforts are worthwhile because they would allow us to increase comparability of our outcomes across studies in research studies and more easily synthesize the findings across smaller studies to provide more definitive conclusions. For example, Outcome Measures in Rheumatology (OMERACT) meets regularly to discuss standardization of outcome measures in rheumatology (Beaton et al., 2009; Boonen et al., 2009). These efforts would help therapists select measures that are most likely to have comparative data and establish measurement properties.

Regardless, it will always be necessary for therapists as part of their interaction with a patient to make decisions about how they will monitor the impact of that interaction. Selecting an outcome measure requires us to consider all of the issues discussed previously. In particular, we wish to think about the following:

- What is my conceptual basis for understanding how I can impact on the outcome, quality of life, or health of this patient?
- What is my current measurement need with respect to evaluating this patient (i.e., diagnosis/discrimination, evaluation of change, prediction)?
- What conceptual basis or priorities affect how my patient views his current problem and preferred outcome?
- What evidence-based interventions will I use? And what will be their direct impact?
  - What indicators would tell me that the intervention is appropriately targeted and dosed?
  - What indicators would tell me that the intervention is having the overall impact on the patient that meets the rehabilitation goals?
- What outcome measures fulfill my measurement needs and are feasible for me to perform?

The following example, Case Example 1, illustrates how outcome measures were selected using these principles for one specific patient problem.

> A 46-year-old male, who works in auto manufacturing, has right lateral elbow pain when he moves his arm. This pain is usually "achy" after activity or at the end of the day but occasionally a "sharper pain" occurs with certain activities. These pain-provoking activities include using tools at work, wringing out a wet towel, and carrying a heavy pot. After his full examination, you conclude that he has "tennis elbow" and want to select outcome measures to monitor the response to your interventions.

In this case, the first step was to search the literature to identify outcome measures that were used in clinical studies on rehabilitation of lateral epicondylalgia, or tennis elbow. A full table of interventions and outcome measures used was available in a systematic review on rehabilitation of lateral spondylitis (Trudel et al., 2004). In addition, there is information from a practice survey that reported on the outcome measures that were currently being used (MacDermid et al., 2010). This highlighted a lack of consensus on appropriate standardized outcome measures. Furthermore, a number of nonstandardized measures are commonly used practice. Despite this setback, it was evident that some core constructs were being evaluated in clinical studies, including pain, muscle strength, and function.

Because the evidence indicated that education and exercise were important components of treatment, as rehabilitation therapists we decided that we wanted outcome to detect changes in the impairments this patient was experiencing and that would be addressed by our interventions (pain and loss of strength). As rehabilitation professionals, we are interested not only in body structure but also in function and participation, and our case highlights that these are also important concerns for the patient.

Next, we decided to differentiate short-term and long-term outcome constructs that were clinically relevant because that is consistent with how we set goals. In the shorter term, outcome evaluations would emphasize impairments so that we can determine whether the interventions we select lead to expected changes in symptoms and structural changes in the tendon itself. In other words, we need to know whether the interventions are targeted correctly and dosed appropriately, and this is best determined by seeing that the expected changes in impairments are occurring. This information is critical to modifying our interventions. We know that we can enhance recovery using strengthening exercises, but the literature also indicates that it is difficult to determine the optimal dosage based on current evidence (Raman, MacDermid, & Grewal, 2011). We rely on our foundational knowledge, which tells us that the size of the tendon is related to the size of the muscle and that the ability to resist future muscle strains will depend on the tensile strength of the tendon. Hence, we need an indicator of muscle strength. We also recognize that the patient has a primary concern of achieving pain relief. Reviewing the evidence about the impact of interventions can also help us determine at what time points we should be measuring. We decided to measure short-term outcomes at baseline and at 2 and 4 weeks following our initial intervention.

In the longer term, we would be concerned that our patient resumes valued participation (safe and productive work) and with preventing future reoccurrences. We should select outcome measures that reflect these concepts and emphasize these as measures to track with respect to achieving long-term goals.

Once we established a framework for what we want to measure, we searched for measures that would fit these criteria and have appropriate measurement properties. This creates a short list for an outcomes strategy:

- Pain relief could be measured using either the Patient-Rated Tennis Elbow Evaluation (PRTEE; Altan, Ercan, & Konur, 2010; Blanchette & Normand, 2010; MacDermid, 2005; Newcomer, Martinez-Silvestrini, Schaefer, Gay, & Arendt, 2005; Rompe, Overend, & MacDermid, 2007), a visual analog scale, or numeric pain rating scale.

- Patient function could be measured using self-report scales that include a functional subscale. These include the PRTEE, Disabilities of the Arm, Shoulder, Hand (DASH), or the Quick DASH.

- Muscle function can be measured using quantitative measures of isometric strength.

  ○ Functional grip—Pain-free grip strength (Stratford, Levy, & Gowland, 1993) is the most responsive and easily performed because most clinics would have quantitative grip devices. We recognize that this measure indicates irritability of the muscle rather than maximal strength, but this is an advantage for our purposes.

  ○ Musculotendinous capacity—Wrist extensor strength would be the most direct functional measurement of tendon physiological function and could easily be measured using a hand-held dynamometer (depending on equipment availability).

  ○ Endurance for activity—A standardized test has yet to be described that quantifies wrist muscle endurance, although a variety of functional tests would tap into this domain. Given the lack of specificity of these tests to our problem and potential problems with validity, we would not implement this measure at this time.

We decided to measure longer-term outcomes at baseline, discharge, and in 6-month follow-up (the latter to be performed by e-mail and telephone survey). Because we know that tennis elbow tends to recur and that we want our patient to maintain his return to valued activity, we might focus on these as long-term outcomes (if resources allow).

The following outcomes measured include:

- Recurrence of symptoms
    - Pain/function (Patient-Rated Forearm Scale; MacDermid, 2005; Newcomer et al., 2005; Overend, Wuori-Fearn, Kramer, & MacDermid, 1999) or pain-free function (Stratford, Levy, Gauldie, Levy, & Miseferi, 1987)
    - Need for additional treatment
- Work outcomes (work status or lost time, or the Work subscale of the DASH; Beaton, Katz, et al., 2001; Solway, Beaton, McConnell, & Bombardier, 2002) or a scale similar to the Work Limitation Questionnaire (Lerner et al., 2001; Lerner, Reed, Massarotti, Wester, & Burke, 2002), which describes the difficulty at work. In clinical practice, we would likely focus on simple indicators of work such as whether the patient was able to maintain regular work duties. In clinical research we might collect more time-consuming measures including work status and presenteeism, because we know that many people who return to work do not return to full productivity (Roy, Desmeules, & MacDermid, 2011; Roy, MacDermid, et al., 2011).
- Resumption of valued regular recreational activity. We would select a patient-specific measure to monitor this such as the COPM (Carswell et al., 2004; Law et al., 1990, 1994, 1998; McColl, Paterson, Davies, Doubt, & Law, 2000) or Patient-Specific Functional Scale (Chatman et al., 1997; Westaway, Stratford, & Binkley, 1998). The COPM takes longer to perform but tends to be used as an integral part of treatment, whereas the Patient-Specific Functional Scale is quicker.

The list has now become much more manageable and we are close to an outcome strategy that applies to this patient and the majority of our future patients with lateral epicondylitis. At this point, we would implement our outcome evaluation strategy on this individual patient and potentially a series of patients to fine-tune our approach in the future.

How to Use Outcome Measures to Help Make Clinical Decisions on Individual Patients

Once an outcome measure and associated administration time table has been established, this template can be used across successive patients as standard practice. There is inherent value in asking patients standardized questions regarding their perceived status as a component of clinical evaluation. Patients appreciate when their perspective is central to the treatment process. There is also inherent value in looking at the individual items scored to identify specific treatment difficulties or targets for functional goals. The benefit of using standardized outcome measurement is achieved as clinicians examine the variance in patients' outcomes and learn more about how to incorporate the actual scores into their clinical decision making. The following example, Case Example 2, shows how that can be approached.

> A male patient, 55 years of age, attends your clinic for the first time with a diagnosis of shoulder pain from a referring general practitioner. The patient has a diagnostic ultrasound report indicating a partial thickness tear of the supraspinatus tendon. Recently, your clinic has added the DASH self-report outcome measure to its clinic assessment protocol. The patient's score is 44 at this visit.

This simple scenario provides an opportunity to examine some of the typical questions one might ask when using outcome measures to evaluate the impact of an evidence-based decision. We should understand how outcome measures fit into our conceptual framework of health and quality of life but, ultimately, quantitative decisions on the meaning of scores are required. Data from reliability and validity studies can help make judgments and define benchmarks for goal setting and reevaluation. This example can be used as a template. If you have not yet refreshed your basic statistical knowledge (variability, normal curve, etc.) and definitions on the properties of clinical measurement, see the definitions at the end of the text on outcome measures. Doing so might make it easier to feel comfortable with adapting the concepts to your practice needs. In our experience, few people understand clinical measurement properties unless they apply them to see their usefulness first-hand. You may wish to go back and forth between reviewing and applying these concepts until you become comfortable with both. The fundamental questions posed are as follows:

- What does the score on this outcome measure tell me about the patient's status?
- What is the error associated with the measured value?
- How much will the score need to change on subsequent assessments so that I can be confident a real change has occurred?
- How much will the score need to change on a subsequent assessment so that I can be confident an important amount of change has occurred?
- What is my long-term treatment goal and how does it relate to a score on its outcome measure?

What Does the Score on This Outcome Measure Tell Me About the Patient's Status?

The DASH (American Academy of Orthopaedic Surgeons, 2002; Beaton, Katz, et al., 2001; Solway et al., 2002; Upper Extremity Collaborative Group, 1996, 1999) was designed to reflect the disability a person experiences as a result of problems with his or her upper extremity. Reliability and validity data are excellent and substantial comparative data that are available for use, including a user manual. This provides confidence that the DASH is a valid measure of upper extremity disability. When looking at the items (the DASH can be obtained from the Web site: www.dash.iwh.on.ca), you will note that some items address symptoms, others specific activities, and others participation in normal life roles. The DASH is scored as a one-dimensional scale and does not separate components of the ICF model of disability, but incorporates items across its dimensions. Similarly, the DASH includes aspects of both psychosocial and physical health. We might consider the DASH to be a valid indicator of functional disability in persons with physical disorders of the upper extremity.

Clinicians develop the ability to "have a feel for" how patients should respond to measures they routinely use. Thus, you can expect a learning curve when you first implement self-report measures in your practice. With continued use, you will achieve a level of comfort with the scores so that you develop an intuitive understanding of what different scores represent. Understanding the scores that we would expect from a typical patient can help us to understand the severity of this particular patient's problem. You should collate published comparative data obtained from populations of interest (in Case Example 2 on p. 86, rotator cuff tear) at different points in clinical recovery to have data for making comparisons. With relatively little clinical experience using outcome measures and a few of these "cheat sheets," most people quickly develop a feel for whether scores reported by a given patient are within an expected range considering the pathology and point in clinical recovery in a very short period of time.

Normative data for the DASH are published on the American Academy of Orthopaedic Surgeons' Web site (American Academy of Orthopaedic Surgeons, 2002) and in the user's manual. The average 55-year-old male or female in the general population reports a DASH score of 12. That is because by this age many people have some problems in their shoulder. Atroshi, Gummesson, Andersson, Dahlgren, and Johansson (2000) reported a mean DASH score of 43 for patients awaiting shoulder surgery compared to a mean score of 35 for nonsurgical patients. Skutek,

Gremerey, Zeichen, and Bosch (2000) reported a mean preoperative DASH score of 49 for persons with rotator cuff tears awaiting surgery. Thus, our exemplar patient—whose DASH score of 44—is consistent with that of other persons reporting substantial disability due to rotator cuff pathology. This can be an important piece of information when planning a rehabilitation program because we know that patients with high levels of disability are likely to have poor rehabilitation outcomes. Furthermore, payers often want to know if what patients are reporting is consistent with the pathology report.

What Is the Error Associated With the Measured Value?

To be confident that a measured value is useful in clinical decision making, we must have some idea of the consistency of the score. In other words, we need to know the amount of error associated with the score that we achieve when we assess our patients. The standard error of mean (SEM) can be used to describe the error associated with a reported value expressed in the original units of the measure. The SEM is related to the variability of the underlying population and the reliability of the scores on that particular outcome measure in a similar group. Although there are several methods for calculating the SEM, the most popular method is as follows:

$$\text{SEM} = (\text{sample standard deviation}) \sqrt{1 - \text{reliability coefficient}}$$

Though the DASH has been shown to have high reliability coefficients across a broad number of conditions, the standard deviation can be expected to vary between different conditions and even within conditions over time as the level of disability changes. Thus, the SEM is an estimate. When faced with a lack of data indicating the SEM appropriate to our patient's condition and level of disability, we can extrapolate from data that most closely approximate our patient. When one is interested in estimating the error associated with a score at a single point in time, internal consistency coefficients are used to indicate stability.

Once you determine the SEM, you must decide on the level of precision of your estimate. One SEM is associated with a 68% confidence interval (for a description of the sampling distribution and z-values, see any standard statistical text). To obtain higher confidence levels, the SEM can be multiplied by z-values associated with different confidence levels. For example, 1.65 is the z-value associated with the 90% confidence level and 1.96 is the z-value associated with the 95% confidence level. By multiplying the SEM for the measures taken by this level of confidence (z-value), you can establish a range within which a patient's true score is likely to lie, at the specified confidence level. By tradition, research studies often use a 95% confidence interval. However, in clinical practice we are often happy with a 90% level for estimation because this is high confidence, but not so rigorous that we would establish very wide confidence intervals that would not be practical in clinical practice.

A SEM (for one point in time) of 4.4 points has been reported for the DASH. Multiplying the SEM of 4.4 points by the z-value of 1.65 provides a 90% confidence level and yields a value of 7.3 points. The interpretation is that at the time of assessment, there is a 90% chance that a patient's true score is within 7.3 points of the measured score.

How Much Will the Score Need to Change on Subsequent Assessments so I Can Be Confident That a Real Change Has Occurred?

One reason for reassessing patients is to determine whether they have changed as a result of implementing an intervention. If we measure a change that exceeds the error associated with the measurement process, then we can be reasonably certain that a true change has occurred. Often, the term *minimal detectable change* (MDC) is used to specify this value. The MDC can be useful when setting short-term goals because it can establish a reasonable target for where there should be a real change in status. It can also assist with establishing reassessment intervals because the therapist should reassess at an interval where an expected change should exceed the MDC.

To obtain the minimal level of detectable change at a specified confidence (MDC_{CL}), $SEM_{test\text{-}retest}$ is multiplied by the z-value associated with the confidence level of interest and by the square root of 2. For example, MDC at a 90% confidence level, designated MDC_{90}, is obtained as follows:

$$MDC_{90} = SEM_{test\text{-}retest} \times z\text{-value} \times \sqrt{2}$$

Estimates of MDC_{90} for the DASH vary, with 11 being a typical value. The interpretation of MDC_{90} is that 90% of stable patients are likely to display a difference on retest less than the value of MDC_{90}. Thus, for the described patient vignette, a change of 11 or more DASH points is required to be reasonably certain that a true change has occurred. If our initial score is 44, the short-term goal (target) becomes 33.

How Many Points Does a Score Need to Change Before We Could Confidently Say That an Important Change Has Occurred?

Clinicians, payers, and other stakeholders (including patients) are not usually concerned with the least detectable difference but rather an important difference—one that makes a difference in the life of patient. The term *clinically important difference* (CID) or *minimal clinically important difference* (Beaton, Boers, & Wells, 2002; Beaton, Bombardier, Katz, Wright, Wells, et al., 2001; Guyatt, Walter, & Norman, 1987; Jaeschke, Singer, & Guyatt, 1989) is often used to describe this quantity. Estimates of the CID require that studies evaluate how much change on a measure is of importance to the patient. There are a variety of clinical measurement analyses that can be used to establish CID. These will not be discussed. Given limitations of the methods and the variability between populations, one might expect to find variations of the CID in the literature. In fact, some studies show that the CID can be the same or lower than the MDC. In reality, the amount of improvement related to the CID will vary according to where a person is on the measure (less so if the scale has been developed using Rasch). A reasonable CID for the DASH has most consistently been reported to be about 15 points and, thus, we would use this as our benchmark for longer-term treatment goals.

What Score Is Required to Meet Our Long-Term Treatment Goals for This Patient?

In EBP decision making and, hence, goal setting, we must consider the following:

- ○ The patient's preferences and expectations.
- ○ Clinical data on the expected effect sizes with the type of intervention we are using.
- ○ Factors that might mediate the treatment response.
- ○ Our personal experience with respect to the expected treatment responses.

These factors determine how this evidence can be applied or extrapolated to the patient. When using standardized outcome measures to set and evaluate progress toward long-terms goals, it is important to have data on patients who have had varying levels of disability to help us set realistic goals. In this case, we are interested in return to work and obtain data on DASH scores that are consistent with return to work. Data obtained by Beaton et al. on scores for working and working patients help us make a reasonable prognosis in this regard. They reported a mean DASH score of 50.7 for persons unable to work because of their upper extremity problem compared to a mean score of 26.8 for persons able to work with an upper extremity problem, albeit with some difficulty of discomfort. In setting a long-term predicted DASH change—for example, patient prognosis—we would want to meet the lower score. Clinicians consider both the CID and the value reported to achieve meaningful participation when setting long-term goals.

Measures can also be used to assist with prognosis. There is an increasing body of literature about what cutoffs on outcome instruments mean in terms of predicting future scores or other outcomes like return to work or satisfaction. For example, by looking at different cutoffs for grip and pinch strength recovery following wrist fracture rehabilitation, it was determined that patients were most satisfied if they had recovered 65% of their grip, 87% of their pinch strength, and 95% of their motion (Chung & Haas, 2009). This knowledge can be discussed with the patient and be reflective in goal setting. Having summary tables of these types of data about outcome measures that apply to your practice can facilitate evidence-based prognosis and reporting.

HOW TO USE OUTCOME MEASURES TO HELP MAKE CLINICAL DECISIONS ON REHABILITATION PROGRAMS

Many clinicians can readily see the benefit of using outcome measures on individual patients but are unsure as to how to use them to evaluate their clinic outcomes. Outcomes research, program evaluation, and benchmarking share some commonality in that large pools of observational data on outcomes are used to make decisions about services or programs. Some areas such as inpatient rehabilitation have moved toward the use of standard measures that are collected in many centers to facilitate these comparisons (e.g., the FIM). Increasingly, professional associations are providing mechanisms to support databases for outpatient services. For example, both the American Physical Therapy Association (APTA Connect) and American Society of Hand Therapists have partnered with Cedaron Medical to create their own outcomes databases. There is increasing pressure from payers to demonstrate outcomes, making it essential that clinicians be prepared to show that meaningful outcomes were achieved for patients and that those outcomes compare favorably to those reported when alternative health care providers or interventions are selected. For those without access to established databases or software, clinic databases can be established using routine office software. In addition, the "Red Book" of *Physical Rehabilitation Outcome Measures* provides a chapter that assists clinicians with a process for using outcome measures in program evaluation.

With the move toward outcomes databases, it will be important to keep in mind the limitations of observational data. Outcome studies or effectiveness research often depends on observational data (not randomized studies). Observational data, no matter how meticulously gathered, are at risk of bias. That means that it is always possible that considerations other than the treatment are responsible for the observations in outcomes. Differences between groups may exist because of treatment. However, alternative sources of difference might be driving the observed differences. The reasons or pathway taken for individuals to end up in a certain subgroup may be the real factor(s) that determines the outcomes achieved. These factors are usually called *biases* because they contaminate the ability to ascribe differences between groups to the (treatment) factor. Differences between and among groups drawn from an outcome database may be due to variation in the distribution of these risk factors. Common factors that might vary between subgroups include age (and associated differences in comorbidity and physical demands), sex/gender, severity of the disorder, variations in comorbidity/physical health, occupational demands, access to timely services, and socioeconomic or geographical/environmental factors. When comparisons are made across different health care systems, this can create another source of potential covariation, thus limiting the ability to define a causal relationship between outcomes achieved and interventions provided.

Identifying and Addressing Barriers to Using Outcomes Instruments in Outcome Evaluation

The importance of measuring health outcomes has been recognized by the rehabilitation professions. Concerted effort has been made to transfer available knowledge into practice as a means to provide rigorous evaluation of the impact of rehabilitation interventions. These efforts have included entry-level curriculum additions; national initiatives by the professional associations of both occupational and physical therapists; traditional workshops; published editorials, scientific articles, and textbooks; professional association endorsement; and development of outcomes databases. Though agreement with the need for outcome measures is consistently high in surveyed therapists, utilization has remained low in many areas of practice (Michlovitz, LaStayo, Alzner, & Watson, 2001). It is often not until the use of an outcome measure is required for authorization and reimbursement for therapy that the provider will use such a measure.

Others have documented barriers that exist to implementing outcome measures in practice (Abrams et al., 2006; Dunckley, Aspinal, Addington-Hall, Hughes, & Higginson, 2005; Dunckley, Hughes, Addington-Hall, & Higginson, 2003; Horner & Larmer, 2006). The most consistent barriers identified include lack of time, administrative support, and specific knowledge on how to find and apply measures. In our experience in teaching outcome measurement and in our clinical trial comparing strategies to help clinicians implement outcome measures in rehabilitation practice, we found that a lack of appreciation for how outcome measures can actually benefit patients is a primary barrier. Therapists also often do not appreciate how much using standardized measures can facilitate their own development of expertise. Lack of time is the most commonly cited barrier for most things in life that we do not accomplish. Lack of time really means that the action is not viewed as being a high enough priority to "bump" other activities that take place during that time. In our experience, once clinicians begin using outcome measures in their practice, they continue to use them because they now can appreciate the value to their patients and can find ways to incorporate them in a way that is time efficient. Most therapists find that self-report measures help them to be more patient-centered, more focused and rigorous in clinical decision making, more effective in communication with patients about goals, and more effective in documentation.

Tips from the Authors

We find that most rehabilitation practitioners are interested in outcome measurement and believe that it is important but find it difficult to integrate standardized outcome measurement as routine practice. This difficulty could be reduced by following the steps that have been outlined in this chapter. Many clinicians wait until outcome measures are demanded by insurers and then incorporate them without a clear plan on how they will be collected or used. We have seen a recent trend for external parties to increasingly demand outcome measures, so the rate of utilization of practice is increasing. However, mandated implementation does not often facilitate therapists' understanding on how to incorporate measures into their clinical decision making with individual patients. These measures may be collected as a requirement for payment. This is unfortunate because it represents a substantial lost opportunity to collect data to benefit our patients and to showcase our work. We have learned that a process guided by local therapists is the best for implementing measures in practice. Some clinics may have elaborate databases and high-tech equipment, whereas for others in a sole-charge clinic, a technologically based solution will not work. We note that with the increasing availability of electronic records and low-cost technology (e.g., smart phones), the options to make a feasible routine outcome strategy is increasing. It is wise to develop a plan with reasonable and attainable interim targets to ensure that the process is not abandoned. Working with therapists who have experience with outcome measures is preferable. Like all new clinical skills, some protected time to adapt the new processes to your clinic is the primary element of success.

EMERGING ISSUES IN OUTCOMES MEASURES

- Outcome measures may be mandated and/or linked to pay for performance.
- Increased availability of rehabilitation outcomes measures/databases will bring opportunity and challenges.
- Large efforts are underway to bring a common language to describing disability, establish core sets of measures for areas of practice, and develop banks of appropriate self-report and impairment measures.
- Rasch (item response theory) approaches to clinical measurement evaluation can bring a new perspective to outcome measurement development and evaluation and challenges how we view and use existing measures.
- The ICF may become the bridge that links a common language to different outcome measures.

CONCLUSION

- Outcome measures can be used to assess the impact of EBP.
- Current health models acknowledge the contribution of physical, social, and psychological domains to health.
- The ICF is becoming the international framework and language for communicating about functioning, disability, and health.
- QOL is a broad concept that relates to overall satisfaction with health and/or life; health has a narrower focus that can be measured with generic health instruments.
- Measures are selected for three different measurement purposes: discrimination, evaluation of change, or prediction.
- Outcome measures commonly used in rehabilitation are classified based on rater (clinician versus self-report), underlying theory (psychometric, Rasch, or decision), and scope (generic, disease/symptom, regional/body part, or patient specific).
- Texts, Web sites, and journal articles provide access to information about outcome measures but contacting developers may be necessary to get forms and permissions.
- Short-term treatment goals for measuring change on an outcome measure should meet or exceed the minimal detectable change.
- Long-term goals should include standardized outcome measurement targets that exceed a clinically important difference and the goals should be linked to comparison data or participation goals.
- Published clinical research data can provide comparative data for comparing individual patients to expected progress or outcomes.
- Lack of time during clinical practice, access to computers/organizational processes that support data collection, comfort with basic clinical measurement principles, and difficulty in changing clinical behavior are reported barriers to implementing outcome measures in practiced. These can be mitigated by utilizing the resources/processes reported in this chapter.

TERMS USED IN OUTCOME MEASURES RESEARCH

Reliability

Reliability = Consistency of scores achieved when repeated measurements are taken when the underlying phenomenon has not changed.

- Cautions: There are many different ways to assess reliability. Reliability by itself is not enough to ensure validity or responsiveness, but poor reliability will compromise both validity and responsiveness.
- Types of reliability
  1. Internal consistency—Homogeneity of items or scores within an instrument (usually assessed using Cronbach's alpha)
  2. Interrater—Agreement between different raters
  3. Intrarater—Agreement between repeated measurements made by the same rater
  4. Test–retest—The agreement scores obtained between two occasions

Kappa (κ)—Intraclass correlation coefficient (Cohen, 1968, 1990; Landis & Koch, 1977; Maclure & Willet, 1987; Shreiner, 1980)

- Tells you: The relative reliability—the ability to distinguish between nominal measurements made on patients (group; yes/no)
- Represents: A ratio of percent agreement corrected for agreement that would occur by change given the proportion of yes/no responses in the sample
- Interpretation: Varies from 0 to 1, no units associated
- Cautions: Is affected by rates of yes/no and thus tends to vary as chance agreement changes; may be unstable where chance agreement is high. That is, kappa can seem poor even when percentage agreement is high if change agreement is also high

Intraclass correlation coefficient (Bartko, 1976; Muller & Buttner, 1995; Shrout & Fleiss, 1979)

- Tells you: The relative reliability—the ability to distinguish between patients
- Represents: A ratio of between person variance divided by total variance (between persons + within persons); if variability on repeated measurements is small compared to the variability between people, reliability will be good
- Interpretation: Varies from 0 to 1, no units associated
- Cautions: Can seem good in the face of large errors if group is highly variable or poor where subject variation is small, even though absolute errors are small

Standard Error of Mean

- Tells you: Absolute reliability—consistency of the measure in original units of the measure
- Represents: Is a measure of within-patient variability × internal consistency
- Interpretation: Provides error margins with a defined amount of confidence; less error being preferable
- Cautions: SEM may not be the same across different ranges of scores (at different time points in rehabilitation)

Minimal detectable change

- Tells you: Whether a true change in status has occurred

- Represents: An estimate of the amount of measurement error multiplied by a confidence factor that represents the extent of confidence one wishes to employ in determining whether a measurement has actually changed; for example:

$$MDC_{90} = SEM_{test-retest} \times z\text{-value} \times \sqrt{2}$$

- Interpretation: If the change on outcome measure exceeds the minimal detectable change, then you can be certain, within that specific level of confidence, that it is unlikely that this change in score would have occurred in the absence of a true clinical change
- Cautions: Varies according to variability of patient population (and sample size upon which estimates were made); changes by condition and point in recovery

Validity—Trueness of a Measure

- Tells you: Whether an instrument performs as expected within a given context to provide a true estimate of the underlying phenomenon in that circumstance
- Cautions: Validity is specific to the purpose, context, and clinical population. No single study will establish it. It is an ongoing process. You hope to find that an instrument has been validated in a group of people similar to those you wish to apply it and has been used to make decisions similar to those you wish to make
- Types of validity
  1. Face—The extent to which an instrument appears to be valid (usually determined by expert review)
  2. Content—The extent to which an instrument addresses and samples relevant aspects within the concept being assessed
  3. Criterion—The extent to which an instrument agrees with an external criterion measurement of that concept. Where a definitive external criterion is available, it can be called a gold standard. If a gold standard does not exist, criterion validity is often taken as the extent to which a particular measure relates to other measures similar measures. Convergent validity assesses the extent to which an instrument agrees with similar conceptual scores and divergent validity assesses the test for a lack of correlation with instruments that address concepts that are believed to be distinct
     a. Concurrent—The external criterion is measured at same point in time
     b. Predictive—The external criterion is measured in the future
  4. Construct—The extent to which instrument scores conform to theoretically derived hypotheses. This is usually performed by testing differences or correlations. Known group differences uses statistical tests of difference to detect differences between scores obtained for subgroups that are theorized to be different. Correlational construct validity assesses whether measures are correlated as they should be based on the relationships between the constructs measured. Convergent and divergent validity are forms of construct validity, the former where measures assess a similar construct and the latter where they do not

Pearson's r—Interclass correlation coefficient
- Tells you: The strength of the linear relationship between two variables
- Represents: The sum of the products of the standard scores of the two measures divided by the degrees of freedom

- Interpretation: Varies from –1 to 1, no units associated. Sign indicated the directionality of the relationship (a negative correlation reflects that scores change in the opposite directions to each other, a positive correlation indicates that scores change in the same direction); for validity, the strength of the association should be based on a priori hypothesis of expected relationships.

- Cautions: It is important to be careful about the spectrum on which association are measured; association may not hold true when generalized outside of this range. Association does not mean agreement; therefore, Pearson correlations are not generally considered acceptable as a reliability indicator. Do not always assume higher is better in validation; the key is that the correlation should support the concepts and hypothesis upon which the measure is framed/ evaluated.

Detection of Clinical Change

Responsiveness—A special kind of validity that reflects the ability of an instrument to detect (real) change over time (Beaton, 2000; Beaton, Bombardier, Katz, & Wright, 2001; Schmitt & Di Fabio, 2004)

- Cautions: There are different ways of measuring change or important change; responsiveness depends on the properties of the instrument, as well as the underlying properties of change being measured in the clinical construct.

Clinically Important Difference

- Tells you: Change in a score indicating a change that is important to the patient

- Represents: An estimate of the amount of change required to attain a clinically important change in status. Usually considers a confidence factor that represents the extent of confidence one wishes to employ in determining whether a measurement has actually changed importantly.

- Interpretation: Is used as a comparator or benchmark to which changes in outcomes are compared to determine whether a clinically relevant outcome has been achieved

- Cautions: There is no gold standard way to determine what important change is; estimates of important change will vary by methods that define important difference and the context in which the study was conducted. Global rating of change may be used as the external criterion of change despite limitations. The number should be considered as a general estimate, not a hard rule. Also called the minimally important (clinical) difference.

Effect size

- Tells you: A standardized rate of change

- Represents: Mean change divided by the standard deviation of the baseline score (as well as other methods)

- Interpretation: When comparing competing measures, the one with a larger effect size will have been more able to detect clinical change

- Cautions: Comparability across studies should be performed with caution given that sample size, the underlying clinical construct, and the time points in which measurements are taken will affect observed effect sizes; methods of separating stable from changed patients can be controversial

SRM

- Tells you: A standardized rate of change

- Represents: Mean change divided by the standard deviation of the change score

- Interpretation: When comparing competing measures, the one with a larger SRM will have been more able to detect clinical change
- Cautions: Comparability across studies should be performed with caution given that sample size, the underlying clinical construct, and the time points in which measurements are taken will affect observed SRM; methods of separating stable from changed patients can be controversial

Receiver Operator Curve

- Tells you: The ability of a measure to distinguish a clinically important change versus detecting that it does not occur
- Represents: The ability to distinguish between two health states using methodology usually applied to diagnostic test validity—the ability of the instrument to detect change, sensitivity (*y*-axis), is plotted against 1 – specificity (*x*-axis)
  - *Sensitivity* is the number of patients correctly identified as having undergone a clinically important change based on their outcome measures score divided by the total number of patients who truly underwent a clinically important change (as per diagnostic terminology, this would represent true positives)
  - *Specificity* is the number of patients correctly identified as not having achieved a clinically important change (based on their outcome measures score) divided by the total number of patients who truly did not undergo a clinically important change (as per diagnostic terminology, this would represent true negatives)
- Interpretation: Area under the curve can be interpreted as the probability of correctly identifying a patient who has undergone a clinically important change versus those who have not undergone an important change
- Cautions: Can be more difficult to interpret; the ideal cutoff can be unstable in small studies. Methods of separating stable from changed patients can be controversial

LEARNING AND EXPLORATION ACTIVITIES

1. Go to the ICF online and look up codes for some common impairments that you measure.
2. Explore the ICF training materials.
3. Following the model of Case Example 1 (p. 84), select an outcomes approach for a patient from your own caseload and discuss with others.
4. Using the Clinical Measurement Study (Appendix A), evaluate one study on a measure of relevance to your caseload—list any terms or methods that you do not understand and consult clinical measurement texts or experts to refine your understanding.
5. Using the Evaluation Instrument (Appendix B), evaluate the measure you selected.
6. Search the Web databases listed in the following table to find measures relevant to your practice.
7. Choose a measure that you use (or plan to) and compile a list of comparative scores that you might use to help make clinical decisions with your chosen scale using studies that reported that measure.
8. Using Case Example 2 (p. 86) as an exemplar, work through the clinical decision-making questions using your outcome measure and patient scenario.
9. Identify one barrier in your clinical practice that might be a challenge to implementing this measure routinely in your practice and develop a plan to resolve it.

TOOLS INCLUDED IN THIS BOOK (APPENDICES A AND B)

1. Critical Appraisal of Study Quality for Psychometric Articles Evaluation Form (MacDermid)—This form and interpretation guide allow user to evaluate individual articles on outcome measures.

2. Outcome Measure Rating Form (Law)—Can be used to summarize the information on an outcome measure as a means of deciding on its value and application.

Outcome Measures Web Sites

WEB/URL	DESCRIPTION
www.nihpromis.org	The official site of PROMIS
www.who.int/classifications/icf/en	This Web site provides information about the new *International Classification*
www.canchild.ca/en/canchildresources/cricitalreviewformsandguidelines.asp	A site that provides information on outcome measures and products developed by CanChild researchers
www.tbims.org/combi	A site that provides information on outcome measures for brain injuries
www.caretrak-outcomes.com	A site that provides tools for evaluating spinal injuries and diseases (30-day free trial, paid subscription required)
www.sf-36.org	A community site that provides news, descriptive information, and demos on the SF tools and products
www.dash.iwh.on.ca	The official Web site of the DASH outcome measure
www.proqolid.org	An online database developed by the Mapi Research Institute that provides descriptive information on quality of life outcome instruments
www.euroqol.org	The official Web site of the EuroQOL instrument
www.rand.org/health/surveys_tools.html	A site that provides information on surveys and tools developed by RAND Health
http://phi.uhce.ox.ac.uk	A site by the National Centre for Health Outcomes Development with a searchable database that provides information and guidance on the selection of patient-reported health measurements
www.cebp.nl/?NODE=77	A site by the Centre for Evidence-Based Physiotherapy that provides descriptions and copies of outcome measures used in physiotherapy
http://onlinestatbook.com	Free online stats textbook
http://statpages.org	Free online stats calculations
http://nilesonline.com/stats	Easy reading stats textbook

Books That Focus on Outcome Assessment/Measures

Bolton, B. (Ed.). (2001). *Handbook of measurement and evaluation in rehabilitation* (3rd ed.). Aspen Publications.

Dittmar, S., & Gresham, G. (Eds.). (2005). *Functional assessment and outcome measures for rehabilitation.* PRO-ED.

Enderby, P., John, A., & Petheram, B. (2006). *Therapy outcome measures for rehabilitation professions: Speech and language therapy, physiotherapy, occupational therapy* (2nd ed.). John Wiley & Sons.

Fayers, P., & Hays, R. (2005). *Assessing quality of life in clinical trials* (2nd ed.). Oxford University Press.

Finch, E., Brooks, D., Stratford, P., & Mayo, N. (2002). *Physical rehabilitation outcomes measures: A guide to enhanced clinical decision-making.* Lippincott Williams & Wilkins.

Hawkins, R. P., Mathews, J. R., & Hamdan, L. (1998). *Measuring behavioral health outcomes: A practical guide.* New York, NY: Kluwer Academic/Plenum Publishers.

Hutchinson, A., McColl, E., Christie, M., & Riccalton, C. (Eds.). (1996). *Health outcome measures in primary and out-patient care.* Amsterdam, The Netherlands: Harwood Academic Publishers.

IsHak, W. W., Burt, T., & Sederer, L. (2002). *Outcome measurement in psychiatry: A critical review.* Washington, DC: American Psychiatric Publishing.

Johnson, C. E., & Danhauer, J. L. (2002). *Handbook of outcome measures in audiology.* Clifton Park, NY: Thomson Delmar Learning.

Laurent, D., Lynch, J., Ritter, P., Gonzalez, V., Stewart, A., & Lorig, K. (1996). *Outcome measures for health education and other health care interventions.* Thousand Oaks, CA: Sage.

Law, M., Baum, C., & Dunn, W. (Eds.). (2005). *Measuring occupational performance* (2nd ed.). Thorofare, NJ: SLACK Incorporated.

Lenderking, W. R., & Revicki, D. A. (2005) *Advancing health outcomes research methods and clinical applications.* McLean, VA: Degnon Associates, Inc.

McDowell, I. (2006). *Measuring health: A guide to rating scales and questionnaires* (3rd ed.). New York, NY: Oxford University Press.

REFERENCES

Abrams, D., Davidson, M., Harrick, J., Harcourt, P., Zylinski, M., & Clancy, J. (2006). Monitoring the change: Current trends in outcome measure usage in physiotherapy. *Manual Therapy, 11*, 46–53.

Altan, L., Ercan, I., & Konur, S. (2010). Reliability and validity of Turkish version of the Patient Rated Tennis Elbow Evaluation. *Rheumatology International, 30*, 1049–1054.

Alviar, M. J., Olver, J., Brand, C., Hale, T., & Khan, F. (2011). Do patient-reported outcome measures used in assessing outcomes in rehabilitation after hip and knee arthroplasty capture issues relevant to patients? Results of a systematic review and ICF linking process. *Journal of Rehabilitation Medicine, 43*, 374–381.

American Academy of Orthopaedic Surgeons. (2002). DASH normative scoring documentation and scores. Retrieved from http://www3.aaos.org/research/normstdy

Atroshi, I., Gummesson, C., Andersson, B., Dahlgren, E., & Johansson, A. (2000). The Disabilities of the Arm, Shoulder and Hand (DASH) outcome questionnaire: Reliability and validity of the Swedish version evaluated in 176 patients. *Acta Orthopaedica Scandinavica, 71*, 613–618.

Bakker, C. H., Rutten van Molken, M., van Doorslaer, E., Bennett, K., & van der Linden, S. (1993). Health related utility measurement in rheumatology: An introduction. *Patient Education and Counseling, 20*, 145–152.

Bartko, J. J. (1976). On various intraclass correlation coefficients. *Psychological Bulletin, 83*, 762–765.

Beaton, D. E. (2000). Understanding the relevance of measured change through studies of responsiveness. *Spine, 25*, 3192–3199.

Beaton, D. E., Boers, M., & Wells, G. A. (2002). Many faces of the minimal clinically important difference (MCID): A literature review and directions for future research. *Current Opinion in Rheumatology, 14*, 109–114.

Beaton, D. E., Bombardier, C., Escorpizo, R., Zhang, W., Lacaille, D., Boonen, A., et al. (2009). Measuring worker productivity: Frameworks and measures. *Journal of Rheumatology, 36*, 2100–2109.

Beaton, D. E., Bombardier, C., Katz, J. N., & Wright, J. G. (2001). A taxonomy for responsiveness. *Journal of Clinical Epidemiology, 54*, 1204–1217.

Beaton, D. E., Bombardier, C., Katz, J. N., Wright, J. G., Wells, G., Boers, M., et al. (2001). Looking for important change/differences in studies of responsiveness. OMERACT MCID Working Group. Outcome measures in rheumatology. Minimal clinically important difference. *Journal of Rheumatology, 28*, 400–405.

Beaton, D. E., Katz, J. N., Fossel, A. H., Wright, J. G., Tarasuk, V., & Bombardier, C. (2001). Measuring the whole or the parts? Validity, reliability, and responsiveness of the Disabilities of the Arm, Shoulder and Hand outcome measure in different regions of the upper extremity. *Journal of Hand Therapy, 14*, 128–146.

Bilbao, A., Kennedy, C., Chatterji, S., Ustun, B., Barquero, J. L., & Barth, J. T. (2003). The ICF: Applications of the WHO model of functioning, disability and health to brain injury rehabilitation. *NeuroRehabilitation, 18*, 239–250.

Blanchette, M. A., & Normand, M. C. (2010). Cross-cultural adaptation of the Patient-Rated Tennis Elbow evaluation to Canadian French. *Journal of Hand Therapy, 23*, 290–299.

Boadella, J. M., Sluiter, J. K., & Frings-Dresen, M. H. (2003). Reliability of upper extremity tests measured by the Ergos work simulator: A pilot study. *J Occupational Rehabilitation, 13*, 219–232.

Boonen, A., Stucki, G., Maksymowych, W., Rat, A. C., Escorpizo, R., & Boers, M. (2009). The OMERACT-ICF Reference Group: Integrating the ICF into the OMERACT process: Opportunities and challenges. *Journal of Rheumatology, 36*, 2057–2060.

Carswell, A., McColl, M. A., Baptiste, S., Law, M., Polatajko, H., & Pollock, N. (2004). The Canadian Occupational Performance Measure: A research and clinical literature review. *Canadian Journal of Occupational Therapy, 71*, 210–222.

Chatman, A. B., Hyams, S. P., Neel, J. M., Binkley, J. M., Stratford, P. W., Schomberg, A., et al. (1997). The Patient-Specific Functional Scale: Measurement properties in patients with knee dysfunction. *Physical Therapy, 77*, 820–829.

Chung, K. C., & Haas, A. (2009). Relationship between patient satisfaction and objective functional outcome after surgical treatment for distal radius fractures. *Journal of Hand Therapy, 22*, 302–307.

Cieza, A., Geyh, S., Chatterji, S., Kostanjsek, N., Ustun, B., & Stucki, G. (2005). ICF linking rules: An update based on lessons learned. *Journal of Rehabilitation Medicine, 37*, 212–218.

Cohen, J. (1968). Weighted kappa: Nominal scale agreement with provision for scaled disagreement or partial credit. *Psychological Bulletin, 70*, 213–220.

Cohen, J. (1990). A coefficient of agreement for nominal scales. *Educational and Psychological Measurement, 20*, 37–46.

Coldwells, A., Atkinson, G., & Reilly, T. (1994). Sources of variation in back and leg dynamometry. *Ergonomics, 37*, 79–86.

Colquhoun, H., Letts, L., Law, M., MacDermid, J., & Edwards, M. (2010). Routine administration of the Canadian Occupational Performance Measure: Effect on functional outcome. *Australian Occupational Therapy Journal, 57*, 111–117.

Colquhoun, H., Letts, L., Law, M., MacDermid, J., & Edwards, M. (2012). Administration of the Canadian Occupational Performance Measure: Effect on practice. *Canadian Journal of Occupational Therapy*.

Deathe, A. B., Wolfe, D. L., Devlin, M., Hebert, J. S., Miller, W. C., & Pallaveshi, L. (2009). Selection of outcome measures in lower extremity amputation rehabilitation: ICF activities. *Disability & Rehabilitation, 31*, 1455–1473.

Dunckley, M., Aspinal, F., Addington-Hall, J. M., Hughes, R., & Higginson, I. J. (2005). A research study to identify facilitators and barriers to outcome measure implementation. *International Journal of Palliative Nursing, 11*, 218–215.

Dunckley, M., Hughes, R., Addington-Hall, J., & Higginson, I. J. (2003). Language translation of outcome measurement tools: Views of health professionals. *International Journal of Palliative Nursing, 9*, 49–55.

Feeny, D., Blanchard, C. M., Mahon, J. L., Bourne, R., Rorabeck, C., Stitt, L., et al. (2004). The stability of utility scores: Test–retest reliability and the interpretation of utility scores in elective total hip arthroplasty. *Quality of Life Research, 13*, 15–22.

Finch, E., Mayo, N. E., & Stratford, P. W. (2002). *Physical rehabilitation outcome measures: A guide to enhanced clinical decision-making* (2nd ed.). Lippincott Williams & Wilkins.

Finger, M. E., Cieza, A., Stoll, J., Stucki, G., & Huber, E. O. (2006). Identification of intervention categories for physical therapy, based on the international classification of functioning, disability and health: A Delphi exercise. *Physical Therapy, 86*, 1203–1220.

Forhan, M., Vrkljan, B., & MacDermid, J. (2009). A systematic review of the quality of psychometric evidence supporting the use of an obesity-specific quality of life measure for use with persons who have class III obesity. *Obesity Reviews*.

Fritz, J. M., Delitto, A., & Erhard, R. E. (2003). Comparison of classification-based physical therapy with therapy based on clinical practice guidelines for patients with acute low back pain: A randomized clinical trial. *Spine, 28*, 1363–1371.

Geertzen, J. H., Rommers, G. M., & Dekker, R. (2011). An ICF-based education programme in amputation rehabilitation for medical residents in The Netherlands. *Prosthetics and Orthotics International, 35*, 318–322.

Grill, E., Stucki, G., Boldt, C., Joisten, S., & Swoboda, W. (2005). Identification of relevant ICF categories by geriatric patients in an early post-acute rehabilitation facility. *Disability & Rehabilitation, 27*, 467–473.

Grimby, G., & Smedby, B. (2001). ICF approved as the successor of ICIDH. *Journal of Rehabilitation Medicine, 33*, 193–194.

Guyatt, G., Walter, S., & Norman, G. (1987). Measuring change over time: Assessing the usefulness of evaluative instruments. *Journal of Chronic Disease, 40*, 171–178.

Harris, S. R., Swanson, M. W., Andrews, M. S., Sells, C. J., Robinson, N. M., Bennett, F. C., et al. (1984). Predictive validity of the "Movement Assessment of Infants." *Journal of Developmental and Behavioral Pediatrics, 5*, 336–342.

Harty, M., Griesel, M., & van der Merwe, A. (2011). The ICF as a common language for rehabilitation goal-setting: Comparing client and professional priorities. *Health and Quality of Life Outcomes, 9*, 87.

Hemmingsson, H., & Jonsson, H. (2005). An occupational perspective on the concept of participation in the *International Classification of Functioning, Disability and Health*—Some critical remarks. *American Journal of Occupational Therapy, 59*, 569–576.

Hickson, L., & Scarinci, N. (2007). Older adults with acquired hearing impairment: Applying the ICF in rehabilitation. *Seminars in Speech and Language, 28*, 283–290.

Hoang-Kim, A., Pegreffi, F., Moroni, A., & Ladd, A. (2011). Measuring wrist and hand function: common scales and checklists. *Injury, 42*, 253–258.

Horner, D., & Larmer, P. J. (2006). Health outcome measures. *New Zealand Journal of Physiotherapy, 34*, 17–24.

Jaeschke, R., Singer, J., & Guyatt, G. H. (1989). Measurement of health status. Ascertaining the minimal clinically important difference. *Controlled Clinical Trials, 10*, 407–415.

Jette, A. M. (1999). Disentangling the process of disablement. *Social Science & Medicine, 48*, 471–472.

Jette, A. M., & Keysor, J. J. (2002). Uses of evidence in disability outcomes and effectiveness research. *Milbank Quarterly, 80*, 325–345.

Kamath, V., & Stothard, J. (2003). A clinical questionnaire for the diagnosis of carpal tunnel syndrome. *Journal of Hand Surgery, 28*, 455–459.

Kaplan, R. M., Alcaraz, J. E., Anderson, J. P., & Weisman, M. (1996). Quality-adjusted life years lost to arthritis: Effects of gender, race, and social class. *Arthritis Care and Research, 9*, 473–482.

Katz, J. N., & Stirrat, C. R. (1990). A self-administered hand diagram for the diagnosis of carpal tunnel syndrome. *Journal of Hand Surgery, 15*, 360–363.

Kuipers, P., Foster, M., Smith, S., & Fleming, J. (2009). Using ICF-environment factors to enhance the continuum of outpatient ABI rehabilitation: An exploratory study. *Disability & Rehabilitation, 31*, 144–151.

Landis, J. R., & Koch, G. G. (1977). The measurement of observer agreement for categorical data. *Biometrics, 33*, 159–174.

Law, M., Baptiste, S., Carswell, A., McColl, M., Polatajko, H., & Pollock, N. (1998). *Canadian Occupational Performance Measure* (3rd ed.) Ottawa, ON: CAOT Publications.

Law, M., Baptiste, S., McColl, M., Opzoomer, A., Polatajko, H., & Pollock, N. (1990). The Canadian occupational performance measure: An outcome measure for occupational therapy. *Canadian Journal of Occupational Therapy, 57*, 82–87.

Law, M., Baum, C., & Dunn, W. (2005) *Measuring Occupational Performance: Supporting Best Practice in Occupational Therapy.* (2nd ed). Thorofare NJ: Slack Incorporated.

Law, M., Polatajko, H., Pollock, N., McColl, M. A., Carswell, A., & Baptiste, S. (1994). Pilot testing of the Canadian Occupational Performance Measure: Clinical and measurement issues. *Canadian Journal of Occupational Therapy, 61*, 191–197.

Lerner, D., Amick, B. C., III, Rogers, W. H., Malspeis, S., Bungay, K., & Cynn, D. (2001). The Work Limitations Questionnaire. *Medical Care, 39*, 72–85.

Lerner, D., Reed, J. I., Massarotti, E., Wester, L. M., & Burke, T. A. (2002). The Work Limitations Questionnaire's validity and reliability among patients with osteoarthritis. *Journal of Clinical Epidemiology, 55*, 197–208.

Leyshon, R. T., & Shaw, L. E. (2008). Using the ICF as a conceptual framework to guide ergonomic intervention in occupational rehabilitation. *Work, 31*, 47–61.

Lohmann, S., Decker, J., Muller, M., Strobl, R., & Grill, E. (2011). The ICF forms a useful framework for classifying individual patient goals in post-acute rehabilitation. *Journal of Rehabilitation Medicine, 43*, 151–155.

MacDermid, J. C. (2005). Update: The Patient-Rated Forearm Evaluation Questionnaire is now the Patient-Rated Tennis Elbow Evaluation. *Journal of Hand Therapy, 18*, 407–410.

MacDermid, J. C., Ramos, J., Drosdowech, D., Faber, K., & Patterson, S. (2004). The impact of rotator cuff pathology on isometric and isokinetic strength, function, and quality of life. *Journal of Shoulder and Elbow Surgery, 13*, 593–598.

MacDermid, J. C., Walton, D. M., Avery, S., Blanchard, A., Etruw, E., Mcalpine, C., et al. (2009). Measurement properties of the neck disability index: A systematic review. *Journal of Orthopaedic & Sports Physical Therapy, 39*, 400–417.

MacDermid, J. C., Wojkowski, S., Kargus, C., Marley, M., & Stevenson, E. (2010). Hand therapist management of the lateral epicondylosis: A survey of expert opinion and practice patterns. *Journal of Hand Therapy, 23*, 18–29.

Maclure, M., & Willet, W. C. (1987). Misinterpretation and misuse of the kappa statistic. *Journal of Epidemiology, 126*, 161–168.

Maini, M., Nocentini, U., Prevedini, A., Giardini, A., & Muscolo, E. (2008). An Italian experience in the ICF implementation in rehabilitation: Preliminary theoretical and practical considerations. *Disability & Rehabilitation, 30*, 1146–1152.

Marx, R. G., Bombardier, C., & Wright, J. G. (1999). What do we know about the reliability and validity of physical examination tests used to examine the upper extremity. *Journal of Hand Surgery, 24A*, 185–193.

Marx, R. G., Hogg-Johnson, S., Hudak, P., Beaton, D., Shields, S., Bombardier, C., et al. (2001). A comparison of patients' responses about their disability with and without attribution to their affected area. *Journal of Clinical Epidemiology, 54*, 580–586.

Mauthe, R. W., Haaf, D. C., Hayn, P., & Krall, J. M. (1996). Predicting discharge destination of stroke patients using a mathematical model based on six items from the Functional Independence Measure. *Archives of Physical Medicine and Rehabilitation, 77*, 10–13.

McColl, M. A., Paterson, M., Davies, D., Doubt, L., & Law, M. (2000). Validity and community utility of the Canadian Occupational Performance Measure. *Canadian Journal of Occupational Therapy, 67*, 22–30.

Michlovitz, S. L., LaStayo, P. C., Alzner, S., & Watson, E. (2001). Distal radius fractures: Therapy practice patterns. *Journal of Hand Therapy, 14*, 249–257.

Mokkink, L. B., Terwee, C. B., Gibbons, E., Stratford, P. W., Alonso, J., Patrick, D. L., et al. (2010). Inter-rater agreement and reliability of the COSMIN (COnsensus-based Standards for the selection of health status Measurement Instruments) checklist. *BMC Medical Research Methodology, 10*, 82.

Morrey, B. F., An, K. N., and Chao, E. Y. S. Functional evaluation of the elbow. In: B. F. Morrey. *The Elbow and Its Disorders, Second Edition.* Philadelphia, PA: W. B. Saunders; 1993:86-97.

Muller, R., & Buttner, P. (1995). A critical discussion of intraclass correlation coefficients. *Statistics in Medicine, 13*, 2465–2476.

Newcomer, K. L., Martinez-Silvestrini, J. A., Schaefer, M. P., Gay, R. E., & Arendt, K. W. (2005). Sensitivity of the Patient-Rated Forearm Evaluation Questionnaire in lateral epicondylitis. *Journal of Hand Therapy, 18,* 400–406.

Oltman, R., Neises, G., Scheible, D., Mehrtens, G., & Gruneberg, C. (2008). ICF components of corresponding outcome measures in flexor tendon rehabilitation—A systematic review. *BMC Musculoskeletal Disorders, 9,* 139.

Overend, T. J., Wuori-Fearn, J. L., Kramer, J. F., & MacDermid, J. C. (1999). Reliability of a patient-rated forearm evaluation questionnaire for patients with lateral epicondylitis. *Journal of Hand Therapy, 12,* 31–37.

Post, M. W., de Witte, L. P., & Schrijvers, A. J. (1999). Quality of life and the ICIDH: Towards an integrated conceptual model for rehabilitation outcomes research. *Clinical Rehabilitation, 13,* 5–15.

Raman, J., MacDermid, J. C., & Grewal, R. (2011). Effectiveness of different methods of resistance exercises in lateral epicondylosis—A systematic review. *Journal of Hand Therapy.*

Reed, G. M., Leonardi, M., Ayuso-Mateos, J. L., Materzanini, A., Castronuovo, D., Manara, A., et al. (2009). Implementing the ICF in a psychiatric rehabilitation setting for people with serious mental illness in the Lombardy region of Italy. *Disability & Rehabilitation, 31*(Suppl. 1), S170–S173.

Reinhardt, J. D. (2011). ICF, theories, paradigms and scientific revolution. Re: Towards a unifying theory of rehabilitation. *Journal of Rehabilitation Medicine, 43,* 271–273.

Rimmer, J. H. (2006). Use of the ICF in identifying factors that impact participation in physical activity/rehabilitation among people with disabilities. *Disability & Rehabilitation, 28,* 1087–1095.

Rompe, J. D., Overend, T. J., & MacDermid, J. C. (2007). Validation of the Patient-Rated Tennis Elbow Evaluation Questionnaire. *Journal of Hand Therapy, 20,* 3–10.

Roy, J. S., Desmeules, F., & MacDermid, J. C. (2011). Psychometric properties of presenteeism scales for musculoskeletal disorders: A systematic review. *Journal of Rehabilitation Medicine, 43,* 23–31.

Roy, J. S., MacDermid, J. C., Amick, B. C., III, Shannon, H. S., McMurtry, R., Roth, J. H., et al. (2011). Validity and responsiveness of presenteeism scales in chronic work-related upper-extremity disorders. *Physical Therapy.*

Roy, J. S., MacDermid, J. C., & Woodhouse, L. J. (2009). Measuring shoulder function: A systematic review of four questionnaires. *Arthritis and Rheumatism, 61,* 623–632.

Roy, J. S., MacDermid, J. C., & Woodhouse, L. J. (2010). A systematic review of the psychometric properties of the Constant-Murley score. *Journal of Shoulder and Elbow Surgery, 19,* 157–164.

Russell, L. B., Gold, M. R., Siegel, J. E., Daniels, N., & Weinstein, M. C. (1996). The role of cost-effectiveness analysis in health and medicine. Panel on Cost-Effectiveness in Health and Medicine *Journal of the American Medical Association, 276,* 1172–1177.

Sackett, D. L., & Torrance, G. W. (1978). The utility of different health states as perceived by the general public. *Journal of Chronic Disease, 31,* 697–704.

Schmitt, J. S., & Di Fabio, R. P. (2004). Reliable change and minimum important difference (MID) proportions facilitated group responsiveness comparisons using individual threshold criteria. *Journal of Clinical Epidemiology, 57,* 1008–1018.

Shreiner, S. C. (1980). Agreement or association: choosing a measure of reliability for nominal data in the 2 × 2 case—A comparison of phi, kappa, and G. *International Journal of Addiction, 15,* 915–920.

Shrout, P. E., & Fleiss, J. L. (1979). Intraclass correlations: Uses in assessing rater reliability. *Psychological Bulletin, 86,* 420–428.

Skutek, M., Fremerey, R. W., Zeichen, J., & Bosch, U. (2000). Outcome analysis following open rotator cuff repair. Early effectiveness validated using four different shoulder assessment scales. *Archives of Orthopaedic and Trauma Surgery, 120,* 432–436.

Smith, R. & Dobson, M. (1993). Measuring utility values for QALYs: Two methodological issues. *Health Economics, 2,* 349–355.

Soberg, H. L., Finset, A., Roise, O., & Bautz-Holter, E. (2008). Identification and comparison of rehabilitation goals after multiple injuries: An ICF analysis of the patients', physiotherapists' and other allied professionals' reported goals. *Journal of Rehabilitation Medicine, 40,* 340–346.

Solway, S., Beaton, D. E., McConnell, S., & Bombardier, C. (2002). *The DASH Outcome Measure user's manual* (2nd ed.). Toronto, ON: Institute for Work and Health.

Steiner, W. A., Ryser, L., Huber, E., Uebelhart, D., Aeschlimann, A., & Stucki, G. (2002). Use of the ICF model as a clinical problem-solving tool in physical therapy and rehabilitation medicine. *Physical Therapy, 82,* 1098–1107.

Stineman, M. G., Ross, R. N., Fiedler, R., Granger, C. V., & Maislin, G. (2003). Functional independence staging: Conceptual foundation, face validity, and empirical derivation. *Archives of Physical Medicine and Rehabilitation, 84,* 29–37.

Stratford, P. W., Levy, D. R., Gauldie, S., Levy, K., & Miseferi, D. (1987). Extensor carpi radialis tendonitis: A validation of selected outcome measures. *Physiotherapie Canada, 39,* 250–255.

Stratford, P. W., Levy, D. R., & Gowland, C. (1993). Evaluative properties of measures used to assess patients with lateral epicondylitis at the elbow. *Physiotherapie Canada, 45*(3), 160–164.

Stucki, G., Cieza, A., Ewert, T., Kostanjsek, N., Chatterji, S., & Ustun, T. B. (2002). Application of the *International Classification of Functioning, Disability and Health* (ICF) in clinical practice. *Disability & Rehabilitation, 24,* 281–282.

Stucki, G., Cieza, A., & Melvin, J. (2007). The *International Classification of Functioning, Disability and Health* (ICF): A unifying model for the conceptual description of the rehabilitation strategy. *Journal of Rehabilitation Medicine, 39,* 279–285.

Stucki, G., Ewert, T., & Cieza, A. (2002). Value and application of the ICF in rehabilitation medicine. *Disability & Rehabilitation, 24,* 932–938.

Stucki, G., Ewert, T., & Cieza, A. (2003). Value and application of the ICF in rehabilitation medicine. *Disability & Rehabilitation, 25,* 628–634.

Stucki, G., Maksimovic, M., Davidovic, D., & Jorga, J. (2007). New International Classification of Functioning, Disability and Health. *Srpski Arhiv Za Celokupno Lekarstvo, 135,* 371–375.

Tempest, S., & McIntyre, A. (2006). Using the ICF to clarify team roles and demonstrate clinical reasoning in stroke rehabilitation. *Disability & Rehabilitation, 28,* 663–667.

Terwee, C. B., Mokkink, L. B., Knol, D. L., Ostelo, R. W., Bouter, L. M., & de Vet, H. C. (2011). Rating the methodological quality in systematic reviews of studies on measurement properties: A scoring system for the COSMIN checklist. *Quality of Life Research.*

Thorborg, K., Holmich, P., Christensen, R., Petersen, J., & Roos, E. M. (2011). The Copenhagen Hip and Groin Outcome Score (HAGOS): Development and validation according to the COSMIN checklist. *British Journal of Sports Medicine, 45,* 478–491.

Tieman, B. L., Palisano, R. J., Gracely, E. J., & Rosenbaum, P. L. (2004). Gross motor capability and performance of mobility in children with cerebral palsy: A comparison across home, school, and outdoors/community settings. *Physical Therapy, 84,* 419–429.

Torrance, G. W. (1987). Utility approach to measuring health-related quality of life. *Journal of Chronic Disease, 40,* 593–603.

Trudel, D., Duley, J., Zastrow, I., Kerr, E. W., Davidson, R., & MacDermid, J. C. (2004). Rehabilitation for patients with lateral epicondylitis: A systematic review. *Journal of Hand Therapy, 17,* 243–266.

Turchin, D. C., Beaton, D. E., & Richards, R. R. (1998). Validity of observer-based aggregate scoring systems as descriptors of elbow pain, function, and disability. *Journal of Bone and Joint Surgery, 80,* 154–162.

Upper Extremity Collaborative Group. (1996). Measuring disability and symptoms of the upper limb: A validation study of the DASH questionnaire. *Arthritis & Rheumatism 39*(9), S112.

Upper Extremity Collaborative Group. (1999). Development of an upper extremity outcome measure: The "DASH" (Disabilities of the Arm, Shoulder and Hand). *American Journal of Industrial Medicine, 29,* S112.

Verhoef, J., Toussaint, P. J., Putter, H., Zwetsloot-Schonk, J. H., & Vliet Vlieland, T. P. (2008). The impact of introducing an ICF-based rehabilitation tool on staff satisfaction with multidisciplinary team care in rheumatology: An exploratory study. *Clinical Rehabilitation, 22,* 23–37.

Ware, J. E., Jr. (2003). Conceptualization and measurement of health-related quality of life: Comments on an evolving field. *Archives of Physical Medicine and Rehabilitation, 84,* S43–S51.

Ware, J. E., Jr., Gandek, B., Kosinski, M., Aaronson, N. K., Apolone, G., Brazier, J., et al. (1998). The equivalence of SF-36 summary health scores estimated using standard and country-specific algorithms in 10 countries: Results from the IQOLA Project. International Quality of Life Assessment. *Journal of Clinical Epidemiology, 51,* 1167–1170.

Ware, J. E., Jr., Kosinski, M., Gandek, B., Aaronson, N. K., Apolone, G., Bech, P., et al. (1998). The factor structure of the SF-36 Health Survey in 10 countries: Results from the IQOLA Project. International Quality of Life Assessment. *Journal of Clinical Epidemiology, 51,* 1159–1165.

Ware, J. E., Jr., & Sherbourne, C. D. (1992). The MOS 36-item short-form health survey (SF-36). I. Conceptual framework and item selection. *Medical Care, 30,* 473–483.

Weigl, M., Cieza, A., Harder, M., Geyh, S., Amann, E., Kostanjsek, N., et al. (2003). Linking osteoarthritis-specific health-status measures to the International Classification of Functioning, Disability, and Health (ICF). *Osteoarthritis and Cartilage, 11,* 519–523.

Werneke, M. W., & Hart, D. L. (2004). Categorizing patients with occupational low back pain by use of the Quebec Task Force Classification system versus pain pattern classification procedures: Discriminant and predictive validity. *Physical Therapy, 84,* 243–254.

Westaway, M. D., Stratford, P. W., & Binkley, J. M. (1998). The patient-specific functional scale: Validation of its use in persons with neck dysfunction. *Journal of Orthopaedic & Sports Physical Therapy, 27,* 331–338.

World Health Organization. (1980). *International Classification of Impairments, Disabilities and Handicaps. A manual of classification relating to the consequences of disease.* Geneva, Switzerland.

Young, N. L., Williams, J. I., Yoshida, K. K., Bombardier, C., & Wright, J. G. (1996). The context of measuring disability: Does it matter whether capability or performance is measured? *Journal of Clinical Epidemiology, 49,* 1097–1101.

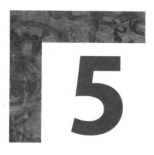

ASKING CLINICAL QUESTIONS AND SEARCHING FOR THE EVIDENCE

Jennie Q. Lou, MD, MSc, OTR and Paola Durando, BA, MLS

LEARNING OBJECTIVES

After reading this chapter, the student/practitioner will be able to:

- Explain the origin of clinical research questions and identify the constituent elements of successful questions.
- Develop skills in formulating answerable clinical questions when searching for evidence.
- Determine the nature and extent of the information needed relevant to a particular question or aspect of professional practice.
- Identify and understand the distinctions between various sources of evidence.
- Critically evaluate information found on the Internet.
- Select appropriate journal citation databases for information needs.
- Describe the characteristics of efficient and effective literature search strategies.
- Employ current awareness tools to keep up to date with topics or journals of interest.

In our daily clinical practice, questions about the best care for our clients arise frequently. As the current best evidence on a given topic changes at an unpredictable rate, even the most experienced practitioners cannot assume that they know the answer without looking into the most current literature. It has become increasingly obvious that the pace of development of new evidence from research is too rapid for standard textbooks to be dependable. When questions do arise, it is unlikely that they will be answered by these textbooks accurately and quickly. Fortunately, the advent of better research, better information resources, and better information technology makes it possible for us to respond to these challenges by learning some basic literature search skills and acquiring access to key evidence resources in the hospital, in the clinic, or at home. Figure 5-1 illustrates the steps in acquiring the evidence. This chapter will describe some of the skills and resources for answering questions of relevance concerning the care of clients in occupational and physical therapy practice.

Law M., & MacDermid, J. C.
*Evidence-Based Rehabilitation: A Guide
to Practice, Third Edition* (pp 105–128).
© 2014 SLACK Incorporated.

Figure 5-1. Steps of acquiring the evidence.

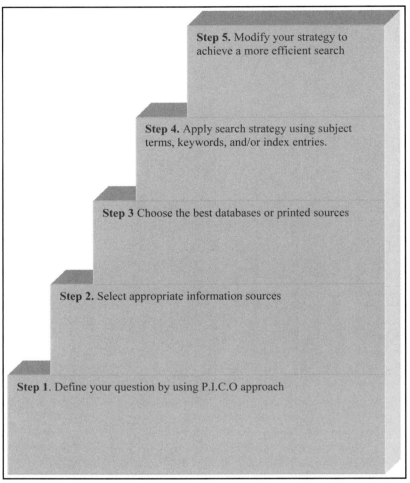

Step 5. Modify your strategy to achieve a more efficient search

Step 4. Apply search strategy using subject terms, keywords, and/or index entries.

Step 3 Choose the best databases or printed sources

Step 2. Select appropriate information sources

Step 1. Define your question by using P.I.C.O approach

DEFINE YOUR QUESTION BY USING A P.I.C.O. APPROACH

The first step for any evidence search is to formulate a "well-built question." This entails identifying a question that is important to the client's well-being, is interesting to you, and that you are likely to encounter on a regular basis in your practice. For practical purposes, it is sometimes more efficient if you seek the advice of consultants for questions that you seldom address in your practice. The process of developing an answerable question is a very critical step because the more clearly you can state your question the more likely you will be able to obtain answers that are directly relevant to your clinical situation.

Where Does the Question Originate?

The most common origin of questions is professional practice. For example, you may have a client who has a specific visual perceptual problem and you do not know how to treat him or her and none of your colleagues are able to help. You could develop a clinical question based on the situation, such as what is the most appropriate intervention for your client. Another common source for questions is professional trends. For example, in occupational therapy there is a push to understand "the form, function, and meaning of occupation" (Zemke & Clark, 1996). From this knowledge, you could form a question to develop a better understanding of a particular occupation. You may also develop a question from the existing published research. For example, reading an article in an occupational or physical therapy journal might raise more questions for you. You could use one of these questions to further explore the literature. Alternatively, you might read a body of literature, realize that there are gaps in your knowledge, and develop a question to explore one of these gaps in more detail. Existing theory is another area where questions can be developed. For example, you might use a particular model and frame of reference in practice and want to critically compare it to what happens in the real world. You could develop a question based on your own curiosity. For the purpose of this book, the following discussion will focus on questions that are generated from clinical practice.

How to Formulate an Answerable Question

Formulating a structured research question points you in a specific direction, helps build your literature search strategy, improves your retrieval, and gives you a way of evaluating answers. One of the benefits of having a well-conceptualized and focused question is that it makes the search for evidence easier. The well-built question makes it relatively straightforward to elicit and combine the appropriate search terms for your literature search. When you develop the question, you are therefore also preparing a checklist or planning a search strategy for your literature search.

To be answerable, the question must be specified clearly so that it includes (a) a specific client group or population; (b) the assessment, treatment, or other clinical issues that you are addressing; (c) the comparison; and (d) the outcome in which you are interested.

In practice, well-built clinical questions usually contain four elements—client/population (P), intervention or exposure (I), comparison (C), and outcome (O). This is a way of breaking down a clinical problem into a question that can be answered. P.I.C.O. is a mnemonic used to describe these four elements; we sometimes refer to this as the anatomy of a question. If you use this "anatomy," it will help you clearly define the question you are trying to answer and facilitate in identifying elements that are of particular importance. Clinical Scenario #1 is used as an example to take you through the question-developing process.

CLINICAL SCENARIO #1
Recently, several older clients have suffered falls, leading to hospital admissions and surgery. The clients, although frail, had all been self-caring before their falls. Getting them back to their own homes was a slow process and two have ended up in long-term institutional care. You wonder whether there is a benefit in initiating a program to prevent older clients from falls at homes.

Patient/Population/Problem

Who or what is your question about? In evidence-based practice, this involves defining the client/patient as a member of a population in terms of the most important characteristics of the patient/population/problem, such as disease, age, sex, ethnic group, etc. But it could also deal with any aspect of health care delivery (e.g., how do we manage our appointments system?). Remember that the articles you search for should be explicit in describing the criteria used to select their subjects. In real life, however, you would be very lucky to find a study that selected exactly the sort of situation with which you are dealing. Therefore, you always need to keep this question in mind, "Are the subjects in this study so different from my situation that I cannot generalize its findings?"

P	I	C	O
Older clients who live independently at home			

Intervention

Intervention is what you wish to do. This covers anything you plan to do. It also involves what you may be doing at present and wish to assess. This would be therapy (e.g., choice of specific intervention), assessments (e.g., which specific assessment tool is more appropriate to use for your client with visual perceptual deficits), preventative measures (e.g., counseling on lifestyle or risk factors), and/or management (e.g., when to refer your client to a cardiac rehabilitation program). You may wish to look for a comparison of two or more interventions, particularly to see whether some innovative intervention is better than your current practice or beats the accepted gold standard.

P	I	C	O
Older clients who live independently at home	Fall prevention program		

Comparison

Is there an alternative intervention to compare, or a no-treatment control group? Please note that your clinical question does not have to always have a specific comparison.

P	I	C	O
Older clients who live independently at home	Fall prevention program	Education on safety at home upon discharge from acute care	

Outcomes

Outcomes are what you wish to achieve. This may also include possible adverse effects that you wish to avoid or minimize. Prevention of disability; recovery of function; and saving of time, money, and effort are some examples of outcomes. Remember that outcomes should define something that is important to the client such as recovery of function (e.g., combing hair), rather than merely an outcome that is of interest to health care providers, such as controlling upper extremity spasticity.

P	I	C	O
Older clients who live independently at home	Fall prevention program	Education on safety at home upon discharge from acute care	Decreased incidence of falls at home

Once you have listed the three (or four) elements of the question, the question should be fairly straightforward.

P	I	C	O
Older clients who live independently at home	Fall prevention program	Education on safety at home upon discharge from acute care	Decreased incidence of falls at home

Question 1: Is a fall prevention program more effective than education upon discharge from acute care in decreasing the incidence of falls in older clients who live independently at home?
Or, if you do not use a comparison,
Question 2: Does a fall prevention program decrease the incidence of falls in older clients who live independently at home?

When developing your question, remember that it should be *relevant, direct, clear*, and *focused*. A common mistake that clinicians often make is to seek answers to questions about a whole process of care rather than a focused clinical issue. Searching for an answer to a generic question is often very difficult. Rather than asking, "What is the impact of a rehabilitation program on the quality of life for my clients?" the clinician may ask, "Can the incidence of falls be decreased by a fall prevention program?" Another example would be instead of asking, "Is occupational therapy effective in treating children with autism?" the clinician may ask, "Does sensory integration improve social behavior in children with autism?" Questions do not have to relate specifically to intervention but can also address issues of prevention, prognosis, or diagnosis. For example, "Does a chronic disease self-management program prevent falls for older adults?"

More recently, an alternative question framing structure known as PESICO (for person, environments, stakeholders, intervention, comparison, outcome) was introduced by Schlosser and colleagues (Schlosser, Koul, & Costello, 2007; Schlosser & O'Neil-Pirozzi, 2006). PESICO incorporates all of the P.I.C.O. elements, and adds *environments*—the contexts in which the problem occurs—and *stakeholders*—those with an interest in the outcome, including the client/patient in the question.

APPROPRIATE INFORMATION SOURCES

Now that you have developed an answerable question, you will need to identify different sources for your search. During your search, you must be able to evaluate and organize the information that you have obtained. A big part of this process is distinguishing relevant from irrelevant information and deciding which source contains the best and most credible information. This can be a daunting task for people who are relatively unfamiliar with scholarly publications. The purpose of the following section is to help you identify different types of scholarly publications and to give you some guidelines for determining their relative merit.

Types of Scholarly Publications

There are three basic types of scholarly publications—books, non-peer-reviewed journals and professional magazines, and peer-reviewed journals.

Books

Books can be focused on a single specialty topic (e.g., activity analysis) or they can be more general in nature (e.g., aging in Canadian society). Books may or may not be peer-reviewed. The credibility of books may be judged by the credentials of the author(s); the reputation of the publisher; the reputation of the author of the preface; the reviews of the book from other reputable sources; the targeted audience (general public versus specific professionals); and the quality, currency, and extent of the citations.

Non-Peer-Reviewed Journals and Professional Magazines

In non-peer-reviewed publications, an author submits a paper and it may or may not be reviewed by the editorial staff of the publication. Though many non-peer-reviewed publications are of high quality, it is unwise to depend solely on these sources for the evidence to answer to your clinical question. Non-peer-reviewed publications tend to have faster turnover of papers (i.e., they get into print faster); therefore, though they can be useful for learning about current trends and controversies in your field of interest, they may not meet the same scientific scrutiny of peer-reviewed papers. Remember that non-peer-reviewed publications can be biased toward a targeted audience.

Peer-Reviewed Journals

Generally speaking, the articles published in peer-reviewed journals are considered more accurate and relevant. They are usually of a higher quality than those in non-peer-reviewed publications. All of the articles, usually with the exception of editorials, have been scrutinized by experts in the field for accuracy of content, quality of research, and relevance to the field. It should also be realized that some peer-reviewed journals are considered to be of higher quality than others.

Most peer-reviewed journals are only available by paid subscription. However, the open access movement is growing. As a result, some entire journals, or journals' archived issues, are freely available. The Directory of Open Access Journals, located at www.doaj.org, lists free, full-text, quality-controlled scientific and scholarly journals.

Types of Articles in Peer-Reviewed Journals

- Short reports: Short reports tend to describe new or developing programs, projects, or treatment techniques. They are also used to present results of research pilot studies and preliminary results from ongoing research. These reports tend to provide the latest advances in a particular area.

- Editorials: In many peer-reviewed journals, editorials are invited papers written by experts in the field. They tend to raise important issues for the field, offer perspectives on controversial subjects, suggest gaps in current knowledge, or propose visionary directions for the future. Because editorials are usually written by an expert in the field, they tend to be useful when developing a background or rationale for proposals. However, these need to be assessed with great care because there are many editorials written that oppose each other even in the most prestigious journals.

- Systematic reviews: Generally speaking, systematic reviews are full-length articles that undergo full peer review. They can be critical reviews of the literature or meta-analyses of existing research. A systematic review is an overview of primary research studies that reach specific standards in terms of methodology. These reviews should be explicit about how the reviewers located the studies and which exclusion and inclusion criteria they used. A meta-analysis is a mathematical synthesis of the results of two or more primary studies that address the same research question and that use comparable methodologies. Systematic reviews usually provide broad background information and preappraised material for your question. They can be a very efficient and effective way to find an answer to your clinical question; however, you need to be aware of the limitations of systemic reviews (e.g., reviewer's bias, missing evidence). When there is any chance it may be available, clinicians should seek a high-quality systematic review rather than the primary studies addressing their clinical question. You can read more information about systematic reviews in Chapter 7.

- Book and technology reviews: Book and technology reviews are usually invited critiques of new resources that are available. Generally speaking, the authors have some degree of expertise in the field specific to the content of the reviewed resource. These reviews provide information on the newest resource materials in a particular area. However, like any review, even distinguished scholars may have opposing views.

- Research articles: There are many types of research articles and many topologies to describe them. Other chapters in this book provide details on the format of research articles and how to evaluate their quality. These articles provide information on the newest scientific findings and advances in a particular area.

Electronic Bibliographic Databases and the Internet

It is very important to distinguish between electronic bibliographic database searches and general Internet searches. Bibliographic databases are indexes to published research, scholarly articles, books, government reports, newspaper articles, etc. Citations often include abstracts. There are many different databases and each database has a particular focus. For example, MEDLINE is an index of medical and biomedical publications, CINAHL focuses on publications from the allied health professions, and ERIC focuses on materials from the field of education. It is important to know what databases are available and on what topics they focus. The information can usually be obtained from your librarian or by reviewing the "Help" or "About" section of the database. Most electronic bibliographic databases are international in scope and, as a result, will provide you with publications that are written in English as well as other languages.

In comparison to an electronic bibliographic database, the World Wide Web (Internet) is made up of interconnected documents that are available through the Internet. The Internet contains a vast amount of information on just about any subject. Searching the Internet will not limit you only to published articles. Although you may find an article published on the Internet, you will also find program descriptions, personal opinions, government documents, information on businesses, organizations, and agencies, etc.

There are many different types of information available on the Internet, but most Web pages can be categorized into types such as news and current events, business and marketing, informational, advocacy, or personal. Table 5-1 provides the function and examples of different types of Web sites. Remember that Web browsers, such as Internet Explorer and Firefox, simply go to Web addresses and are search engines that simply look for the terms that you designate. It is crucial for you to understand that they do not evaluate the accuracy or value of the Web sites and that there are sites that contain inaccurate, out-of-date, or false information. You are responsible for determining the usefulness of the sites. Figure 5-2 presents three steps for evaluating Web sites. Many of the

Table 5-1
<center># Types of Web Sites and Their Function</center>

TYPE OF SITES	FUNCTION AND EXAMPLES
News and current events	• Provide extremely up-to-date information • Include news centers, newspapers, and other periodicals • Examples include CBC, CNN, and the *New York Times*
Business/marketing	• Usually are published by companies or other commercial enterprises • Primary purpose is to promote the company or to sell products • Often include a mixture of information, entertainment, and propaganda • For U.S.-based sites, the URL or Web address usually ends in .com • Examples include Microsoft (www.msn.com) and Indigo (www.indigo.ca)

Informational	• Often provided by government (.gov) or educational institutions (.edu)
	• Provide factual information on a particular topic
	• May include reference materials, research reports, databases, calendars of events, statistics, etc.
	• Examples include the following:
	  ◦ The National Institute of Health (www.nih.gov)
	  ◦ National Library of Medicine (www.nlm.nih.gov)
	  ◦ Canadian Occupational Therapy Association (www.caot.org)
	  ◦ Harvard University (www.harvard.edu)

Advocacy	• Usually are published by an organization with the purpose of influencing public opinion • Examples: Disabled Woman's Network (http://dawn.thot.net/) and Advocacy Center for Canadian Seniors (www.advocacycentreelderly.org/)
Personal	• Are published by individuals who may or may not be part of a larger group or organization • May include almost any type of information including biographical data, information on work, hobbies, etc. • For U.S.-based sites, the URL often includes a tilde (~) • Examples include individual or family home pages, individual faculty or students at a university, member pages from an Internet service provider, and blogs
Other	• Such as entertainment

same criteria for judging library databases and resources can also be used for Web sites. Relevancy has been important in judging other kinds of information sources, and the relevance of Web sites accessed is also important when searching the Internet. In addition to relevancy, you need to evaluate the Web site for its authority, accuracy, objectivity, currency, and commercialism. Table 5-2 provides a checklist of the questions you can ask yourself at each step as you evaluate a Web page.

You probably have noticed that the greatest advantage of the Internet is that some portion of the world's literature has been made conveniently available to you. You also need to keep in mind that a major disadvantage is that quality control simply does not exist. There are two major problems with searching the Internet as part of a literature review. The first problem is narrowing your search

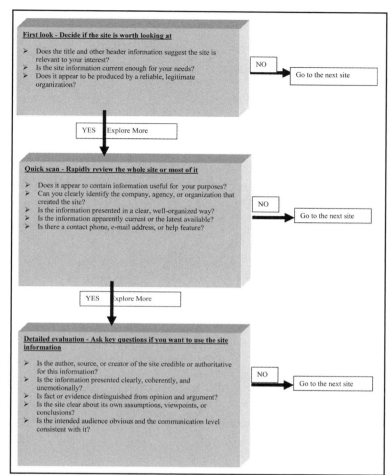

Figure 5-2. Three steps for evaluating Web sites.

enough to find useful information, and the second problem is identifying which sites are credible. Anyone can have a Web site. Not all information found on the Internet can be considered credible, reliable, or even correct. As a result, it is important to have strict criteria for selecting sites to review. Generally speaking, it is a good idea to limit your searches initially to government, university, and professional association Web sites.

Health on the Net (HON) is an independent organization that certifies sites whose policies and procedures meet standards for ethics, accuracy, sourcing, and content quality. Look for the HON logo, which indicates that the Web site complies with the HON code standard for trustworthy health information.

Google Scholar, located at http://scholar.google.com, is a free search engine that is useful for discovering, browsing, and quickly locating highly cited articles. For complete literature searches and literature reviews, you will obtain more current, comprehensive, and relevant results using bibliographic citation databases.

Table 5-2

Checklist of Questions You Can Ask Yourself
at Each Step as You Evaluate a Web Page

AUTHORITY—*Check who is responsible for the page and what their qualifications and associations are*
- Who is sponsoring the site? Authors and creators of Web sites should be clearly stated within the sites and means should be included for contacting them and/or the Webmaster. Any commercial or organizational affiliations should also be included.
- What are the goals and/or values of the person/organization?
- What makes the author(s) an authority on this subject?
- Does the author(s) cite his or her experience/credentials?
- Are they accredited or endorsed by a reputable organization?
- If the site contains articles, do they contain footnotes? If so, does material taken from other sources appear to be fully credited?

ACCURACY—*Try to determine what the sources for the information at the site are*
- Are the facts verifiable?
- Are the sources of information cited, and are individual articles signed and attributed?
- How is the information presented (e.g., fact, opinion, propaganda, etc.)? If presented as fact, is it accurate?

OBJECTIVITY—*Look for the presence of bias and consider the impact of any stated affiliations on the possible attitudes about the topic*
- What is the purpose of the site? Consider the six types of Web pages listed previously and consider whether the page is trying to entertain, inform, persuade, or advertise.
- Is there a bias (cultural, political, religious, etc.)? If so, is the bias clearly stated?

CURRENCY—*Consider how old the information is*
- Is the date of the last revision posted anywhere on the page?
- What is the date of the last revision?
- How frequently is it updated?
- Is some of the information out of date?

SCOPE, COVERAGE, AND RELEVANCE—*Consider the scope of the site is and what it focuses on*
- What kind of information does it have and does it meet your needs? Who is the intended audience (general, specialized readership, scholars, etc.)?
- What is the level of the material (basic, advanced, etc.)?
- What time period is covered?
- What geographical area is covered?
- Is this information a subset of a more comprehensive source?

COMMERCIALISM
- Is the presenter selling something—a product, a philosophy, himself/herself?
- Does the page have a corporate sponsor?
- Are there any hidden costs?
- Do you have to enter personal identification in order to proceed?

Conducting a Literature Search

Ways of Searching

Once you have formulated a clinical question, you are ready to plan a literature search strategy to find specific information that will answer your question. After identifying your search sources, it is effective to identify your search terms (subject headings and keywords) before you begin to search the bibliographic databases. Search terms can come from your clinical scenario and from background reading (e.g., books, Web sites, review articles). If necessary, you can use exclusion criteria or limiters to reduce the database search results to a small list of relevant citations.

Evidence searching is done primarily by using the following methods/tools:

- Searching electronic bibliographic databases (e.g., MEDLINE, CINAHL, Healthstar, PsycINFO, ERIC, OTseeker, PEDro, etc.)
- Manually searching through specific journals (e.g., a journal that you know publishes materials in your areas of interest)
- Retrieving articles listed in the reference lists of articles that you already have on your topic of interest
- Searching the Internet

A comprehensive literature search will probably use all of these methods/tools in an iterative fashion. There are two main goals to always keep in mind when you perform your searches:

- Increase the likelihood of retrieving relevant items—*sensitivity*
- Increase the likelihood of excluding irrelevant items—*specificity*

If you are doing a search and it yields an unmanageably large number of results, you probably need to increase the specificity of your search. On the other hand, if you get too small a number of results, you probably need to increase sensitivity or to broaden your search. Table 5-3 provides some tips on increasing specificity and sensitivity in your searches. Remember, an effective evidence search is not an aimless and tangential hunt with the hopes of finding something that might be useful—systematic, explicit, and reproducible are the guiding principles!

An effective search is all of the following:

- Guided by a specific answerable question or series of questions
- Completed in a systematic and methodological manner
- Documented explicitly
- Reproducible on subsequent days or by other people

Different Databases

There are numerous electronic bibliographic databases that can be used to conduct a search. Some are available on the "open Web" for free, whereas others are commercial and must be accessed through an institutional (library, university, hospital, professional association, etc.) or individual paid subscription.

MEDLINE

What Is MEDLINE?

MEDLINE is an electronic bibliographic database produced by the U.S. National Library of Medicine. Updated almost daily, it is widely recognized as the premier source for bibliographic and abstract coverage of a wide range of literature. MEDLINE encompasses the fields of medicine, nursing, rehabilitation therapy, allied health, dentistry, veterinary medicine, the health care system, and the preclinical sciences. More than 18 million records from more than 5,500 biomedical journals are indexed. Abstracts are included for more than 80% of the records. Although the majority of the records in MEDLINE relate to journal articles, the database also includes bibliographic details of systematic reviews, randomized controlled trials, and guidelines. Because the database is so large and comprehensive, MEDLINE is often a good place to start a search, because you will usually find something on your topic of interest.

Table 5-3

Strategies for Effectively Searching Electronic Databases

Too many articles—you can increase *specificity* by narrowing or refining your search
- Narrow your question
- Use more specific search terms
- Search using subject headings (controlled vocabulary) rather than keywords (free-text/textword searching)
- Apply subheadings to subject headings to limit results to certain aspects of your topic
- Combine terms using "AND" to represent other aspects of the question
- Apply limiters such as English language, human subject, age group, publication type (e.g., review articles, randomized controlled trials, etc.), country, or years of publication

Too few articles—you can increase *sensitivity* by broadening your search
- Broaden your question
- Find more search terms from relevant records
- Try different combinations of terms
- Use truncation (* or $) in keyword searching to retrieve variant word endings
- Add synonymous and related terms and combine them using "OR"
- Use both subject heading and keywords as search terms
- Use the explode feature of subject heading searches
- Apply all subheadings (or qualifiers) to subject headings
- Search further back in time
- Include all publication types

Do not forget to use the "Help" function of the database to increase your searching effectiveness!

MEDLINE can be accessed through the Web site of most health sciences libraries and coverage dates back to 1947. The U.S. National Library of Medicine provides free access to MEDLINE through PubMed at www.ncbi.nlm.nih.gov/pubmed. Because MEDLINE content is sold to various database providers, you may find that the MEDLINE database looks different depending on where you use it because libraries offer different interfaces for database searching. Generally speaking, the information is the same and it is only the interface (i.e., the way you interact with the database) that differs.

How to Search MEDLINE

There are basically two ways of searching databases like MEDLINE: keyword or subject heading. Keyword searching, also known as textword or free-text searching, is a method of searching using words and phrases from the title, abstract, and keywords of references. There are some problems with this method of searching because the database will search for only exactly what you type in and does not automatically allow for variant spellings, plurals, and so on. In a keyword search, the database scans its records to see whether any contain that exact term; therefore, if you enter the word *therapy*, you will retrieve citations containing the word therapy but not *therapist* or *therapeutic*.

Compare the following journal article titles:
- "Development of a Protocol for Improving the Clinical Utility of Posturography as a Fall-Risk Screening Tool"
- "Contribution of Muscle Weakness to Postural Instability in the Elderly"
- "Multifactorial Intervention With Balance Training as a Core Component Among Fall-Prone Older Adults"
- "Disequilibrium and Its Management in Elderly Patients"

These four journal articles discuss the same general topic of postural balance; however, the authors used different words to express this concept. Using a keyword search, you would need to search for these items using all the possible synonyms such as musculoskeletal equilibrium, postural equilibrium, postural instability, etc. On the other hand, using the Medical Subject Heading (MeSH), "Postural balance" would retrieve all of these journal articles regardless of the titles or authors' choice of wording.

Most databases have some form of indexing system. MEDLINE's is called MeSH. This is a bit like the index at the back of a book. It attempts to solve the problems of different authors using different terms to describe the same concept or process. MeSH contains over 26,000 subject headings. Each of these subject headings, or descriptors, represents a single concept appearing in the health care literature. A new MeSH is created as new terms appear in emerging areas of research. For example, the MeSH "Independent living" and "Patient positioning" were added in 2010. When a new citation is added to MEDLINE, indexers and subject specialists choose and apply the appropriate MeSH (usually 10 to 20) to represent the contents of the article.

You do not need to know the MeSH for your topic when you start a MEDLINE search. When you enter a keyword in MEDLINE, the interface will intuitively suggest an appropriate MeSH. Another technique for finding MeSH is to look at what subject headings were assigned to relevant articles on your topic. Although using MeSH terms is a more precise and complete way of searching, there may be times when there is no MeSH available for the subject you are searching and you will need to search using keywords; for example, the proper noun "Cybex" is a fitness equipment manufacturer. MeSH are arranged into hierarchical structures called *trees*, starting with broad terms that branch off and become increasingly narrower with more specific terms. The tree structure of MeSH allows you to explode your search. This means that you can search for a MeSH plus all of its narrower terms simultaneously. For example, if you wanted to run a comprehensive search for citations relating to acupuncture, you could explode the MeSH "Acupuncture" to include all narrower terms:

- Acupuncture
  - Acupuncture analgesia
  - Acupuncture, ear
  - Electroacupuncture
  - Meridians
  - Acupuncture points
  - Moxibustion

The hierarchical trees allow you to select broader terms if your retrieval is too small and narrower or more specific terms if your retrieval is too large.

How to Refine Your Search

Some MEDLINE searches are very precise and neat. You may have a very specific MeSH term that retrieves a small and very well-focused set of citations that you can scan for applicability. Most of the time, it is not that simple and you will have to plan and execute a search strategy. To show that MEDLINE can become overwhelming, perform a MeSH search on Alzheimer's disease and see how many citations come up. Now try something different. Before you run the search, scroll down to the "Limits" tick boxes. There are a number of limiters, or filters, here that allow you to restrict the citations to those in English, those with an abstract, or those dealing with human subjects. How many of the articles on Alzheimer's disease that are in English, contain an abstract, and deal with human studies now appear? You can also choose the years you wish to search, and you can restrict to certain age group (e.g., infants, adolescents, adults), language, male or female study participants, and publication types (e.g., review articles or randomized trials). By adding the limits, you are decreasing

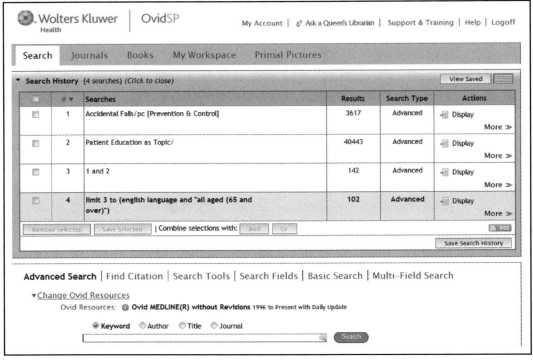

Figure 5-3. Subject heading search results.

your search results. This can be especially useful if you are not doing a comprehensive literature review. See Table 5-3 for some tips on how to narrow or broaden your search. Aside from subject or topical searches, you can also search for specific authors, journal titles, or article titles.

Typically, though, you will be searching for more than one concept. Let us say you were searching a database to identify citations to articles on patient education for fall prevention. You would search each concept separately and then combine the sets of results using "AND" to obtain the overlap between two sets, resulting in a smaller retrieval. In the example shown in Figure 5-3, the retrieval is further reduced once the "English" and "Adult over 65" limits are applied to the combined set of results.

The Cumulative Index to Nursing and Allied Health

The Cumulative Index to Nursing and Allied Health (CINAHL) database is owned by EBSCO Publishing. Located at www.ebscohost.com/cinahl or through institutional subscription, it provides authoritative coverage of the literature related to nursing and allied health including physical therapy, occupational therapy, and health education. More than 3,000 journals are indexed either in their entirety or on a selected basis. CINAHL uses CINAHL subject headings to index its literature, and over 70% of CINAHL subject headings are the same as MeSH. The other CINAHL headings were developed to reflect the terminology used by nursing and allied health professionals.

Ovid

Ovid, which is located at www.ovid.com, is a commercial database provider for a collection of health and life sciences databases. Depending on an institution's subscription, it may include MEDLINE, EBM Reviews, the Cochrane Database of Systemic Reviews (CDSR), EMBASE Drugs & Pharmacology, Health and Psychosocial Instruments (HAPI), HealthSTAR, and other databases. Although you may simultaneously search several Ovid databases, it is inadvisable to do so because subject headings may differ between databases.

The Cochrane Library

The Cochrane Library is a primary source for clinical effectiveness information. It is available through institutional subscription. The best-known Cochrane resource is the CDSR. Cochrane systematic reviews provide the best available source of information about the efficacy of health care interventions. It contains the full text of systematic reviews undertaken by the Cochrane Collaboration, an international network of individuals and institutions committed to preparing, maintaining, and disseminating systematic reviews of the effects of health care. All reviews are updated as new studies are identified. CDSR contains completed reviews and protocols of reviews in progress.

OTDBASE

OTDBASE, located at www.otdbase.org, is a small occupational therapy journal literature search service that contains abstracts from 23 international occupational therapy journals dating back to 1970. Its creator is Canadian occupational therapist Marilyn Conibear. It is accessible to individuals, institutions, and professional associations for a modest annual subscription fee.

OTSearch

OTSearch, located at www1.aota.org/otsearch, is an occupational therapy bibliographic database maintained by the American Occupational Therapy Association. It covers literature in occupational therapy and its related subject areas. Books, proceedings, reports, selected journals, and newsletters are indexed. OTSearch is available through individual or institutional subscription.

OTSeeker

OTSeeker, located at www.otseeker.com, is a free database started in 2002 as a collaboration between Australian universities and associations. It contains abstracts of systematic reviews and randomized controlled trials relevant to occupational therapy. It is an evidence-based resource, because trials have been critically appraised and rated. OTSeeker was modeled on PEDro. In addition to keyword searching, users can search using intervention and diagnosis drop-down menus.

Physiotherapy Evidence Database

Physiotherapy Evidence Database (PEDro), is located at www.pedro.org.au. It is a free database of over 18,000 randomized trials, systematic reviews, and clinical practice guidelines in physiotherapy. It is an evidence-based resource, because all trials are independently assessed for quality. PEDro is produced by the Centre for Evidence-Based Physiotherapy at the George Institute for Global Health.

National Rehabilitation Information Center

RehabDATA, located at www.naric.com/research, contains 70,000 abstracts of books, reports, articles, and audiovisual materials relating to disability and rehabilitation research. It is produced by the National Rehabilitation Information Center in Maryland and is free.

Center for International Rehabilitation Research Information & Exchange

The Center for International Rehabilitation Research Information & Exchange (CIRRIE) is located at http://cirrie.buffalo.edu. At the University at Buffalo, State University of New York, CIRRIE's mission is to facilitate the sharing of information and expertise in rehabilitation research between the United States and other countries. CIRRIE is free and includes the in-process *International Encyclopedia of Rehabilitation*.

Occupational Therapy Critically Appraised Topics

Occupational Therapy Critically Appraised Topics (OT CATs) is located at www.otcats.com. OT CATs is supported by the University of Western Sydney. CAT stands for critically appraised topic, a short, less rigorous version of a systematic review. CATS, a free resource, has not been formally peer reviewed other than by the site developer.

APPLY SEARCH STRATEGY USING SUBJECT HEADINGS AND KEYWORDS

Step-by-Step Searching for Evidence for Clinical Scenario #1 Using The Cumulative Index to Nursing and Allied Health

First, there are some questions you need to ask yourself at the beginning of your search:

- How far back in the literature do I wish to go?
- Do I want only articles available either in online full text or in print at my library, or will I use an interlibrary loan service for articles not locally available?
- What sort of articles will be useful: recent research, overviews, or systematic reviews?
- Are there any languages beyond my own that I would consider retrieving?
- Do I only want articles that have an online abstract?

We will search the CINAHL database for journal articles on fall prevention. Before we look for journal articles that address our specific research question, we may want to do some background reading in review articles to obtain a sense of the current state of research on fall prevention. Using the accidental falls/prevention and control heading/subheading combination, 3,656 citations are retrieved articles. This is obviously way too many articles to retrieve or to review! Next, we will use search limits to narrow our search on fall prevention to English-language review articles published since the year 2005. We can further limit our results by age group 65+, reducing our final set of results to 8 citations (Figure 5-4).

The clinical question formulated earlier in this chapter asks whether patient education upon discharge from acute care is effective in preventing accidental falls in older clients who live independently at home. This time we will perform a database search that includes the intervention, patient education.

When we view the subject term *patient education* in its subject hierarchy, we decide to also search the more specific term *patient discharge education* (Figure 5-5).

Once we combine sets 1 and 2 using "AND" to get the overlap between both sets, apply the English language and age 65+ limits and published since 2005 limits, we are left with 58 citations (Figure 5-6). That is a manageable amount of evidence with which to start!

To obtain a more comprehensive retrieval, search additional databases such as the ones described in this chapter.

When you need to do a comprehensive literature search, you may wish to ask a health sciences librarian to help you plan and document your searches. It is helpful to print or save the search history of each database you search. Your search strategy will therefore be transparent to others and reproducible at a later date.

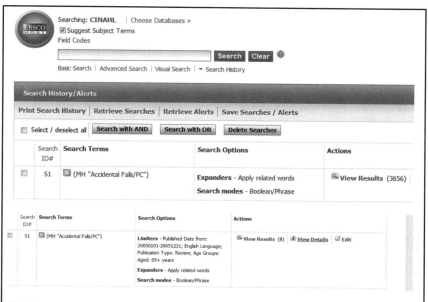

Figure 5-4. CINAHL search example.

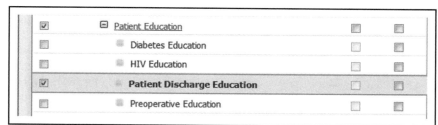

Figure 5-5. Keyword search results.

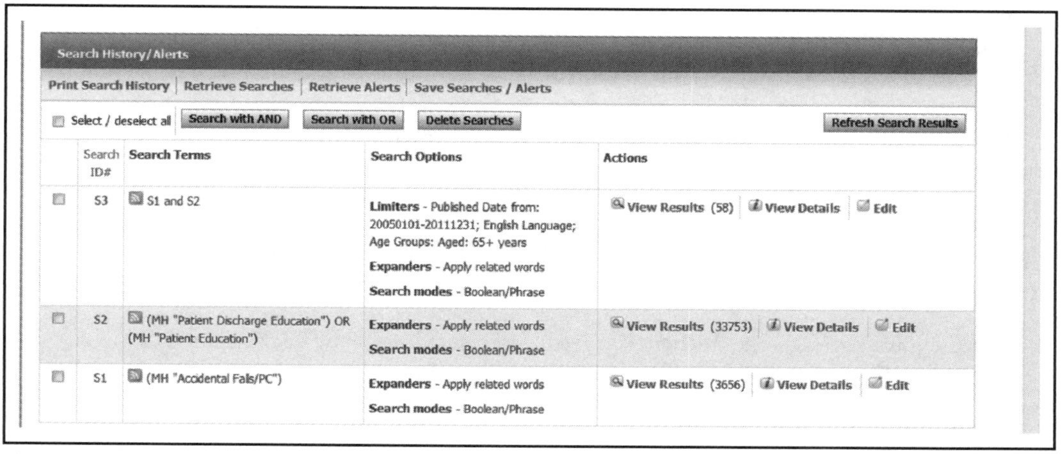

Figure 5-6. Combination search results.

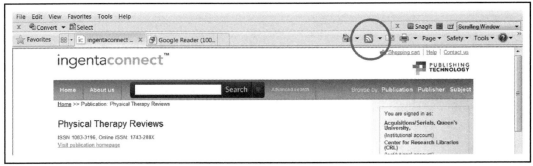

Figure 5-7. Example of an RSS feed.

Current Awareness Services

Once you have developed an effective search strategy in a database and retrieved relevant journal articles, you can set up a Search Alert Service. This will alert you every time a new citation is added to the database that matches your search strategy. A search alert could also notify you whenever a journal publishes a new issue, and its table of contents will be displayed.

Current awareness services are tools that enable you to easily keep up with the professional literature in your field of interest. Current awareness tools save you time and are free. These services were traditionally provided through e-mail alerts but now are often offered through Really Simple Syndication (RSS) feeds. RSS feeds push updates of Web pages to your RSS reader so that you can easily see when your subscribed Web pages have been updated without having to check individual Web sites and without cluttering your e-mail inbox.

An RSS reader is a tool that regularly checks the feeds you have subscribed to for fresh content. If new content is found, your RSS reader will alert you; generally this is done by bolding the title of the feed. Most up-to-date Internet browsers have built-in RSS readers. However, accessing your feeds will be limited to the computer that you saved them on. You can also use Web-based RSS readers, such as Google Reader located at www.google.com/reader.

Web-based RSS readers allow you to access your feeds from any computer with an Internet connection. The disadvantage of Web-based RSS readers is that you need to set up an account and remember your password.

How will you know if there is an RSS feed on a Web site? You will see one of the icons shown in Figure 5-7 on the Web site. In Internet Explorer 8, the feed icon at the top of your browser window will become orange, instead of grey (see Figure 5-7).

Creating an RSS Feed for a Journal Table of Contents Using Your Web Browser

Visit the journal's Web site. If there is a feed, you can subscribe by clicking the RSS icon.

When you click on the feed icon, you will be taken to the page for that feed. To subscribe to the feed in your browser, click on the "Subscribe to This Feed" link. This will add the Web site to the Feeds Folder in your Internet Explorer Favorites tab.

TicTocs Journal Table of Contents Service, located at www.tictocs.ac.uk, is a convenient free site for quickly obtaining journals' RSS feeds. It lists over 14,000 scholarly journals' table of contents from over 750 publishers.

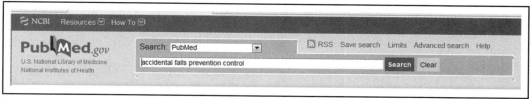

Figure 5-8. Setting up a search alert—Step 1, search keywords.

Creating an RSS Feed for Database Search Results Using Your Web Browser

Just as you can set up Table of Contents Alerts, you can set up Search Alerts. PubMed is useful for subscribing to search results because PubMed is free and you do not need to create an account in order to create search alerts.

Let us do this step-by-step.

- Run your search in PubMed. For example, enter "accidental falls prevention and control" in the search box. Click on "Search" (Figure 5-8).

- Clear the search box. Enter "patient education" and click on "Search." Go to the advanced "Search" tab. Combine the two sets using "AND" as shown in Figure 5-9. Click on "Search" (see Figure 5-9).

- Click on the orange RSS icon to open up the options box. Choose the number of citations to display and name your feed (Figure 5-10).

- Click on "Create RSS." An orange icon will appear in the same box. Click it to go the feed page. Subscribe to the feed using your browser-based RSS reader.

Search Alerts Using a Web-Based Reader

Google Reader is one of the best-known Web-based RSS readers. If you do not have a Google account, set one up (it is free) and log into your account. You can add, or search for, an RSS feed from within Google Reader. You can also view database search results feeds using Google Reader.

The next step is selecting the relevant articles from the search results.

SELECTING RELEVANT ARTICLES FROM THE LITERATURE SEARCH: MODIFY YOUR STRATEGY TO ACHIEVE A MORE EFFICIENT SEARCH

Once you have obtained a copy of an article, you will want to see whether it is suitable for answering your question. You will want to judge its validity, reliability, and—most important of all—applicability. The following are the questions you need to ask yourself:

- Are the results of the article valid (validity)?

- What are the results (reliability)?

- Will the results help me in caring for my clients (applicability)?

You may find it helpful to use a checklist to assess whether it meets these three conditions. See Chapter 6 for more information about critically reviewing articles.

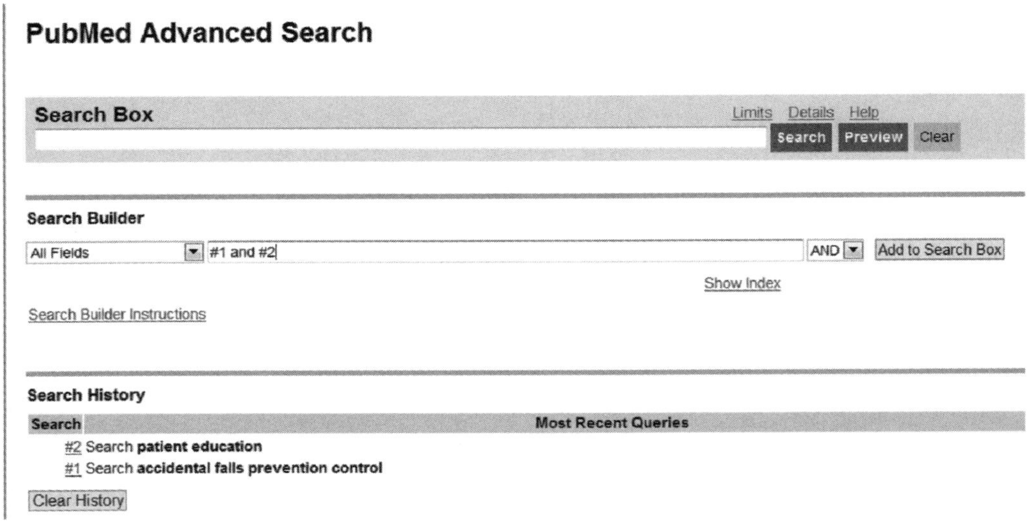

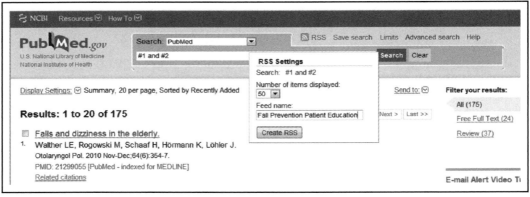

Figure 5-9. Setting up a search alert—Step 2, combine searches.

Figure 5-10. Setting up a search alert—Step 3, create RSS.

TAKE-HOME MESSAGES

Asking Questions

✓ A well-built question originates from professional practice, professional trends, existing published research, or existing theory.

✓ Answerable questions should include the following:

- Specific client group or population
- Intervention (assessment, treatment, or other clinical issues)
- Outcome
- Comparison

✓ Good questions are relevant, direct, clear, and focused.

Different Sources of Evidence

✓ Books: Important to judge their credibility.

✓ Non-peer-reviewed journals or professional magazines: Good for learning about current trends but do not carry absolute credibility.

✓ Peer-reviewed journals: Considered more accurate and relevant; usually of a higher quality.

Electronic Bibliographic Databases and the Internet

✓ Electronic bibliographic databases are compilations of published research, scholarly articles, books, etc., each with a different focus (e.g., MEDLINE, CINAHL, RehabDATA).

✓ Internet—Researcher is responsible for judging relevancy, authority, accuracy, objectivity, currency, and commercialism; difficult to narrow search parameters to the degree needed to find relevant and useful information.

Conducting a Literature Search

✓ Adjust search parameters in accordance with sensitivity (to increase the likelihood of retrieving relevant items) and specificity (to increase the likelihood of excluding irrelevant items).

✓ All effective literature searches should be the following:

- Systematic
- Explicit
- Reproducible

Learning and Exploration Activity 1: Developing an Answerable Question

YOUR CLINICAL SCENARIO
Write down a clinical scenario that you have encountered in your own experience.

Step 1—Identify the situation you are in.

P			
Patient/Population/Problem			

Stop 2—List the intervention—What do you wish to do?

P	I		
Patient/Population/Problem	Intervention		

Step 3—List the comparison, if any.

P	I	C	
Patient/Population/Problem	Intervention	Comparison	

Step 4—Identify the outcome you wish to achieve.

P	I	C	O
Patient/Population/Problem	Intervention	Comparison	Outcome

Step 5—Write out the question using the three key (or four) elements now.

P	I	C	O
Patient/Population/Problem	Intervention	Comparison	Outcome
Question:			

Congratulations! You should have an answerable question now. Remember that your question should always be *relevant*, *direct*, *clear*, and *focused!*

LEARNING AND EXPLORATION ACTIVITY 2: SEARCHING FOR AN EVIDENCE QUESTION

- List the key words in your question you developed from Reader Exercise 1. These key words should be grouped by P.I.C.O. concepts.

	P	I	C	O
	Patient/Population/Problem	Intervention	Comparison	Outcome
Keywords & Subject Headings				

- Select databases (remember to use the ones you can access easily first)
- Narrow or broaden your search by using some of the strategies listed in Table 5-3.
- Set screening criteria to pick out the articles that are relevant to your original question.

FINAL WORD

The best way to get skilled at evidence searching is to practice!

REFERENCES

Schlosser, R. W., Koul, R., & Costello, J. (2007) Asking well built questions for evidence-based practice in augmentative and alternative communication. *Journal of Communication Disorders, 40*, 225–238.

Schlosser, R. W., & O'Neil-Pirozzi, T. (2006). Problem formulation in evidence-based practice and systematic reviews. *Contemporary Issues in Communication Sciences and Disorders, 33*, 5–10.

Zemke, R., & Clark, F. (1996). *Occupational science: An evolving discipline.* Philadelphia, PA: F. A. Davis.

SUGGESTED READINGS

Booth, A. (1996). In search of the evidence: Informing effective practice. *Journal of Clinical Effect, 1*, 25–29.

Centre for Evidence-Based Medicine. (2004). Formulating answerable clinical questions. Retrieved from http://www.cebm.utoronto.ca/practise/formulate

Finlayson, M., & Lou, J. Q. (1999). *Practical steps to critical appraisal: A foundation for evidence-based practice.* Ft. Lauderdale, FL: Nova Southeastern University.

Guyatt, G. H., & Rennie, D. (1993). Users' guides to the medical literature [Editorial]. *Journal of the American Medical Association, 270*, 2096–2097.

Hunt, D. L., Jaeschke, R., & Mckibbon, K. A. (2000). Users' guides to the medical literature, XXI: Using electronic health information resources in EBP. *Journal of the American Medical Association, 283*, 1875–1879.

Oxman, A. D., Sackett, D. L., & Guyatt, G. H. (1993). Users' guides to the medical literature. I. How to get started. The Evidence-Based Medicine Working Group. *Journal of the American Medical Association, 270*, 2093–2095.

Richardson, W. S., Wilson, M. C., & Nishikawa, J. (1995). The well-built clinical question: A key to evidence-based decisions. *ACP Journal Club, 123*, A12–A13.

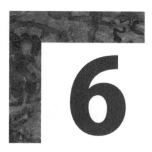

EVALUATING THE EVIDENCE

Joy C. MacDermid, PhD, PT Reg (Ont), FCAHS and
Mary Law, PhD, OT Reg (Ont), FCAHS

LEARNING OBJECTIVES

This chapter will assist you in being able to:

- Select the types of research evidence needed to address different types of clinical questions.
- Define principles of quality in quantitative and qualitative evidence.
- Identify levels of evidence and variations in evidence-ranking systems.
- Find and select appropriate tools to critically appraise clinical evidence.
- Use critical appraisal tools and concepts to evaluate qualitative or quantitative evidence.
- Have a systematic process for selecting the best evidence to answer a clinical question.

Evaluating the quality and truthfulness of clinical research evidence is one of the hallmarks of evidence-based practice (EBP). After identifying a clinical question and formulating and completing a search of the literature, the next step is evaluating the articles retrieved. Evaluating the evidence means examining and analyzing the available research to decide what findings are valid and clinically useful. This step is important because our confidence in the conclusions made in clinical research is dependent on the quality of the research design.

HISTORICAL BACKGROUND

Although health care providers have used clinical evidence to inform their decision making throughout history, the advent of what is now called *evidence-based practice* has evolved in the late 20th century. Dr. Archie Cochrane, a Scottish epidemiologist, promoted the need for rigorous research as a basis for treatment and developed the Cochrane Center, which later evolved into the Cochrane Collaboration (Winkelstein, 2009). The Cochrane Collaboration is a diffuse international collaboration that collects and synthesizes the world's clinical evidence on different clinical topics and develops standards for how to evaluate evidence. Dr. David Sackett, a clinical epidemiologist and physician, taught evidence-based medicine in a problem-based format during the 1960s at McMaster University. He is generally acknowledged as a founder of the evidence-based approach to evaluating evidence and applying it to patients. His classic textbook on evidence-based medicine

Law M., & MacDermid, J. C.
Evidence-Based Rehabilitation: A Guide
to Practice, Third Edition (pp 129–156).
© 2014 SLACK Incorporated.

helped move these methods into entry-level medical training and thereafter into other health disciplines (Sackett, 2000; Sackett, Straus, Richardson, Rosenberg, & Haynes, 2000). Dr. Sackett published one of the earliest levels of evidence and, later at Oxford University, contributed to the "levels of evidence" that remain most commonly used (Cohen, 1996). Although the science of how we evaluate evidence continues to evolve, the basic tenants of these early steps remain.

THE NEED TO BE A CRITICAL CONSUMER OF RESEARCH

The volume of research is increasing beyond what any individual person can process. Thus, filtering information is a critical skill during training and to maintain competency. When we evaluate evidence we are concerned with detecting biases and differentiating between higher and lower quality studies. The need to differentiate the best evidence has led to the development of processes for appraising and ranking clinical research studies. The importance of critical appraisal in EBP has led to the development of systems, processes, tools, and support systems for rating clinical research evidence. In this chapter, we will focus on how the practitioner can appreciate different approaches to research and use quality appraisal or risk of bias assessment to appraise individual research studies. We will discuss ranking systems and how appraisal of the quality and validity of clinical research contributes to both evidence-based recommendations and personal decisions about implementing evidence in practice. In subsequent chapters, we will focus on appraising synthesized knowledge that comes from systematic reviews or practice guidelines.

An important premise in evaluating the quality of clinical research evidence is understanding that different study designs may be needed for different types of clinical questions and over the course of investigation of new ideas or interventions (Fritz, MacDermid, & Snyder-Mackler, 2011). It is important to understand different types of research evidence, how they can inform practice, and their inherent limitations.

AN APPRECIATION FOR RESEARCH PARADIGMS AND DESIGNS

Research that can inform our practice crosses a spectrum of research paradigms and designs. In Figure 6-1 we illustrate how the type of research question and associated research design might evolve over the course of investigating an issue. We can think about our evolving understanding of the clinical phenomenon as being a series of questions. Initially, we might want to understand a clinical phenomenon such as a health characteristic, problem, disease/disorder, patient perspective/experience, intervention, adverse event, or clinical process. The type of research design needed to study these phenomena will vary according to the characteristics of the phenomenon and the stage of emerging knowledge (see Figures 6-1 and 6-2). Early on, we may pursue descriptive or hypothesis-generating research in order to understand the phenomenon. For example, we might start with a simple qualitative description to understand who, what, where, and when. Or we might need bench research to describe the mechanisms. As these studies inform a deeper understanding of the phenomenon and why/how it operates, we may develop theories. Once theories are in place it is possible to test them. Testing of theoretical constructs can happen in labs or in qualitative research or quantitative research.

Once we know what the phenomenon is, we may be interested in describing the incidence/prevalence of the phenomenon on a larger scale. When starting to conduct clinical research (on patients), it is important to be able to identify (diagnostic studies) and measure the clinical phenomenon (clinical measurement studies). Once diagnosis and measurement are in place, we will be able to find factors that can help us predict its intensity or change (e.g., prognostic studies) or which interventions best affect change (treatment effectiveness). Effectiveness studies can be designed to look into

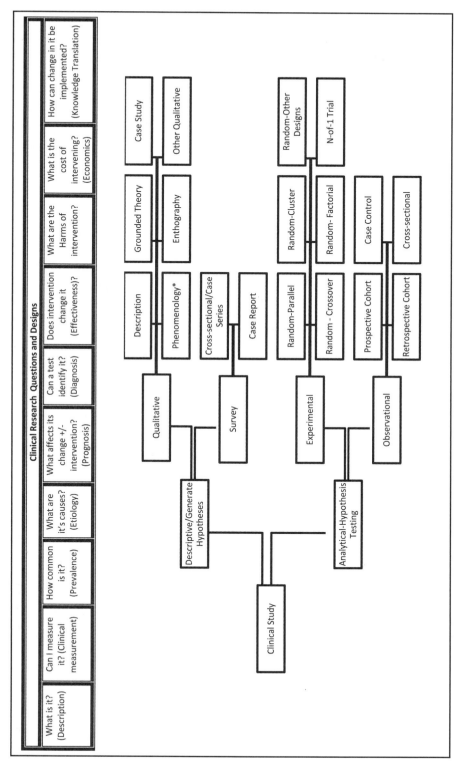

Figure 6-1. This figure illustrates how research questions might evolve over the course of understanding a clinical issue (along the top) and some of the types of design that might be seen in published studies. Earlier in the understanding of an issue we tend to see more descriptive designs and later we may see more studies that are designed for hypothesis testing. Note although we have created a summary of this in this figure, the alignment between design and analysis are not always this clear. For example, phenomenology* is more about theory testing than other types of qualitative research.

Figure 6-2. Moving from your clinical question to your appraisal of studies. This figure illustrates the critical link between the clinical question that drives your search for the right evidence and the process that you use to evaluate the quality of that evidence.

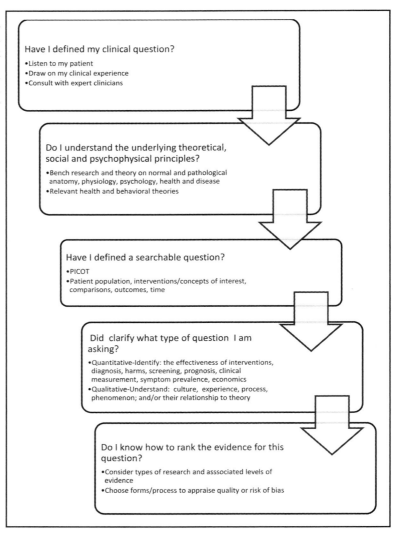

whether treatments work under ideal circumstances (efficacy trials) or in routine clinical practice situations (effectiveness trials). Once we know that treatments are effective under ideal conditions we may be more interested in effectiveness research that informs our understanding of how they work in practice. We may return to qualitative or bench methods at multiple points to explain the phenomena that arise from clinical research or observations. Once treatments are implemented it becomes important to have research that informs our understanding of potential harms from those interventions (monitoring for adverse events). Once we know the benefits and harms, we will be interested in research on how much it costs (cost-effectiveness research) and how it can be transferred into practice (knowledge translation).

Research does not always progress linearly along this continuum, because different research teams may be focusing on different elements of a problem. However, this cycle of evolving knowledge is important because it helps us appreciate different forms of evidence. Although descriptive research will ultimately be classified as a lower level of evidence in EBP rating systems, this work is often foundational to achieving higher levels of evidence. Lower levels of evidence are important foundational blocks but are insufficient to provide confidence when used to make clinical decisions about what to do with an individual patient. Qualitative findings may be important throughout the research cycle. Early on they help us understand what a phenomenon is; later they inform the process of change or deepen our theoretical basis. Ultimately, EBP does require quantitative evidence about the nature and size of effects that can be expected when enacting a clinical test or intervention. This accounts for the emphasis on quantitative clinical research to support practice.

In the research tree in Figure 6-1, we have divided descriptive and analytical hypothesis-driven research. Descriptive research, whether qualitative or quantitative, aims to describe or explain. Descriptive research may be used to develop a theory or hypothesis that is later tested in analytical research. Analytical research is based on asking testable research questions and answering those questions with a certain level of confidence through hypothesis testing. Hypothesis testing implies the use of inferential statistics. In this text we are not able to provide details on the many different quantitative and qualitative research designs because entire textbooks are devoted to each, but we will try to emphasize key types and concepts as they relate to EBP. Figure 6-2 provides a broad overview of the types of research designs commonly used in rehabilitation research.

QUALITATIVE METHODS IN EVIDENCE-BASED PRACTICE

Rehabilitation professionals inherently value qualitative research because it aligns with our approach. Many qualitative researchers are concerned that it is not adequately considered in EBP, which has primarily emphasized quantitative designs. EBP is increasingly recognizing the importance of qualitative research (Broeder & Donze, 2010; Thorne, 2006) and mixed methods (Flemming, 2007; Shaw, Connelly, & Zecevic, 2010) and is learning how to integrate qualitative evidence with quantitative evidence. Although qualitative researchers agree that rigor is important in qualitative research, not all agree on how that should be evaluated or whether it is even possible to establish levels of evidence for this type of research (Cesario, Morin, & Santa-Donato, 2002; Hammersley, 2007). It is our view that qualitative evidence should be appraised for quality, but ranking quality is less important than assuring relevancy.

It is clear that qualitative findings can enrich our understanding of clinical phenomenon and provide a perspective not achieved through quantitative evidence. For example, the effectiveness of an intervention is best determined using a randomized controlled clinical trial because we need to be confident that the intervention will deliver a specific and quantifiable outcome to a majority of people. However, treatments do not affect all people equally and the reasons why people did or did not accept, or respond to, a treatment may require qualitative methods. The experience of living in the community with a newly acquired disability or in access to care may be critical in implementing new interventions and may be best studied using qualitative methods. Mixed methods that combine qualitative and quantitative methods can build on the strengths of each and can be powerful when mixed methods research (Creswell & Plano Clark, 2011) is carefully applied.

Appraisal of Qualitative Research

With the proliferation of qualitative research in rehabilitation, there is increased awareness of the aspects of quality that pertain to this form of inquiry. Rigorous quality manifests itself in different ways than in quantitative research. Appraisal guides for qualitative methods are now available (see Appendix D). Kuper, Lingard, and Levinson (2008) suggested that users of qualitative research ask themselves six questions in appraising whether the results can be trusted and applied to their own practice settings.

1. Was the sample used in the study appropriate to its research question?
2. Were the data collected appropriately?

3. Were the data analyzed appropriately?

4. Can I transfer the results of this study to my own setting?

5. Does the study adequately address potential ethical issues, including reflexivity?

6. Overall: is what the researchers did clear?

These are appropriate questions, but a knowledge of the qualitative paradigm is often necessary to answer them. Issues to pay particular attention to when evaluating qualitative research are described in the following sections and in the appraisal guide for the Letts et al. Qualitative Research Tool (see Appendix D).

Qualitative Study Design Issues

There are many different types of research designs that in qualitative terms methodology are framed more as approaches or traditions. Different forms of qualitative research can have different perspectives on what is the truth and how it is viewed. Qualitative research can serve different purposes, ranging from pure description (Sandelowski, 2000, 2010) to development and testing of theory (Avis, 2003; Mitchell & Cody, 1993; Sandelowski, 1993). Five major approaches or designs are used in qualitative research: narrative, ethnography, phenomenology, grounded theory, and case study (Creswell, 2012). Of these approaches, case study, ethnography, phenomenology, and grounded theory are most often seen in the rehabilitation literature and will be discussed in more detail here.

- A case study is an in-depth study of a bounded system such as a process, activity, event, program, or interaction. Researchers gain access to the situation through a gatekeeper and rationale for the case is directly linked to the purpose of the study. A case study can use multiple sources of data such as interviews, observation, documents, artifacts, etc. It is often analyzed through description of the case, classification of the case information, and the themes that arise from it. The authors often attempt to provide an in-depth picture of the case using text/narrative, tables, and figures.

- Ethnography is a qualitative research approach that arose in the field of anthropology. The purpose is to study a particular culture or group of people to identify their daily life patterns, meanings, and beliefs. Ethnography has been used to study cultural groups, as well as groups of people with specific health problems or disabilities. Ethnography is often performed through observation and interviews and may involve collecting multiple sources of information over an extended period of time (i.e., field research). Sampling is intended to locate representatives of the "culture-sharing group." Data are analyzed for themes and pattern regularities that describe the culture shared by the group and how culture sharing works within the group. The purpose is to interpret and make sense of how the group works.

- The purpose of phenomenology is to understand the lived experience, interpret that experience, and provide information that can be shared with and used by others. In phenomenology, the researcher focuses on finding people who have experienced a particular phenomenon of interest. Interviewing is the most common method of data collection. Data are analyzed for significant statements, meaning of units, and textural and structural description with a focus on describing the essence of the experience. The study attempts to delineate what happened and how was it experienced.

- Grounded theory design is used when generating or verifying theoretical concepts. Themes that emerge from research are used to develop an understanding and theoretical explanation of the social world of the people being studied. Sampling locates multiple, homogeneous, theory-linked individuals who participated in a central phenomenon. Data collection is typically through interviews. Qualitative coding techniques focus on creating or confirming a theory. Authors often develop a conditional matrix and present a visual model or theory and discuss propositions around the theoretical framework.

Qualitative Methods

Achieving descriptive clarity is a very important characteristic for a qualitative research study. Authors of qualitative studies should include clear descriptive information about the participants, the study site, and the researcher so that readers develop a strong understanding of the context of the research.

Sampling

The purpose of sampling in qualitative research is quite different from quantitative methods. Participants are not selected randomly but, rather, for a specific purpose—purposive sampling. For example, participants may be chosen because they are of a certain age or culture or have experienced specific events important to the study. The sampling strategies used in a study should be well described and justified by the authors. Sample size of qualitative studies is generally smaller than in quantitative studies and there are no specific formulae to calculate appropriate sample size. Rather, sampling in a qualitative study is continued until sampling redundancy or theoretical saturation of the data is achieved. In other words, qualitative researchers are more concerned that they have completely heard their audience rather than seeking statistical power. Miles and Huberman (1994) have described a typology for sampling in qualitative inquiry.

Data Collection and Analysis

All data collection procedures should be explicitly described including specific methods, training of data gatherers, the length of time for the study, and the data collected. There are a variety of methods for sampling and collecting data in qualitative research and these must be appropriate for the purpose and qualitative paradigm. Interviews based on semi-structured interview guides are the most common, but many other forms of evidence including verbal records, text, direct observation, records, and artifacts can be used. Qualitative researchers often use multiple methods to enhance the trustworthiness of their findings. The use of multiple methods is one type of triangulation, a group of strategies used to ensure the rigor of a qualitative research study. The researcher may be completely separate or have some level of involvement or connection to the participants or issue. Often in qualitative research it is expected that this will be defined and considered in interpretation.

Qualitative analysis can be conducted for simple description (Sandelowski, 2000, 2010) but more often defines the content or meaning of phenomena (Creswell, 2012). A variety of methods for managing, describing, classifying, coding, and interpreting data are used, and how this is done depends on the research paradigm. A qualitative textbook can provide more detail on these techniques (Creswell, 2012; Creswell & Plano Clark, 2011). Most qualitative research contains methods to ensure the trustworthiness of the data (whereas in quantitative research we think about reliability and validity). Procedures to enhance the rigor of the study such as triangulation (cross-referencing multiple sources), member checking (asking participants to verify the findings), and consistency of coding themes (examining whether different interpreters agree) should be described.

Appraisal of Qualitative Studies

There is debate among qualitative researchers whether appraisal forms can be used in qualitative research. The Critical Appraisal Skills Programme evaluation form starts off with two screening questions that check whether there was a clear statement of the aims and that the methods were appropriate to those aims (Public Health Resource Unit, 1997). Only if these are fulfilled is a more detailed appraisal conducted. Our view is that the open-ended format developed by our colleagues at McMaster provides the right balance of giving direction to the appraisal process while providing sufficient latitude to critique according to context (www.srs-mcmaster.ca/Portals/20/pdf/ebp/qualreview_version2.0.pdf). We suggest that learners work through appraisal using this form and companion guide and a study relevant to their area of practice to gain appreciation of the qualitative appraisal process.

In contrast, others have provided a structured and quantitative assessment of the level of evidence of qualitative research (Cesario et al., 2002), providing specific criteria in five different categories that are evaluated criteria and scored. The five categories evaluated included descriptive vividness, methodological congruence, analytical preciseness, theoretical connectedness, and heuristic relevance. We are not convinced that assigning a level of evidence should be the goal of qualitative appraisal; rather, when reading these studies you should determine whether the findings are credible and relevant before determining how they might enhance the interpretation or application of evidence into your practice.

Quantitative Evidence

Quantitative research is the main focus in EBP. Quantitative evidence can define how accurate a diagnostic test is or how big a treatment effect is expected. Quantitative studies can be descriptive (see Figure 6-2) but often test hypotheses to make conclusions. Testing hypotheses about clinical tests and interventions is how we operationalize confidence in evidence-based clinical decision making. Quantitative research design knowledge is needed to understand and operationalize EBP. Textbooks on this topic should be consulted as needed when performing critical appraisal (Portney L.G. & Watkins, 2009). We cannot describe all designs or the issues that improve their internal validity (trueness) in this textbook but a few key issues will be highlighted.

Erroneous conclusions about the direction or size of effects observed in research studies can arise for a variety of reasons. Two broad categories of error in quantitative research are random error (leads to imprecision) or systematic error (bias).

Random Error

Quantitative studies are based on a sample of people who are used to represent the population (i.e., people to whom the findings might apply). It is always possible that, by chance, a sample does not provide an accurate representation of the population from which it is drawn (random error). Smaller samples are less likely to represent the population than larger samples. Statistics deals with random error by calculating confidence intervals around estimates and by considering sample size in the calculation of error terms. Random error contributes to a lack of precision, sometimes termed *wide confidence intervals*. When studies are underpowered (the sample size is too small), error margins are quite large and can result in a failure to detect true differences. Sample size is often considered a critical issue during the critical appraisal process.

Systematic Error or Bias

Systematic error in quantitative research is a serious concern because it can result in false conclusions and can be more difficult to detect than random error. If individuals in one study group are handled differently than the other study group, these differences, not treatment, might be the reason for group differences. There are many types of potential bias (Hartman, Forsen, Jr., Wallace, & Neely, 2002), and research textbooks should be consulted on this issue (Portney & Watkins, 2009). In general, biases can arise from how participants are entered into studies (sampling/selection bias), how interventions are provided, how outcomes are measured (measurement bias), or how data are analyzed (Coughlin, 1990; Goetghebeur & Loeys, 2002; Kleinbaum, Morgenstern, & Kupper, 1981; Sackett, 1979; Tripepi, Jager, Dekker, Wanner, & Zoccali, 2008). For example, intervention bias can arise if participants in a study control group are able to access the active intervention (contamination) or a different intervention (co-intervention), if the treatments are not provided according to plan (proficiency bias or treatment fidelity), or if adherence varies. Measurement biases can arise when instruments are not properly calibrated, expectations of the evaluator or patient affect their responses (expectation bias), and when information is differentially remembered (recall bias). Content knowledge in your field about the disorders, patient groups, and measurement tools will help you detect bias within clinical studies.

EBP requires us to consider the direction and size of effects when applying evidence to individual patients. There are many strategies for improving the truthfulness of the conclusions and the accuracy of the estimated size of effects. The most important ones include randomization, concealment of randomization, blinding, and intention to treat analyses.

Randomization is the single most powerful tool for discounting the effects of factors that could potentially bias study findings. When a sufficient number of people are randomized, all covariates should be equally distributed across the groups. By balancing these factors, they do not contaminate our conclusions. In assessing the quality of studies we look for randomization and when it is present we look for assurances that it was conducted properly.

Concealment of allocation means that the allocation sequence and individual assignments are withheld from those involved in a trial until the participant has consented to participate in the study (Akobeng, 2005; Berger, 2010; Berger & Do, 2010; Doig & Simpson, 2005; Viera & Bangdiwala, 2007). It is designed to keep people conducting the research from influencing which participants are assigned to a given intervention group by knowing the current or upcoming assignments. Clinicians and patients often have opinions about which intervention might work better for specific patients— even when their overall position qualifies as being equipoise. Clinicians may not offer the trial to certain patients if they know what allocation will be (Schulz & Grimes, 2002). Ideally, allocation is timed close to the intervention to minimize any potential for differential early dropouts.

Blinding is an important issue in clinical studies because it protects against a number of biases that are difficult to detect. People can introduce bias into studies in a multitude of ways; for example, how they investigate cases, how they implement treatments, how they interact with participants, or how they determine outcomes. Therefore, blinding people involved in a study as to which treatment has been allocated/implemented is an important mechanism for reducing potential sources of bias. The most important people to blind are often considered the health care provider and the patient— which is often termed *double-blind*. However, blinding can and should extend beyond these individuals because many other people involved in trials can potentially affect the results (Devereaux et al., 2002). The following groups should be blinded to treatment: participants, health care providers, data collectors, outcome assessors, and data analysts. In the most rigorous circumstances, personnel writing the manuscript are blinded to allocation until the final stages of completing the manuscript. Tests of the success of blinding should be used (Kolahi & Abrishami, 2009).

Another major concern is differential loss of subjects over the course of study so that final comparisons do not provide a valid reflection of the group differences. We do not know the outcomes of people who drop out, and they can be systematically different than those who remain in the study. For example, in some studies participants drop out because they are fully functional and no longer have time to participate in research. In other cases, the outcomes are so bad (death being the worst-case scenario) that the participants are unable to participate. An intention-to-treat analysis that includes dropouts or crossovers in the analysis according to their original assignment is one strategy that is used to circumvent this concern (Fergusson, Aaron, Guyatt, & Hebert, 2002; Kruse et al., 2002). During quality appraisal, we look for high retention of participants as being a quality indicator. Studies use a variety of approaches to mitigate missing data and lost to follow-up including imputation of missing values and sensitivity analysis (Streiner & Geddes, 2001).

Approaches to Appraisal of Quantitative Research

There are a number of ways to evaluate the quality of quantitative evidence. The variety of research designs, appraisal methods, and tools can be a challenge. Ultimately, no single evidence classification is absolutely right or wrong, but the use of critical appraisal tools and supports can help therapists incorporate quality assessment into their use of clinical research. Rather than looking for the ultimate critical appraisal tool, it is preferable for therapists to understand the inherent principles of research design and how rigor is introduced when designing and executing clinical research. Then therapists can pick the right appraisal tool and process for their specific needs.

Critical appraisal can be performed using simple classification systems (i.e., level of evidence) or more detailed appraisal instruments. Critical appraisal instruments range from very structured tools that contain specific questions and defined response categories to open-ended scales where the assessor is guided to make judgments about specific issues. A structured tool like those developed by the chapter author is preferable when learning critical appraisal because it provides direction.

Different depths of critical appraisal are appropriate depending on the context. For example, it may be appropriate to do a quick scan of the literature and retrieve the one or two best papers when answering an urgent clinical question. Understanding the levels of evidence may help you to quickly locate the best quality studies in such a situation. When you are planning to implement a new intervention into your practice, you should delve more deeply into the available research studies to understand a range of issues that might affect the validity or usefulness of the research across different patients.

The availability of preappraised evidence is increasing and provides an option to gain an appreciation of a scope of best evidence without doing all the "heavy lifting." Sources like McMaster PLUS (Haynes et al., 2006) and rehabilitation versions (http://plus.mcmaster.ca/rehab/Default.aspx) make EBP more practical by sending out preappraised targeted evidence. As developers of these resources, we are highly supportive of the need for preappraised evidence. However, we also caution clinicians against being solely reliant on others for appraisal, because it will not always be possible to access preappraised, synthesized evidence for all research questions relevant to your practice. Nevertheless, it is fair to say that the need to appraise primary clinical research studies in order to conduct EBP has dramatically decreased with the development of better evidence synthesis resources.

Types of Appraisal of Quantitative Research

There are three basic approaches to evaluating published quantitative research:

1. Instruments that assess the methodological quality of studies.
2. Instruments that assess the quality of the reporting of clinical studies.
3. Tools/processes for assessing the risk of bias.

These approaches share similarities, but have different purposes.

The Cochrane Collaboration uses a "risk of bias" tool to assess the potential for the conclusions or estimates from clinical research studies to be wrong (biased) in the estimation of the size and direction of the effect (Table 6-1; Higgins & Green, 2008). It is important to separate this type of assessment of internal validity from that of external validity (generalizability or applicability) and precision (the extent to which study results are free from random error). *Applicability* is determining whether a study result can be applied to a certain situation. *Precision* is dependent on the sample size and outcome measurement properties. For example, a small trial with a low risk of bias may provide imprecise results. Conversely, a large trial may be precise (narrow confidence interval) but have a high risk of bias if internal validity is poor. Risk of bias assessment focuses on issues that are most likely to introduce bias and may pay little attention to aspects of research design that are considered in quality assessment. For example, ethical approval and calculating sample size are not directly

Table 6-1

The Cochrane Collaboration's Tool for Assessing Risk of Bias

DOMAIN	SUPPORT FOR JUDGMENT	REVIEW AUTHORS' JUDGMENT
Selection Bias		
Random sequence generation	Describe the method used to generate the allocation sequence in sufficient detail to allow an assessment of whether it should produce comparable groups.	Selection bias (biased allocation to interventions) due to inadequate generation of a randomized sequence.
Allocation concealment	Describe the method used to conceal the allocation sequence in sufficient detail to determine whether intervention allocations could have been foreseen in advance of, or during, enrollment.	Selection bias (biased allocation to interventions) due to inadequate concealment of allocations prior to assignment.
Performance Bias		
Blinding of participants and personnel—Assessments are made for each main outcome (or class of outcomes)	Describe all measures used, if any, to blind study participants and personnel from knowledge of which intervention a participant received. Provide any information relating to whether the intended blinding was effective.	Performance bias due to knowledge of the allocated interventions by participants and personnel during the study.
Detection Bias		
Blinding of outcome assessment—Assessments are made for each main outcome (or class of outcomes)	Describe all measures used, if any, to blind outcome assessors from knowledge of which intervention a participant received. Provide any information relating to whether the intended blinding was effective.	Detection bias due to knowledge of the allocated interventions by outcome assessors.
Attrition Bias		
Incomplete outcome data—Assessments are made for each main outcome (or class of outcomes)	Describe the completeness of outcome data for each main outcome, including attrition and exclusions from the analysis. State whether attrition and exclusions were reported, the numbers in each intervention group (compared with total randomized participants), reasons why attrition/exclusions were reported, and any re-inclusions in analyses performed by the review authors.	Attrition bias due to amount, nature, or handling of incomplete outcome data.
Reporting Bias		
Selective reporting	State how the possibility of selective outcome reporting was examined by the review authors and what was found.	Reporting bias due to selective outcome reporting.
Other Bias		
Other sources of bias	State any important concerns about bias not addressed in the other domains.	Bias due to problems not covered elsewhere in the table.

From "The Cochrane Collaboration's Tool for Assessing Risk of Bias in Randomised Trials" by J. P. T. Higgins, D. G. Altman, & P. C. Gøtzsche, 2011, *British Medical Journal,* 343:d5928. Adapted with permission.

related to the risk of bias, although they do indicate study quality. Conversely, a study may use the best possible research methods but still be biased. For example, even well-designed, high-quality rehabilitation trials have potential for bias when lack of blinding cannot be instituted.

Risk of bias assessment requires judgments about potential sources of bias. This requires knowledge of the trial methods and a judgment about the extent to which these constitute risk and, thus, may be best performed by experienced raters. The risks/issues that might introduce bias are often context dependent. For example, when evaluating crossover trials, it would be important to consider washout as a source of bias. Another difference between quality rating and risk of bias assessment is that quality rating is performed at the level of the study, whereas risk of bias is assessed for each individual study outcome. For example, within the same study, assessments performed by a therapist may have a higher potential for bias than assessments that were self-reported.

This risk of bias assessment involves consideration of the six features of potential risk of bias as outlined in Table 6-1 (Higgins, Altman, Sterne, Cochrane Statistical Methods Group and the Cochrane Bias Methods Group, 2012). Raters decide on each element and indicate either a low risk of bias, a high risk of bias, or "unclear." This tool is typically used for trials and cohort studies. There is controversy about the use of risk of bias versus quality assessment tools. The Cochrane Collaboration favors risk of bias assessment (Higgins et al., 2012). However, the reliability of the risk of bias assessment has been shown to be low even among experienced evaluators (Hartling et al., 2012), which raises concerns about its appropriateness for clinicians practicing EBP.

Reporting guidelines or checklists are focused on improving the standards for reporting research. Because quality appraisals or risk of bias assessments are based on the written research report, such efforts are needed to improve the accuracy of these assessments. The first and perhaps most well known is the Consolidated Standards of Reporting Trials (CONSORT) criteria, developed for reporting of clinical trials (Hopewell et al., 2008; Moher et al., 2012; Schulz, Altman, & Moher, 2010). A variety of reporting guidelines have now been published for many different research designs and have now been reported in a Web-based repository (www.equator-network.org/index.aspx?o=1032). These tools are not appraisal tools but monitor and encourage better reporting, which eventually improves the validity of quality assessments.

Quality appraisal tools evaluate at the level of the study and are generally multidimensional scales that focus on elements of design and conduct of the study. Quality appraisal tools can be generic or specific to the type of research design, structured, or open-ended. A systematic review of such tools concluded that there is considerable variability in intent, components, construction, and psychometric properties of these tools (Katrak, Bialocerkowski, Massy-Westropp, Kumar, & Grimmer, 2004). However, no superior tool has been identified (Katrak et al., 2004). Quality appraisal tools can be very useful to gain an appreciation for research design and guide the appraisal process, but ultimately the therapist decides whether he or she has sufficient confidence in the evidence to change his or her practice. Quality appraisal tools often focus on research design elements such as randomization, allocation, recruitment, retention, sample size, blinding, and statistical analyses. We have provided critical appraisal tools for quantitative and qualitative research in Appendices C and D.

LEVELS OF EVIDENCE FOR INDIVIDUAL RESEARCH STUDIES

Prior to the advent of EBP, bench research was often viewed as the necessary proof to move innovations into practice. A primary contribution of EBP has been to make it clear that observations on patients that are rigorous and free of bias are the best evidence upon which to base clinical decision making. Thus, bench research is ranked low in this regard. The concept of ranking levels of evidence is based on the principle that certain study designs have more rigor and provide more

Table 6-2

Early Levels of Evidence System (1979)

Level 1: Evidence obtained from at least one properly randomized controlled trial

Level 2-1: Evidence obtained from well-designed cohort or case-control analytic studies, preferably from more than one center or research group

Level 2-2: Evidence obtained from comparisons between times or dramatic results in uncontrolled experiments

Level 3: Opinions of respected authorities, based on clinical experience, descriptive studies, or reports of expert committees

From "Bias in Analytic Research" by D. L. Sackett, 1979, *Journal of Chronic Disease, 32*, pp. 51–63. Adapted with permission.

confidence for clinical decision making. The best study design varies according to the type of study that is being conducted (see Figure 6-1).

A hallmark of EBP has been the increased focus on the randomized controlled trial (RCT). Why is this? A primary concern of rehabilitation therapists is treatment effectiveness. The RCT is the only experimental design that can ascertain effectiveness. As we discussed, randomization is our primary protection against unknown sources of bias because covariates are equally distributed across the comparison groups. Thus, an RCT provides the strongest confidence that any differences between the groups can be directly attributed to the intervention. This is why RCTs are considered the Level 1 evidence of treatment effectiveness. However, an RCT is susceptible to bias if the execution is poor. Hence, where the critical appraisal process reveals such flaws plan our confidence (and level of evidence) can be reduced.

Early evidence rating systems ranked the RCT as level 1 evidence for treatment effectiveness. As RCTs proliferated, it became necessary to have a mechanism to summarize multiple, sometimes conflicting, RCTs. Hence the emergence of a new methodology: the systematic review. Some rating systems now classify these as the highest quality of evidence. As evidence syntheses have proliferated, reviews of reviews, also called *overviews*, are now used to synthesize multiple systematic reviews. The critical appraisal of systematic reviews is covered in detail in Chapter 7.

One of the earliest published rating systems, the Canadian Task Force on the Periodic Health Examination, was published in 1979 and applied a simple three-level hierarchy of evidence (Canadian Task Force on the Periodic Health Examination, 1979; Table 6-2). The original levels of evidence were further developed to include evidence synthesis (Table 6-3) and are more thoroughly described (www.cebm.net/index.aspx?o=1025). This has become the predominant level of evidence used by journals that report the level of evidence of published studies. The Web site recently revised the levels of evidence and the 2011 version can also be downloaded from that site. This version is not yet widely used and its value remains to be seen.

In the standard CEBM levels of evidence, three potential situations are considered to be sufficiently rigorous to be labeled as Level 1. Level 1A would consist of a systematic review of a number of RCTs, where the studies substantially agree with each other in terms of the direction and approximate size of the effects observed. A Level 1B study would be an individual RCT where the size of the treatment effect was relatively precisely defined, as indicated by a narrow confidence interval. A Level 1C study is a very unusual circumstance in rehabilitation. This occurs when, in the absence of a randomized study, an overwhelmingly dramatic change in outcomes can be demonstrated once a new treatment becomes available. For example, vaccination did not require RCTs to be accepted into practice because they made such an overwhelmingly clear improvement in health outcomes.

Table 6-3

Oxford Centre for Evidence-Based Medicine Standard Levels of Evidence

LEVEL	THERAPY/ PREVENTION, AETIOLOGY/HARM	PROGNOSIS	DIAGNOSIS	DIFFERENTIAL DIAGNOSIS/ SYMPTOM PREVALENCE STUDY	ECONOMIC AND DECISION ANALYSES
1A	SR (with homogeneity) of RCTs	SR (with homogeneity) of inception cohort studies; CDR validated in different populations	SR (with homogeneity) of Level 1 diagnostic studies; CDR with 1B studies from different clinical centres	SR (with homogeneity) of prospective cohort studies	SR (with homogeneity) of Level 1 economic studies
1B	Individual RCT (with narrow confidence interval)	Individual inception cohort study with >80% follow-up; CDR validated in a single population	Validating cohort study with good reference standards; or CDR tested within one clinical center	Prospective cohort study with good follow-up	Analysis based on clinically sensible costs or alternatives; systematic review(s) of the evidence; and including multi-way sensitivity analyses
1C	All or none$	All or none case series	Absolute SpPins and SnNouts	All or none case series	Absolute better-value or worse-value analyses
2A	SR (with homogeneity) of cohort studies	SR (with homogeneity) of either retrospective cohort studies or untreated control groups in RCTs	SR (with homogeneity) of Level >2 diagnostic studies	SR (with homogeneity) of 2B and better studies	SR (with homogeneity) of Level >2 economic studies
2B	Individual cohort study (including low quality RCT; e.g., <80% follow-up)	Retrospective cohort study or follow-up of untreated control patients in an RCT; Derivation of CDR or validated on split-sample only	Exploratory cohort study with good reference standards; CDR after derivation, or validated only on split-sample or databases	Retrospective cohort study, or poor follow-up	Analysis based on clinically sensible costs or alternatives; limited review(s) of the evidence, or single studies; and including multiway sensitivity analyses
2C	"Outcomes" research; ecological studies	"Outcomes" research		Ecological studies	Audit or outcomes research

(continued)

Table 6-3 (continued)

Oxford Centre for Evidence-Based Medicine Standard Levels of Evidence

LEVEL	THERAPY/ PREVENTION, AETIOLOGY/HARM	PROGNOSIS	DIAGNOSIS	DIFFERENTIAL DIAGNOSIS/ SYMPTOM PREVALENCE STUDY	ECONOMIC AND DECISION ANALYSES
3A	SR (with homogeneity) of case-control studies		SR (with homogeneity) of 3B and better studies	SR (with homogeneity) of 3B and better studies	SR (with homogeneity) of 3B and better studies
3B	Individual case control study		Non-consecutive study; or without consistently applied reference standards	Nonconsecutive cohort study, or very limited population	Analysis based on limited alternatives or costs, poor quality estimates of data, but includes sensitivity analyses incorporating clinically sensible variations
4	Case-series (and poor quality cohort and case-control studies)	Case-series (and poor quality prognostic cohort studies)	Case-control study, poor or non-independent reference standard	Case-series or superseded reference standards	Analysis with no sensitivity analysis
5	Expert opinion without explicit critical appraisal, or based on physiology, bench research or "first principles"	Expert opinion without explicit critical appraisal, or based on physiology, bench research or "first principles"	Expert opinion without explicit critical appraisal, or based on physiology, bench research or "first principles"	Expert opinion without explicit critical appraisal, or based on physiology, bench research or "first principles"	Expert opinion without explicit critical appraisal, or based on economic theory or "first principles"

From "Oxford Centre for Evidence-Based Medicine, Standard Levels of Evidence," by B. Phillips, C. Ball, D. Sackett, D. Badenoch, S. Straus, B. Haynes, M. Dawes, 1998, Updated by J. Howick, 2009. Available at: www.cebm.net/index.aspx?o=1025. Reprinted with permission.

SR = Systematic review; CDR = Clinical decision rule; Absolute SpPin = Diagnostic finding whose specificity is so high that a positive result rules in the diagnosis. Absolute SnNout = Diagnostic finding whose sensitivity is so high that a negative result rules out the diagnosis.

§ All patients died before the Rx became available, but some now survive. Some patients died before the Rx became available, but now none die as a result of it.

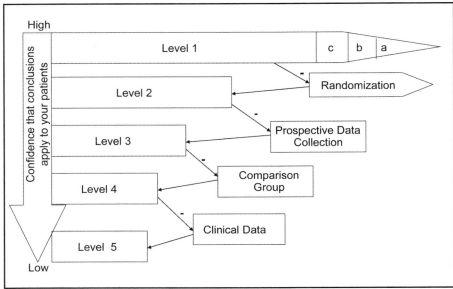

Figure 6-3. Levels of evidence for effectiveness issues that affect confidence in results and lower level of evidence. This figure illustrates how each step-down to a lower level of evidence is attributed a major research design issue.

Level 1 studies are those that provide the highest internal validity, enhancing our confidence that if we select this intervention for our patients, we will be able to achieve similar outcomes.

Figure 6-3 illustrates another way to think about levels of evidence. As we lose important elements of research design, we also lose confidence in the internal validity of the study conclusions. This means we have less confidence that if we use the intervention we will be able achieve similar outcomes for our patients. Level 2 studies differ from RCTs in that we have lost randomization and have less protection against potential biases and confounders. The most positive aspect of a prospective cohort study is that it identifies patients prior to having their outcome and follows them forward in time. This reduces some potential sources of bias such as recall bias. A Level 2A study is a systematic review of cohort (prospective) studies that agree with each other in terms of the direction and approximate size of the effects obtained. A Level 2B study is a single high-quality cohort study with greater than 80% follow-up of patients. There is a substantial emphasis on follow-up in cohort studies because therein lies the greatest potential bias. As we discussed previously, differential dropout can result in biased estimates of treatment effect.

A Level 3A study is a systematic review of case-control studies that agree with each other, whereas a Level 3B is a single individual case-control study. Level 3 evidence for treatment effectiveness occurs when studies are case-controlled. A case-control study design is one where patients are identified for research after exposures (treatments) have been completed. The reason that we have dropped down another level of confidence at this point is because we have lost the potential protection against biases that result from collecting information on patients before their outcomes have been achieved. The primary threat to the internal validity of the case-control study is that the reasons/mechanisms by which patients are available for study may introduce a bias in which patients are included in the study. For example, in studying the effects of a rehabilitation program on total knee arthroplasty conducted in an outpatient setting, patients who died or were too unwell or immobile would be excluded. The sample of patients that remain available to study have a better prognosis and outcome than the entire group. Because we are particularly interested in function in rehabilitation studies, this is a very important potential source of bias, because function may determine whether research subjects can participate.

To drop down another level of evidence, we again lose an important element of research design—our comparison group. Level 4 evidence consists of case series. A case series evaluates the clinical outcomes of a single group of patients. No matter how rigorously we evaluate their outcomes, we remain uncertain as to what would have happened to these patients if an alternate intervention had been selected. Though authors of these studies frequently try to compare the results to those reported in literature in other case series, these comparisons are tentative due to variations in study samples. A case series is a descriptive study because we cannot test hypotheses about differential treatment effects.

Finally, to drop down to our lowest level of evidence, we lose a critical component of research design in an EBP framework—observations made on patients. Level 5 consists of expert opinion without explicit critical appraisal, physiology, bench (lab) research, or first principles (theory). In rehabilitation, it is common for expert opinion to be held in high regard. Some treatment approaches are even named for their developers, indicating the deference provided to the expert. We also rely on numerous conceptual frameworks to support our interventions. Though both experts and conceptual framework should be considered important in hypothesis generating, it is only through hypothesis testing that we are able to establish higher levels of confidence about what we can expect when intervening with real patients. Similarly, although animal research is important foundational knowledge, it needs verification in clinical studies before we can be confident of its application. Though we value foundational research, we should also have a healthy skepticism about these foundations, because a review of the literature can readily identify how many times foundational beliefs have been disproven.

THE LEVEL SYSTEM APPLIED TO OTHER STUDY DESIGNS

Perhaps because treatment effectiveness is such a priority issue for clinicians, the role of the RCT often overshadows other important research designs. The outcomes of interest in trials can be impairments, disabilities, participation, or overall cost-effectiveness. The RCT is the optimal design for questions about interventions including those used to prevent, treat, or rehabilitate. It is important to remember that other designs are needed for other research questions. We have outlined some of these in Figure 6-1. The other four types of studies characterized in the Oxford levels of evidence (see Table 6-3) are prognosis, diagnosis, differential diagnosis/symptom prevalence study, and economic and decision analyses.

The optimal study design varies across different types of clinical studies. For example, the optimal design (Level 1B) for a prognosis study is an inception cohort study with greater than 80% follow-up. The optimal study design for a diagnostic test study consists of a cohort study with good reference standards. For differential diagnosis or symptom prevalence, a single prospective cohort study with good follow-up is a Level 1B study. Finally, in economic and decision analyses, the estimates of effect should be based on clinically sensible costs/alternatives and systematic reviews of the evidence and include multivariate sensitivity analyses. It is important to remember that Level 1 evidence does not always mean an RCT.

Despite differences in the optimal study design and, hence, the specifics of each level, certain consistencies are evident across different types of questions and their associated levels of evidence:

- A systematic review of high-quality studies always provides the highest level of rigor.

- An individual study using the optimal design for that type of clinical question is typically considered high-quality (Level 1) evidence.

Figure 6-4. Embracing qualitative and quantitative evidence to answer clinical questions.

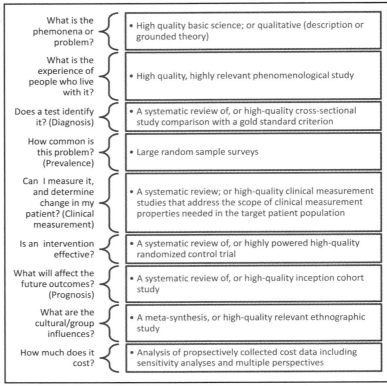

Question	Evidence
What is the phemonena or problem?	• High quality basic science; or qualitative (description or grounded theory)
What is the experience of people who live with it?	• High quality, highly relevant phenomenological study
Does a test identify it? (Diagnosis)	• A systematic review of, or high-quality cross-sectional study comparison with a gold standard criterion
How common is this problem? (Prevalence)	• Large random sample surveys
Can I measure it, and determine change in my patient? (Clinical measurement)	• A systematic review; or high-quality clinical measurement studies that address the scope of clinical measurement properties needed in the target patient population
Is an intervention effective?	• A systematic review of, or highly powered high-quality randomized control trial
What will affect the future outcomes? (Prognosis)	• A systematic review of, or high-quality inception cohort study
What are the cultural/group influences?	• A meta-synthesis, or high-quality relevant ethnographic study
How much does it cost?	• Analysis of propsectively collected cost data including sensitivity analyses and multiple perspectives

- Prospective data collection indicates higher study quality than retrospective data collection.
- Expert opinion, bench research, and conceptual frameworks/theories/first principles are always considered the lowest (Level 5) evidence.

In Figure 6-4, we illustrate how quantitative and qualitative research designs might be integrated across our spectrum of clinical questions.

GRADING OF RECOMMENDATIONS, ASSESSMENT, DEVELOPMENT, AND EVALUATION FOR THE OVERALL QUALITY OF EVIDENCE

In this chapter we have been talking about evaluating individual studies. However, most decision making takes place when we consider multiple studies on a given topic. There are a variety of methods for grading the overall quality of evidence. One that has achieved some level of international consensus is grading of recommendations assessment, development, and evaluation (GRADE; Brozek, Akl, Alonso-Coello, et al., 2009; Brozek, Akl, Jaeschke, et al., 2009; Guyatt et al., 2008). The GRADE system classifies the quality of evidence in one of four levels—high, moderate, low, and very low. Some of the organizations using the GRADE system combine the low and very low categories. Evidence based on RCTs starts as high-quality evidence but may be reduced for compromised quality including study limitations, inconsistency of results (between studies), indirectness of evidence, imprecision (in effect estimates), and reporting bias. GRADE combines considerations about the evidence with other considerations to decide on overall recommendations. These considerations are listed and are discussed further in the chapter on evidence synthesis products in relation to clinical practice guidelines. Further, the *Journal of Clinical Epidemiology* has recently published a detailed series outlining all of the specifics of the GRADE approach (Balshem et al., 2011; Brunetti et al., 2012; Guyatt, Oxman, Akl, et al., 2011; Guyatt, Oxman, Kunz, Atkins, et al., 2011; Guyatt, Oxman, Kunz, Brozek, et al., 2011; Guyatt, Oxman, Kunz, Woodcock, et al., 2011a, 2011b; Guyatt, Oxman, Montori, et al., 2011; Guyatt, Oxman, Santasso, et al., 2012; Guyatt, Oxman, Sultan, et al., 2011; Guyatt, Oxman, Sultan, et al., 2012; Guyatt, Oxman, Vist, et al., 2011). The level of detail in these publications is more appropriate for guideline developers than for users of evidence. For EBP practitioners, GRADE recommendations consider a balance of evidence and focus on the following:

- The quality of evidence
- Uncertainty about the balance between desirable and undesirable effects
- Uncertainty or variability in values and preferences
- Uncertainty about whether the intervention represents a wise use of resources

More details on GRADE will be discussed in relation to clinical practice guidelines.

Alternative Rating Systems

A number of authors have provided alternative rating systems often in an attempt to accommodate additional study designs or types of evidence. No single rating system addresses all study designs or covers all potential types of evidence. When comparing classification systems it becomes apparent that many similarities can be found between evidence ranking systems. In general, evidence rankings should have the same theme: moving from systematic reviews down to more individual assessments. Lower levels of evidence have less control over potential sources of bias.

Levels of evidence classifications have limitations. For example, few address clinical practice guidelines and evidence-based algorithms. None address clinical measurement research, which is an important area of rehabilitation knowledge. Furthermore, how to evaluate or integrate qualitative research is rarely addressed. Finally, though EBP is clear that clinical decisions include patient preferences and clinical expertise, this is not explicitly addressed.

Quality Appraisal Tools

Though it is important to understand the basic principles involved in critical appraisal, the use of tools to provide structure to the process can be invaluable. In this section, we provide critical appraisal tools developed by the chapter authors and provide Web sites where additional forms can be obtained (Table 6-4). Critical appraisal forms, developed by Law and colleagues in the 1990s and refined since then, can be downloaded from the SLACK Incorporated Web site at www.efacultylounge.com or from McMaster University's Centre for Evidence-Based Rehabilitation Web site at www.srs-mcmaster.ca/Default.aspx?tabid=630. Hard copies are in the Appendices. These tools have been used to teach and perform critical appraisal in a variety of rehabilitation and educational contexts. The accompanying guidelines describe the process, as well as key features that should be considered when assessing each element of research design.

Dr. MacDermid has developed critical appraisal forms for effectiveness studies, prognostic studies, diagnostic studies, and clinical measurement studies. These tools have been used to teach and perform critical appraisal and to conduct systematic reviews in rehabilitation. The forms (see Appendices) provide a structure to the critical appraisal process by defining specific criteria that should be addressed to assess quality and by providing an accompanying interpretation guide that clarifies how to assess the criteria. In general, a score of 2 is provided for optimal study design, a score of 1 is suboptimal study design, and a score of 0 is recorded when inappropriate methods were used or the methods were not reported. The forms for effectiveness studies can be used across

Table 6-4

Online Critical Appraisal Tools

WEB SITE URL	TYPE OF STUDIES EVALUATED	NUMBER OF ITEMS
Appraisal of Guidelines for Research & Evaluation* www.agreetrust.org	Clinical practice guidelines	23
Best Evidence Topics www.bestbets.org/links/BET-CA-worksheets.php	Diagnostic test Economic analysis Prognosis Systematic review Qualitative research Clinical practice guidelines	29 34 37 33 40 32
Center for Evidence-Based Emergency Medicine www.ebem.org/analyse.html	Treatment effectiveness Prognosis Diagnostic test Systematic review	13 10 11 12 to 15
Centre for Evidence-Based Medicine, Oxford www.cebm.net/?o=1157	Treatment effectiveness Prognosis Diagnostic test Economic analysis Systematic review Clinical practice guidelines	11 10 8 14 10 18
Centre for Evidence-Based Medicine, Oxford CATmaker www.cebm.net/?o=1216	Treatment effectiveness Prognosis Diagnostic test Systematic review	
Centre for Evidence-Based Medicine, Toronto http://ktclearinghouse.ca/cebm/teaching/worksheets	Treatment effectiveness Prognosis Diagnostic test Systematic review	14 10 9 10
Centre for Evidence-Based Mental Health http://cebmh.warne.ox.ac.uk/cebmh/education_critical_appraisal.htm	Treatment effectiveness Prognosis Diagnostic test Systematic review	9 9 8 9
Centre for Health Evidence* www.jamaevidence.com/resource/520	Treatment effectiveness Diagnostic test Prognosis Clinical practice guidelines Economic analysis Qualitative research	12 9 9 10 10 8
Critical Appraisal Skills Programme* www.sph.nhs.uk/sph-files/casp-appraisal-tools	Diagnostic test Qualitative study Economic analysis Systematic review	12 10 10 10

(continued)

Table 6-4 (continued)

Online Critical Appraisal Tools

WEB SITE URL	TYPE OF STUDIES EVALUATED	NUMBER OF ITEMS
Evidence-Based Medicine, Alberta* www.ebm.med.ualberta.ca/	Treatment effectiveness Prognosis Diagnostic test Economic analysis Systematic review Clinical practice guidelines	11 10 10 10 11 11
Evidence-Based Medicine, Duke http://guides.mclibrary.duke.edu/content. php?pid=274373&sid=2262324	Treatment effectiveness Prognosis Diagnostic test Qualitative study Economic analysis Systematic review Clinical practice guidelines	12 9 9 7 10 10 4
Health Care Practice Research & Development Unit http://usir.salford.ac.uk/12969/	Treatment effectiveness	51
McMaster–Occupational Therapy (has a guide to interpretation) www.srs-mcmaster.ca/Default.aspx?tabid=630	Treatment effectiveness Qualitative study	15 27
Preferred Reporting Items for Systematic Reviews and Meta-Analyses (PRISMA) www.prisma-statement.org/	Systematic review	27

*Includes guide to interpretation.

all levels of evidence, not just RCTs. Separate appraisal forms and guides are provided for clinical measurement, prognostic, effectiveness, and diagnostic test studies (see Appendices).

Other potential critical appraisal tools can be used. There are a variety of resources available on the Internet and some of the tools are highlighted in Table 6-3. The items of the Physiotherapy Evidence Database (PEDro) scale can be used for critical appraisal, and you may be able to cross-check your appraisal scores to those posted (www.pedro.org.au/english/tutorial).

A systematic review addressed 120 different critical appraisal tools appearing in the literature (Katrak et al., 2004). This review found substantial variation between instruments in scope, structure, and scoring. Rehabilitation practitioners may need to bypass scales designed only for use with RCTs (especially those that focus on blinding issues), because these will have limited usefulness in rehabilitation literature.

Strategies for Improving Your Critical Appraisal Skills

Learning critical appraisal is not always the most enjoyable type of professional development. Clinicians often want to focus on practical clinical skills, not appraisal skills. However, critical appraisal is one of those tasks that becomes more enjoyable with experience. Journal clubs—especially ones that include some experienced critical appraisers—can be the most expedient and enjoyable way to learn critical appraisal. Evidence-based journal clubs are a useful means of dedicating time to read, appraise, and make action-based decisions about clinical evidence emerging in the literature. The use of journal clubs in physiotherapy has been studied and indicates substantial variability in the use of problems and evidence, as well as staff enthusiasm (Turner & Mjolne, 2001). Strategies for success include regular meeting times, access to evidence-based resources, a commitment to critical appraisal of all articles, the use of patient-based cases or scenarios to bring meaning to the evidence, and a process to institute change and ongoing evaluation. Web-based journal clubs are starting to become more common and are now offered by some professional associations as a member benefit.

In learning the information we discussed in this chapter it is important to apply the concepts discussed. Thinking about your clinical questions and practicing appraisal of specific studies is a big part of the EBP process. Using the tools provided and articles that have a clinical interest to you is essential to developing your critical appraisal skills. In the beginning you may choose articles based on their clinical interest and see the variation in quality in published rehabilitation research. As time goes on, you will want to quickly screen out lower quality research and focus on better quality studies.

THE ROLE OF STATISTICAL KNOWLEDGE IN CRITICAL APPRAISAL

Lack of confidence in performing critical appraisal is a frequently reported barrier to EBP (Bryar et al., 2003). A variety of strategies can be used to enhance skill and confidence. A number of online statistical texts and critical appraisal Web sites are listed at the end of this chapter. For example, www.statsoft.com/textbook/basic-statistics/?button=1 is a free online textbook that starts with some elementary concepts but has descriptions of even complicated statistics. Another Web resource is *Online Statistics Education: An Interactive Multimedia Course of Study* (http://onlinestatbook.com/). Statisticians seem to be enthusiastic about sharing knowledge on the Web and many useful resources can be found. The *Canadian Medical Association Journal* has published a series of basic-statistics-for-clinicians articles that focus on how to interpret the statistical section of clinical research papers (Guyatt, Jaeschke, et al., 1995a, 1995b; Guyatt, Walter, et al., 1995; Jaeschke et al., 1995).

CONCLUSION

Judging the quality and relevance of research evidence requires knowledge about differences in qualitative, quantitative, and mixed method paradigms. Clinicians must learn about research methods that are designed to reduce potential for random or systematic error in clinical research. These concepts are applied during the process of critical appraisal. Critical appraisal of research evidence requires a structured and thorough evaluation of research to determine which studies provide the most valid conclusions. There are an increasing number of sources of synthesized and appraised evidence that can reduce the burden of critical appraisal. However, clinicians still must be able to perform critical appraisal to fully operationalize EBP. Critical appraisal tools can help clinicians learn the critical appraisal process and conduct systematic evaluations. Clinicians should understand the risk of bias assessment tools and be able to interpret their findings in systematic reviews reported by the Cochrane Collaboration. Critical appraisal skills develop with focused practice. It can be useful to discuss study quality with colleagues through structured journal clubs or informal discussions to develop these skills.

Take-Home Messages

Evaluating the Evidence

✓ EBP requires that clinicians search through preappraised evidence repositories and conduct their own appraisals to determine their confidence in study conclusions.

✓ Different levels of evidence for effectiveness include (in order): systematic reviews or overviews, randomized controlled trials, cohort studies, case-control studies, case series, expert opinion, bench research, or theoretical principles.

✓ Different clinical questions require different study designs, each with their own potential sources of bias and quality appraisals.

✓ Qualitative and mixed methods evidence enriches our understanding of clinical practice and clinical research. Methods for appraisal of qualitative evidence focus on the trustworthiness of the findings and their relevancy.

✓ Therapists must consider research design issues and their potential to introduce bias before implementing the conclusions of research studies.

✓ A variety of structured and semi-structured appraisal tools are available to assist with quality appraisal.

✓ Critical appraisal is a skill that improves with practice. Evidence-based journal clubs provide a useful mechanism to achieve this.

Study Quality Appraisal Instruments Included as Appendices in This Book

1. Form and Guide: Clinical Measurement Studies—Appendix A
2. Form and Guide: Outcome Measures—Appendix B
3. Form and Guide: Qualitative Review—Appendix C
4. Form and Guide: Quantitative Review—Appendix D
5. Form and Guide: Intervention Studies—Appendix E
6. Form and Guide: Prognostic Studies—Appendix F
7. Worksheet: Evaluating Articles About Diagnostic Tests—Appendix G

Web Links

Web/URL	DESCRIPTION
www.srs-mcmaster.ca/Default. aspx?tabid=630	McMaster's Centre for Evidence-Based Rehabilitation Critical appraisal Web page.
The CONSORT Statement www.consort-statement.org/ (home page)	The CONSORT statement lays out a number of guidelines for conducting good RCTs, which are essential for sound SRs. The home page has more detailed information and updates on current work.
Centre for Evidence-Based Medicine Levels of Evidence Classification www.cebm.net/?o=1025	This levels of evidence system is an updated version of the original description of levels of evidence as described by Sackett, Haynes, and others.
Guide to Research Methods: The Evidence Pyramid http://library.downstate.edu/ EBM2/2100.htm	This evidence pyramid was prepared by the Suny Downstate Medical Center. The evidence-based tutorial provides basic definitions and examples of clinical research designs to help the medical student or new clinician understand how the design of a research study may affect whether to accept its findings in caring for a patient.

University of Illinois at Chicago—Is All Evidence Created Equal www.uic.edu/depts/lib/lhsp/ resources/levels.shtml	This site, compiled by the University of Chicago Library, takes an open-ended approach to the topic. Students will likely find the bottom of the page most useful because it discusses the characteristics of specific types of evidence and where to find them.
A New View of Statistics www.sportsci.org/resource/stats/ index.html	An excellent primer or refresher to many aspects of statistics, compiled and created by New Zealander William Hopkins.
http://davidmlane.com/hyperstat/ index.html	Free online statistics textbook.
http://statpages.org/	Free online statistics calculations.
http://nilesonline.com/stats/	Easy reading statistics textbook.
Physiotherapy Evidence Database www.pedro.org.au/	This is a searchable PEDro database that provides bibliographic details, abstracts, and ratings of RCTs, systematic reviews, and evidence-based clinical practice guidelines in physiotherapy.
OTSeeker www.otseeker.com/	This is a searchable database that provides abstracts and ratings of randomized controlled trials and systematic reviews relevant to occupational therapy.
Evidence-Based Medicine Tool Kit www.ebm.med.ualberta.ca/	This site provides critical appraisal tools.
Appraisal of Guidelines for Research & Evaluation www.agreetrust.org	This site provides critical appraisal tools for clinical practice guidelines (Chapter 13).
Best Evidence Topics www.bestbets.org	This site provides a database of critically appraised topics and tools.
Center for Evidence-Based Emergency Medicine www.ebem.org/analyse.html	This site provides critical appraisal tools.
Centre for Evidence-Based Medicine, Oxford www.cebm.net/?o=1157	This site provides a database of critically appraised topics and tools.
Centre for Evidence-Based Medicine, Oxford CATmaker www.cebm.net/?o=1216	This site provides a software tool to help create critically appraised topics.
Centre for Evidence-Based Medicine, Toronto http://ktclearinghouse.ca/cebm/ teaching/worksheets	This site provides critical appraisal tools.
Centre for Evidence-Based Mental Health http://cebmh.warne.ox.ac.uk/cebmh/ education_critical_appraisal.htm	This site provides critical appraisal tools.
Centre for Health Evidence www.jamaevidence.com/ resource/520	This site provides critical appraisal tools.
Critical Appraisal Skills Programme www.sph.nhs.uk/sph-files/ casp-appraisal-tools/	This site provides critical appraisal tools.

Evidence-Based Medicine, Duke http://guides.mclibrary.duke.edu/content.hp?pid=274373&sid=2262324	This site provides critical appraisal tools.
Health Care Practice Research & Development Unit http://usir.salford.ac.uk/12969/	This site provides critical appraisal tools.
McMaster University–Occupational Therapy www.srs-mcmaster.ca/Default.aspx?tabid=630	This site provides critical appraisal tools.
Preferred Reporting Items for Systematic Reviews and Meta-Analyses (PRISMA) www.prisma-statement.org/	This is a checklist for evaluating meta-analyses and randomized controlled trials.
University of Southern Australia www.unisa.edu.au/cahe/resources/cat/default.asp	Provides lists of critical appraisal tools and links to the Web sites where they were developed.

LEARNING AND EXPLORATION ACTIVITIES

The purpose of this chapter was to introduce students to various types of evidence and the different means of classifying this evidence. The following practical exercises are intended to allow the student to become comfortable evaluating the evidence.

1. Pick a clinical issue that interests you and construct a variety of research questions (using Figures 6-1 and 6-2) that would draw upon different types of research evidence. Discuss the pros and cons of this type of evidence with others and decide which ones might have the biggest impact on your practice.

2. Decide upon a treatment of interest (perhaps one you have been studying in class) and perform a search of the literature for articles or studies relating to that treatment. When you find one, attempt to place it in one of the levels of evidence systems cited in this chapter. Justify your answers. Does the level help you have more confidence in the study?

3. Choose a quantitative and/or qualitative article that focuses on a rehabilitation intervention of your choice. Critically review this article using the appropriate form.

4. Find a different critical appraisal form that you could use to evaluate the same article. Appraise your article again. If you are doing a quantitative assessment we suggest that you compare a quality appraisal tool with assessing risk of bias. Contrast and compare the two forms/processes. Which one worked better for you?

5. Design a process for a journal club and conduct a trial run. Discuss barriers and facilitators.

REFERENCES

Akobeng, A. K. (2005). Understanding randomised controlled trials. *Archives of Disease in Childhood, 90*, 840–844.

Avis, M. (2003). Do we need methodological theory to do qualitative research? *Qualitative Health Research, 13*, 995–1004.

Balshem, H., Helfand, M., Schunemann, H. J., Oxman, A. D., Kunz, R., Brozek, J., et al. (2011). GRADE guidelines: 3. Rating the quality of evidence. *Journal of Clinical Epidemiology, 64*, 401–406.

Berger, V. W. (2010). Assessing the quality of randomization and allocation concealment. *Osteoarthritis and Cartilage, 18*, 1361.

Berger, V. W., & Do, A. C. (2010). Allocation concealment continues to be misunderstood. *Journal of Clinical Epidemiology, 63*, 468–469.

Broeder, J. L., & Donze, A. (2010). The role of qualitative research in evidence-based practice. *Neonatal Network, 29*, 197–202.

Brozek, J. L., Akl, E. A., Alonso-Coello, P., Lang, D., Jaeschke, R., Williams, J. W., et al. (2009). Grading quality of evidence and strength of recommendations in clinical practice guidelines. Part 1 of 3. An overview of the GRADE approach and grading quality of evidence about interventions. *Allergy, 64*, 669–677.

Brozek, J. L., Akl, E. A., Jaeschke, R., Lang, D. M., Bossuyt, P., Glasziou, P., et al. (2009). Grading quality of evidence and strength of recommendations in clinical practice guidelines: Part 2 of 3. The GRADE approach to grading quality of evidence about diagnostic tests and strategies. *Allergy, 64*, 1109–1116.

Brunetti, M., Shemilt, I., Pregno, S., Vale, L., Oxman, A. D., Lord, J., et al. (2012). Grade guidelines: 10. Considering resource use and rating the quality of economic evidence. *Journal of Clinical Epidemiology*. 66(2):140-150

Bryar, R. M., Closs, S. J., Baum, G., Cooke, J., Griffiths, J., Hostick, T., et al. (2003). The Yorkshire BARRIERS project: diagnostic analysis of barriers to research utilisation. *International Journal of Nursing Studies, 40*, 73–84.

Canadian Task Force on the Periodic Health Examination. (1979). The periodic health examination. *Canadian Medical Association Journal, 121*, 119–1254.

Cesario, S., Morin, K., & Santa-Donato, A. (2002). Evaluating the level of evidence of qualitative research. *Journal of Obstetric, Gynecologic, and Neonatal Nursing, 31*, 708–714.

Cohen, L. (1996). McMaster's pioneer in evidence-based medicine now spreading his message in England. *Canadian Medical Association Journal, 154*, 388–390.

Coughlin, S. S. (1990). Recall bias in epidemiologic studies. *Journal of Clinical Epidemiology, 43*, 87–91.

Creswell, J. W. (2012). *Qualitative inquiry and research design: Choosing among five traditions.* Thousand Oaks, CA: Sage.

Creswell, J. W., & Plano Clark, V. L. (2011). *Designing and conducting mixed methods research.* Thousand Oaks, CA: Sage.

Devereaux, P. J., Bhandari, M., Montori, V. M., Manns, B. J., Ghall, W. A., & Guyatt, G. H. (2002). Double blind, you have been voted off the island! *Evidence-Based Mental Health, 5*, 36–37.

Doig, G. S., & Simpson, F. (2005). Randomization and allocation concealment: A practical guide for researchers. *Journal of Critical Care, 20*, 187–191.

Fergusson, D., Aaron, S. D., Guyatt, G., & Hebert, P. (2002). Post-randomisation exclusions: The intention to treat principle and excluding patients from analysis. *British Medical Journal, 325*, 652–654.

Flemming, K. (2007). The knowledge base for evidence-based nursing: A role for mixed methods research? *Advances in Nursing Science, 30*, 41–51.

Fritz, J. M., MacDermid, J. C., & Snyder-Mackler, L. (2011). Counting what counts. *Journal of Orthopaedics & Sports in Physical Therapy, 41*, 907–908.

Goetghebeur, E., & Loeys, T. (2002). Beyond intention to treat. *Epidemiologic Reviews, 24*, 85–90.

Guyatt, G., Jaeschke, R., Heddle, N., Cook, D., Shannon, H., & Walter, S. (1995a). Basic statistics for clinicians: 1. Hypothesis testing. *Canadian Medical Association Journal, 152*, 27–32.

Guyatt, G., Jaeschke, R., Heddle, N., Cook, D., Shannon, H., & Walter, S. (1995b). Basic statistics for clinicians: 2. Interpreting study results: Confidence intervals. *Canadian Medical Association Journal, 152*, 169–173.

Guyatt, G., Oxman, A. D., Akl, E. A., Kunz, R., Vist, G., Brozek, J., et al. (2011). GRADE guidelines: 1. Introduction—GRADE evidence profiles and summary of findings tables. *Journal of Clinical Epidemiology, 64,* 383–394.

Guyatt, G., Oxman, A. D., Sultan, S., Brozek, J., Glasziou, P., Alonso-Coello, P., et al. (2012). GRADE guidelines 11—Making an overall rating of confidence in effect estimates for a single outcome and for all outcomes. *Journal of Clinical Epidemiology.*

Guyatt, G., Walter, S., Shannon, H., Cook, D., Jaeschke, R., & Heddle, N. (1995). Basic statistics for clinicians: 4. Correlation and regression. *Canadian Medical Association Journal, 152,* 497–504.

Guyatt, G. H., Oxman, A. D., Kunz, R., Atkins, D., Brozek, J., Vist, G., et al. (2011). GRADE guidelines: 2. Framing the question and deciding on important outcomes. *Journal of Clinical Epidemiology, 64,* 395–400.

Guyatt, G. H., Oxman, A. D., Kunz, R., Brozek, J., Alonso-Coello, P., Rind, D., et al. (2011). GRADE guidelines 6. Rating the quality of evidence—Imprecision. *Journal of Clinical Epidemiology, 64,* 1283–1293.

Guyatt, G. H., Oxman, A. D., Kunz, R., Woodcock, J., Brozek, J., Helfand, M., et al. (2011a). GRADE guidelines: 8. Rating the quality of evidence—Indirectness. *Journal of Clinical Epidemiology, 64,* 1303–1310.

Guyatt, G. H., Oxman, A. D., Kunz, R., Woodcock, J., Brozek, J., Helfand, M., et al. (2011b). GRADE guidelines: 7. Rating the quality of evidence—Inconsistency. *Journal of Clinical Epidemiology, 64,* 1294–1302.

Guyatt, G. H., Oxman, A. D., Montori, V., Vist, G., Kunz, R., Brozek, J., et al. (2011). GRADE guidelines: 5. Rating the quality of evidence—Publication bias. *Journal of Clinical Epidemiology, 64,* 1277–1282.

Guyatt, G. H., Oxman, A. D., Santesso, N., Helfand, M., Vist, G., Kunz, R., et al. (2012). GRADE guidelines 12. Preparing Summary of Findings tables—Binary outcomes. *Journal of Clinical Epidemiology.*

Guyatt, G. H., Oxman, A. D., Sultan, S., Glasziou, P., Akl, E. A., Alonso-Coello, P., et al. (2011). GRADE guidelines: 9. Rating up the quality of evidence. *Journal of Clinical Epidemiology, 64,* 1311–1316.

Guyatt, G. H., Oxman, A. D., Vist, G., Kunz, R., Brozek, J., Alonso-Coello, P., et al. (2011). GRADE guidelines: 4. Rating the quality of evidence—Study limitations (risk of bias). *Journal of Clinical Epidemiology, 64,* 407–415.

Guyatt, G. H., Oxman, A. D., Vist, G. E., Kunz, R., Falck-Ytter, Y., Alonso-Coello, P., et al. (2008). GRADE: An emerging consensus on rating quality of evidence and strength of recommendations. *British Medical Journal, 336,* 924–926.

Hammersley, M. (2007). The issue of quality in qualitative research. *International Journal of Research & Method in Education, 30,* 287–305.

Hartling, L., Hamm, M. P., Milne, A., Vandermeer, B., Santaguida, P. L., Ansari, M., et al. (2012). Testing the risk of bias tool showed low reliability between individual reviewers and across consensus assessments of reviewer pairs. *Journal of Clinical Epidemiology.*

Hartman, J. M., Forsen, J. W., Jr., Wallace, M. S., & Neely, J. G. (2002). Tutorials in clinical research: Part IV: Recognizing and controlling bias. *Laryngoscope, 112,* 23–31.

Haynes, R. B., Holland, J., Cotoi, C., McKinlay, R. J., Wilczynski, N. L., Walters, L. A., et al. (2006). McMaster PLUS: a cluster randomized clinical trial of an intervention to accelerate clinical use of evidence-based information from digital libraries. *Journal of the American Med Informatics Association, 13,* 593–600.

Higgins, J. P., Altman, D. G., Sterne, A. C., Cochrane Statistical Methods Group, & the Cochrane Bias Methods Group. (2012). Chapter 8: Assessing risk of bias in included studies. In J. P. Higgins & S. Green (Eds.), *Cochrane handbook for systematic reviews of interventions.* The Cochrane Collaboration.

Higgins, J. P., & Green, S. (2008). *Cochrane handbook for systematic reviews of interventions* (Version 5.0.1). Retrieved from www.cochrane-handbook.org/

Hopewell, S., Clarke, M., Moher, D., Wager, E., Middleton, P., Altman, D. G., et al. (2008). CONSORT for reporting randomized controlled trials in journal and conference abstracts: explanation and elaboration. *PLoS Medicine, 5,* e20.

Jaeschke, R., Guyatt, G., Shannon, H., Walter, S., Cook, D., & Heddle, N. (1995). Basic statistics for clinicians: 3. Assessing the effects of treatment: Measures of association. *Canadian Medical Association Journal, 152,* 351–357.

Katrak, P., Bialocerkowski, A. E., Massy-Westropp, N., Kumar, V. S., & Grimmer, K. (2004). A systematic review of the content of critical appraisal tools. *BMC Medical Research Methodology, 4,* 22.

Kleinbaum, D. G., Morgenstern, H., & Kupper, L. L. (1981). Selection bias in epidemiologic studies. *American Journal of Epidemiology, 113*, 452–463.

Kolahi, J., & Abrishami, M. (2009). Multiple-blind: Towards a new blinding protocol for future generations of clinical trials. *Medical Hypotheses, 73*, 843–845.

Kruse, R. L., Alper, B. S., Reust, C., Stevermer, J. J., Shannon, S., & Williams, R. H. (2002). Intention-to-treat analysis: Who is in? Who is out? *Journal of Family Practice, 51*, 969–971.

Kuper, A., Lingard, L., & Levinson, W. (2008). Critically appraising qualitative research. *British Medical Journal, 337*, a1035.

Miles, M. B., & Huberman, A. M. (1994). *Qualitative data analysis* (2nd ed.). Thousand Oaks, CA: Sage.

Mitchell, G. J., & Cody, W. K. (1993). The role of theory in qualitative research. *Nursing Science Quarterly, 6*, 170–178.

Moher, D., Hopewell, S., Schulz, K. F., Montori, V., Gotzsche, P. C., Devereaux, P. J., et al. (2012). CONSORT 2010 explanation and elaboration: updated guidelines for reporting parallel group randomised trials. *International Journal of Surgery, 10*, 28–55.

Portney, L. G., & Watkins, M. P. (2009). *Foundations of clinical research, applications to practice* (3rd ed.). Pearson/Prentice Hall.

Public Health Resource Unit, Institute of Health Science, Oxford. (1997). *Critical appraisal checklist for an article on qualitative research*. Retrieved from www.gla.ac.uk/media/media_64038_en.pdf

Sackett, D. L. (1979). Bias in analytic research. *Journal of Chronic Disease, 32*, 51–63.

Sackett, D. L. (2000). The fall of "clinical research" and the rise of "clinical-practice research." *Clinical and Investigative Medicine, 23*, 379–381.

Sackett, D. L., Straus, S. E., Richardson, W. S., Rosenberg, W., & Haynes, R. B. (2000). *Evidence-based medicine. How to practice and teach EBM* (2nd ed.). Toronto, ON: Churchill Livingstone.

Sandelowski, M. (1993). Theory unmasked: The uses and guises of theory in qualitative research. *Research in Nursing & Health, 16*, 213–218.

Sandelowski, M. (2000). Whatever happened to qualitative description? *Research in Nursing & Health, 23*, 334–340.

Sandelowski, M. (2010). What's in a name? Qualitative description revisited. *Research in Nursing & Health, 33*, 77–84.

Schulz, K. F., Altman, D. G., & Moher, D. (2010). CONSORT 2010 Statement: Updated guidelines for reporting parallel group randomised trials. *Trials, 11*, 32.

Schulz, K. F., & Grimes, D. A. (2002). Allocation concealment in randomised trials: Defending against deciphering. *Lancet, 359*, 614–618.

Shaw, J. A., Connelly, D. M., & Zecevic, A. A. (2010). Pragmatism in practice: Mixed methods research for physiotherapy. *Physiotherapy: Theory and Practice, 26*, 510–518.

Streiner, D., & Geddes, J. (2001). Intention to treat analysis in clinical trials when there are missing data. *Evidence-Based Mental Health, 4*, 70–71.

Thorne, S. (2006). Reflections on "Helping Practitioners Understand the Contribution of Qualitative Research to Evidence-Based Practice." *Evidence-Based Nursing, 9*, 7–8.

Tripepi, G., Jager, K. J., Dekker, F. W., Wanner, C., & Zoccali, C. (2008). Bias in clinical research. *Kidney International, 73*, 148–153.

Turner, P. & Mjolne, I. (2001). Journal provision and the prevalence of journal clubs: A survey of physiotherapy departments in England and Australia. *Physiotherapy Research International, 6*, 157–169.

Viera, A. J., & Bangdiwala, S. I. (2007). Eliminating bias in randomized controlled trials: Importance of allocation concealment and masking. *Family Medicine, 39*, 132–137.

Winkelstein, W., Jr. (2009). The remarkable Archie: Origins of the Cochrane Collaboration. *Epidemiology, 20*, 779.

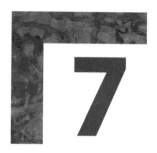

SYSTEMATICALLY REVIEWING THE EVIDENCE

Laura Bradley, MSc OT, OT Reg (Ont) and
Mary Law, PhD, OT Reg (Ont), FCAHS

LEARNING OBJECTIVES

After reading this chapter, the student/practitioner will be able to:

- Understand the difference between narrative reviews, systematic reviews, meta-analyses, and metasyntheses.
- Understand the methods used for conducting a systematic review or metasynthesis.
- Understand the best method for critically appraising a systematic review.
- Understand the best method for critically appraising a metasynthesis.

You are now well on your way to developing the art and science of evidence-based rehabilitation. You have been increasing your skills in finding, assessing, and using the evidence in everyday practice. You are experienced at asking relevant questions and you have an understanding of where to find the information you need. You recognize the importance of reviewing several sources of information, including journals, colleagues, and client choice with your own clinical experience to arrive at clinical decisions. The process is becoming second nature, but you are still left wondering, "Did I get it all?"

With constant demands on the time and resources available to clinicians, the expectation of appraising and understanding all research pertaining to a specific subject matter can be daunting. High-quality literature is being published at too great a rate to be thoroughly analyzed by each practitioner (Klassen, Jadad, & Moher, 1998). Furthermore, it is difficult for a clinician to remain unbiased in the evaluation of literature surrounding his or her question. There is a tendency to appraise or find articles that support what was originally being sought. To address these issues, critical reviews have arisen. A review sets out to analyze and summarize a specific subset of research information and come to a conclusion based on the information included in the review. There are two main categories of quantitative review: narrative and systematic (Table 7-1). A review of research using qualitative methods, or metasynthesis, will be explored later in the chapter.

Law M., & MacDermid, J. C.
Evidence-Based Rehabilitation: A Guide
to Practice, Third Edition (pp 157–174).
© 2014 SLACK Incorporated.

Table 7-1

Differences Between Narrative and Systematic Reviews

FEATURE	NARRATIVE REVIEW	SYSTEMATIC REVIEW
Question addressed	Often broad overview of the topic; but can focus on a particular perspective	A specific research question is posed and drives study methodology
Search strategy	Not usually specified or systematic	A strategy designed to find all relevant research is explicitly stated in the methods
Selection of studies included	Not usually specified	Specific inclusion and exclusion criteria are applied in a standardized way to determine the studies included
Appraisal of study quality or potential for bias	Can absent or integrated in discussion (inconsistent)	Performed on all included papers using a standardized process and tools
Synthesis of evidence across studies	Usually narrative with differential emphasis on different studies	Can be narrative or quantitative
Recommendations	Driven by authors	Considers and communicates strength of the evidence
Inclusion of author expertise, experience, and opinions	Commonly present	Absent

NARRATIVE REVIEW

A narrative review is a gathering of information by an individual who may be considered an expert in the field (Klassen et al., 1998). This type of review differs from a systematic review in that it sets out to answer a research question but lacks the explicit description of an organized approach to gathering the literature (Duffy, 2005). This facet of the narrative review becomes its chief limitation; the decision tree to include or exclude articles is typically not provided for the reader, making it difficult to evaluate the quality of the information contained within the publication.

Recently, a more systematic approach to narrative reviews has developed; these types of reviews are called *scoping reviews*. Although it is recognized that a clear consensus of the definition of scoping reviews has not yet been established (Rumrill, Fitzgerald, & Merchant, 2010), the Canadian Institutes of Health Research defines scoping reviews as "exploratory projects that systematically map the literature available on a topic, identifying key concepts, theories, sources of evidence and gaps in the research" (n.d.). The purpose of scoping reviews is to examine the range of information available on a particular topic or research question, determine the necessity of undertaking a full systematic review, summarize and disseminate research findings, and, finally, identify gaps in the literature surrounding a specific topic (Arskey & O'Malley, 2005). Arskey and O'Malley (2005) proposed six stages to completing a scoping review:

- **Stage 1: Identifying the research question.** At this stage, the researcher determines what he or she is setting out to discover which includes establishing definitions for searching and determining the breadth of coverage (Arskey & O'Malley, 2005; Rumrill et al., 2010).

- **Stage 2: Identify the relevant studies.** The researcher will set out to identify primary studies, both published and unpublished, from electronic databases, reference lists, hand searches, as well as organization and conference literature (Arskey & O'Malley, 2005). Practical issues related to time and resources available must be determined at this stage in order to balance comprehensiveness and feasibility (Levac, Colquhoun, & O'Brien, 2010).

- **Stage 3: Study selection.** Studies are excluded or included based on the original research question and search parameters. At this stage, however, definitions and search criteria may be developed post hoc in order to include information that was captured as the researchers become more familiar with the body of literature (Arskey & O'Malley, 2005).

- **Stage 4: Charting the data.** Material is sorted according to themes and key issues using a data-charting form (Arskey & O'Malley, 2005). No distinction is given to the data's methodological quality or empirical weight (Rumrill et al., 2010).

- **Stage 5: Collating, summarizing, and reporting the results.** An overview of all material captured in the review is presented. Again, the quality of the evidence is not presented, because the purpose of the scoping review is to present a breadth of knowledge in one area (Arskey & O'Malley, 2005).

- **Stage 6: Consultation (optional).** This stage, deemed optional for researchers, sets out to provide "opportunities for consumer and stakeholder involvement to suggest additional references and provide insights beyond those in the literature" (Levac et al., 2010, p. 3).

SYSTEMATIC REVIEW

A systematic review, by contrast, is a summary of the literature that uses clear methods to perform a thorough search and critical appraisal of individual studies on a defined topic area for which there are sufficient studies of a similar design (Cochrane Collaboration, n.d.). This is different from the scoping review in that a scoping review will address broader areas in which a variety of methodologies may exist and does not typically offer an examination of the quality of the included studies (Arskey & O'Malley, 2005). The goal of a systematic review is to investigate a specific research question in ways that minimize bias and random error. Such a review will have clear inclusion and exclusion criteria, with only the most rigorous studies of the pool of literature included. In essence, a systematic review will critically appraise relevant studies for you and provide you with a conclusion that you can then apply to practice. Quantitative systematic reviews, or meta-analyses, contain a statistical summary of at least one outcome in two or more trials.

The completion of a systematic review is time consuming and can be very costly. Various schools of thought on systematic reviews have produced slightly different methodologies for conducting reviews. Although these differences exist, they generally follow a typical pattern. The following path presented, adapted from Duffy (2005), outlines a general process that this may take:

Formulating a review question

↓

Conducting a comprehensive search of the literature

↓

Critically appraising each study

↓

Synthesizing the findings

↓

Reporting the results

Step 1: Formulating a Review Question

Because systematic reviews set out to answer a specific clinical question, the development and clarity of that question is paramount. Ask a poor question and you are likely to have a systematic review of limited use. Ask a clear and specific question and you are likely to have a systematic review that can potentially be applied to clinical practice (Klassen et al., 1998). Questions generally arise from a gap in the literature, clinical encounters, clinician or patient queries, or clinical trends (Akobeng, 2005; Counsell, 1997; Lapier, 2003). At times, questions result from the introduction of a new treatment or technique, which must be compared to the standard treatment of the time. Alternately, different clinics, professionals, or even countries may approach the same situations in different ways. These, too, must be compared to ensure best practice. Finally, different elements of treatment can have different costs associated with them. Questions can set out to examine which treatment is most cost effective for a particular situation. These types of studies, called *cost-effectiveness research*, are discussed in detail in Chapter 8.

Questions for systematic review classically focus on one of the following areas: diagnosis, etiology, prognosis, treatment, or prevention (Mulrow & Cook, 1997). As discussed in earlier chapters, clinical research can be defined on the basis of four elements: population, intervention, comparison, and outcome (P.I.C.O.). A good systematic review question will use these elements to define inclusion and exclusion criteria that direct which articles are retrieved for the review. Recently there have been more innovative applications of the systematic review process. One example is the use of a systematic review process to classify outcome measures into conceptual frameworks such as the *International Classification of Functioning, Disability and Health*. Regardless of the review purpose, the process should find and extract conclusions and make recommendations on the basis of the best possible evidence. To this end, there are types of publications that lend themselves better to answering different review questions (Table 7-2). In the absence of the best levels of evidence, other types of evidence, or lower levels of evidence, may be included.

Step 2: Conducting a Comprehensive Search of the Literature

After the question has been posed and the inclusion and exclusion criteria have been outlined, the reviewers begin the process of combing the literature for relevant articles. This process of searching the evidence is presented in detail in Chapter 5. The systems used to search the evidence should be clearly indicated by the reviewers, as well as the search terms used.

The most common place to begin searching for information is through electronic databases such as CINAHL or EMBASE. Although this seems a fairly straightforward process, it often becomes quite complicated. As you may remember, many of the different databases use different headings and subheadings for the same information. For example, the term *cancer*, which is common in most databases, has the heading *neoplasms* in MEDLINE. Similarly, one database's hyperlink may not exist in another. For example, in CINAHL, the term *occupational therapy* can be exploded and searched independently. In MEDLINE, it can only be searched as a keyword. These differences

Table 7-2

Levels of Evidence in Systematic Reviews

REVIEW TYPE	LEVEL OF BEST EVIDENCE
Treatment and/or prevention	Randomized controlled trials
Diagnostic tests	Comparison to a gold standard
Prognosis	Cohort studies
Review of risk factors	Cohort, case/control, or ecologic studies

From "Formulating Questions and Locating Primary Studies for Inclusion in Systematic Reviews," by C. Counsell, 1997, *Annals of Internal Medicine, 127*(5), pp. 380-387. Adapted with permission.

make it vital for reviewers to include terms that they have searched in order to ensure that relevant articles have not been missed. Many researchers, clinicians, and students make use of methods to save their searches so they can be referenced later on. These methods can include paper-and-pen charting of searches, Refworks lists, and "save search" features within different databases. It is important to record your searches in some way in order to highlight your thought processes while searching, as well as keep track of what has been done to minimize confusion or ensure that all keywords and subheadings have been included in different databases. Regardless of the method chosen, a well-documented search will save time and frustration later on.

After all electronic databases have been exhaustively searched, other techniques can be used to gather relevant sources of information. Reviewers can opt to manually search the reference lists in relevant journals or conference proceedings. Similarly, reviewers can manually search the reference lists of articles already identified for inclusion. Caution in this technique must be used, however, because reference bias can result in more favorable results being referenced more often (Counsell, 1997).

Regardless of the method of choosing articles, the reviewers should state clearly what the method was, relevant search terms used, and the inclusion and exclusion criteria that began the search. See Chapter 5 for detailed information on searching.

Step 3: Critically Appraising Each Study

As in primary research studies, flaws in the data can affect the results of a systematic review. For this reason, each article must be appraised for its relevance to the inclusion criteria, methodological strengths, and potential sources of bias. Publication bias is one area in which reviewers often face difficulty (Akobeng, 2005; Moher, Jadad, & Klassen, 1998). On one hand, articles included for publication in peer-reviewed journals can be viewed as a strong source of evidence. On the other hand, articles with favorable results may be published more often than those with unfavorable results; hence the term *publication bias*. These unpublished papers often provide valuable information but are not included for appraisal by the general public. Some reviewers include these unpublished studies even though they have not been peer reviewed in order to minimize this source of potential bias.

Appraising each article for the review should be undertaken by at least two reviewers with a predetermined set of criteria. In most cases, the reviewers appraise the articles independently, often assigning a score to each article. Common criteria include the level of methodology, the use of blinding, the reporting and treatment of missing data, and the way that subjects who were lost to follow-up were included in the final result (Whitney, 2004). These were addressed in more detail in the previous chapter. The reviewers then get together to compare results. Any discrepancies are discussed and a common ground is found. In some cases, disputed articles are brought to an outside reviewer for appraisal. Researchers may also use predetermined levels of evidence to set criteria for inclusion. Examples of levels of evidence can be found on the Centre for Evidence-Based Medicine's Web site at www.cebm.net/index.aspx?o=1025 and are further discussed in Chapter 6.

As with the previous step, regardless of the way in which the articles were appraised, the method and appraisal criteria should be clearly explained for the reader.

Step 4: Synthesizing the Findings

There is presently no agreed-upon method for synthesizing the items in a qualitative systematic review. Clinical judgment should be used to determine the appropriate combination of the reviewed studies. Were the included studies, in fact, similar enough in methodology, population, or outcome measure to have their findings pooled? Often the reviewers make a statement to this fact before presenting the summary results.

A quantitative systematic review, or meta-analysis, offers a different picture. As you recall, the goal of a meta-analysis is to reach a conclusion through statistical means. At this point, the reviewers have several options available to them. As reported by Moher, Jadad, and Klassen (1998), combination of data through statistical means is an option available to systematic reviewers.

Step 5: Reporting the Results

The final process, reporting the findings, is also the most important to the reader. In this step, all of the work that has been put into the systematic review can be shared with potential readers. The entire process, not just the end result, must be written up. All of the variables and choices made along the way affect how the final outcome emerges. The reviewers must cite any and all possibilities for bias that could have existed both in the original trials and in the secondary work of the systematic review. Here are two examples of completed systematic reviews from the rehabilitation literature:

> Graven, C., Brock, K., Hill, K., & Joubert, L. (2011). Are rehabilitation and/or care co-ordination interventions delivered in the community effective in reducing depression, facilitating participation and improving quality of life after stroke? *Disability & Rehabilitation, 33*(17/18), 1501–1520.

> Blauw-Hospers, C., & Hadders-Algra, M. (2005). A systematic review of the effects of early intervention on motor development. *Developmental Medicine & Child Neurology, 47*(6), 421–432.

META-ANALYSIS

The quantitative approach of a meta-analysis, as mentioned earlier, contains a statistical summary of at least one outcome in two or more trials. These results are presented statistically in graphic form. The graphic form, or *forest plot*, is well known in the evidence-based practice (EBP) world, most commonly as the logo of the Cochrane Collaboration (Figure 7-1). A forest plot shows the reader "information from the individual studies that went into the meta-analysis and an estimate of the overall results" (Akonbeng, 2005, p. 846). Visually, it is a vertical line with a number of horizontal lines running across it. During meta-analysis, each study involved is distilled down to a confidence interval, which states with 95% certainty what the effects of that study were. Thus, a forest plot represents the pooled odds ratios of all the studies in the review. If a (horizontal) confidence interval of a result crosses the (vertical) line of no effect, it means either that a significant difference does not exist between the treatment and the control or that the sample size was too small to allow us to be confident where the true result lies. The diamond represents the pooled data from all the

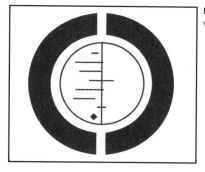

Figure 7-1. Cochrane Collaboration logo. (This logo has been reproduced with kind permission of the Cochrane Collaboration.)

studies in question. In the example of the Cochrane logo, the diamond is to the left of the line of no effect. If this were a true forest plot, we could say that the meta-analysis showed that the treatment in question had no effect. For an example of a forest plot related to a rehabilitation intervention, see:

Pollock, A., Baer, G., Pomeroy, V. M., & Langhorne, P. (2007). Physiotherapy treatment approaches for the recovery of postural control and lower limb function following stroke. *Cochrane Database of Systematic Reviews, 1.*

Meta-analyses are useful because they provide one overall estimate of the effectiveness of an intervention, but they also have some disadvantages. It is important to assess and know the methodological quality of the studies so that biased results are not included. In addition, the recommendations coming from a meta-analysis may not apply to specific clients.

The goal of a systematic review, aside from offering a summary of original articles, is to be published. Much in the same way as original articles, systematic reviews can suffer from publication biases. Many people think that a systematic review finding no significant results from a group of trials is not useful. The truth could not be more contrary. Many clinical misjudgments are made daily because of negative publication bias or the tendency for journals to only publish results that are positive. If practitioners knew about the negative results coming from some systematic reviews, they may change their practice habits. However, negative results are not as interesting as positive ones and therefore get less coverage. Publishing both positive and negative systematic reviews is the only way in which a more complete knowledge of which interventions or treatments are beneficial can be garnered. Through the publication of all research, the health sciences and rehabilitation community can find out which currently practiced treatments deserve to be altered or abandoned.

Using systematic reviews in clinical practice—although in many cases preferable—still contains some inherent risks. Just as in individual studies, there are high- and low-quality systematic reviews. Systematic reviews presenting results of poor-quality studies with questionable methods or an unclear question will still not be of clinical use. The existence of a systematic review on a topic does not replace your ability to look at the literature with a critical eye (Klassen et al., 1998). How, then, can a practitioner know whether a systematic review is of use or of good enough quality to apply to clinical practice?

CRITICALLY APPRAISING SYSTEMATIC REVIEWS

Critically appraising systematic reviews should be considered an art as well as a science. A clinician appraising a systematic review needs to rely as much on clinical judgment as preset review forms. Many methods of evaluating systematic reviews have been proposed; however, it is ultimately a clinician's choice as to which method is most useful. One method, developed by Oxman and Guyatt (1991), has been shown to distinguish between systematic reviews of good and poor quality.

Table 7-3

Guide to Appraising Systematic Reviews

QUESTION	ANSWER		
1. Were the methods used to find primary research studies reported?	No	Partially	Yes
2. Was the search comprehensive?	No	Can't tell	Yes
3. Were the criteria used for deciding which studies to include in the review reported?	No	Partially	Yes
4. Was bias in the selection of studies avoided?	No	Can't tell	Yes
5. Were the criteria used for assessing validity of the studies reported?	No	Partially	Yes
6. Was the validity of all studies assessed using appropriate criteria?	No	Can't tell	Yes
7. Were the methods used to combine findings of the studies to reach a conclusion reported?	No	Can't tell	Yes
8. Were the methods appropriate?	No	Partially	Yes
9. Was the conclusion supported by the data and/or analysis?	No	Partially	Yes
10. What was the overall scientific quality of the review?	Extensive flaws, major flaws, minor flaws, or minimal flaws		

Adapted from "Validation of an Index of the Quality of Review Articles," by A. Oxman, & G. Guyatt, 1991, *Journal of Clinical Epidemiology, 44,* pp. 1271-1278. Adapted with permission.

This method, outlined in Table 7-3, asks the reader to rate specific elements of a systematic review. The scoring, presented in Table 7-4, distinguishes between a systematic review that has minimal (a score of 7), minor (a score of 5 to 6), major (a score of 3 to 4), or extensive (a score of 1 to 2) flaws.

Ultimately, the clinical user will decide what this score will mean (Peach, 2002). For example, a systematic review with a lower score may be used in the absence of other higher quality research. Similarly, a systematic review with a very high score may not be of clinical use if it cannot be applied to the specific population of interest. Worksheets to help clinicians review systematic reviews are offered through the Centre for Evidence-Based Medicine's Web site, available at www.cebm.net/index.aspx?o=1157.

Shea et al. (2007) developed another example of an instrument used to assess the methodological quality of systematic reviews. They created an 11-item tool through a combination of the enhanced Overview Quality Assessment Questionnaire, a checklist created by Sacks, and three elements deemed important to understanding the quality of a review, namely language restriction, publication bias, and publication status. This tool, named AMSTAR (Assessment of Multiple Systematic Reviews), was found to have good face and content validity (Shea et al., 2007). Further information regarding the development of the tool as well as the tool itself can be found at www.biomedcentral.com/1471-2288/7/10.

Another system of critically appraising systematic reviews was presented by the Centre for Evidence-Based Medicine in the University of Alberta. These researchers have compiled a list of questions and a worksheet to help guide researchers through appraising a systematic review. The

Table 7-4		
Scoring of Systematic Reviews		
Step 1	Is the "no" option used for one or more of questions 2, 4, 6, or 8?	No: Go to step 3
		Yes: Go to step 2
Step 2	How often is the "no" option used for questions 2, 4, 6, 8?	Four times: review scores a 1
		Two to three times: review scores a 2
		1 time: review scores a 3
Step 3	Is the "can't tell" option used for one or more of questions 2, 4, 6, or 8?	No: review scores a 7
		Yes: review scores a 4

Adapted from "Validation of an Index of the Quality of Review Articles," by A. Oxman, & G. Guyatt, 1991, *Journal of Clinical Epidemiology, 44*, pp. 1271-1278. Adapted with permission.

information can be found at www.ebm.med.ualberta.ca/SystematicReview.html (questions) and www.ebm.med.ualberta.ca/SystematicReviewWorksheet.html (worksheets). The following sections go through this method of appraisal in more detail. The more questions receiving a "yes" response, the higher the quality of the review (Duffy, 2005). Throughout this section, statistical concepts will be briefly explained. Because the goal of this chapter is not to teach statistics, further information—should it be needed—can be found in any good quality statistical text. All statistical definitions in this section have been taken from the University of Toronto's Center for Evidence-Based Medicine, found at http://ktclearinghouse.ca/cebm/glossary.

Section 1: Are the Results Valid?

1. Did the overview address a focused clinical question? As with any research, reviews that ask a poor question will have a lower quality. Each element of P.I.C.O. should be present in the reviewer's question.

2. Were the criteria used to select articles for inclusion appropriate? It is important to note whether the inclusion and exclusion criteria for the review are appropriate and will serve to answer the question. Without strong, clear, and appropriate inclusion criteria, it is possible that the overall results will be weakened by studies that are not valid to the original question.

3. Is it unlikely that important, relevant studies were missed? What were the reviewers' searching methods? Have they been presented in a way that will allow you to decide whether there are any gaps? The greater the rigor of the original search, the less likely that the final review will suffer from random error and publication bias (Counsell, 1997; Whitney, 2004). Appropriate search strategies were discussed earlier in this chapter.

4. Was the validity of the included studies appraised? *Validity* refers to the study's level of truth, or potential freedom from bias. The higher the validity of each included study, the greater the overall validity of the final review.

5. Were assessments of studies reproducible? There should be some explanation as to how the reviewing team came to include each of the studies. For example, evidence that the reviewers were blinded or that there was a system in place should the reviewers disagree will add strength to the final product.

6. Were the results similar from study to study? This can be examined through tests for homogeneity. *Homogeneity* means that the results of each individual trial are mathematically compatible with the results of any of the others (Greenhalgh, 1997). Reviewers should not be comparing studies that are too different in either population or outcome.

Section 2: What Are the Results?

1. What are the overall results of the review? The results of the review need to be clearly stated in order for you to determine whether it is useful to your situation or may be applied to your practice. If the overall results were not statistically significant, review some of the reasons why this may be in order to determine whether the review is still of clinical significance. A meta-analysis may report the results in terms of an odds ratio (OR) or relative risk (RR). The OR and RR are reported in relation to 1: greater than 1 indicates an increased likelihood of the outcome found in the treatment group and less than 1 indicates the decreased likelihood of the outcome found in the treatment group. An OR or RR of 1 indicates no difference.

    a. Odds ratio: The ratio of the odds of having the target disorder in the experimental group relative to the odds in favor of having the target disorder in the control group (in cohort studies or systematic reviews) or the odds in favor of being exposed in subjects with the target disorder divided by the odds in favor of being exposed in control subjects (without the target disorder).

    b. Relative risk: The ratio of risk in the treated group to the risk in the control group.

2. How precise were the results? The investigator should present his or her results in terms of how precise they are. This is called a *confidence interval* (CI), which quantifies the uncertainty of the measurement.

    a. Confidence intervals: It is usually reported as a 95% CI, which is the range of values within which we can be 95% sure that the true value for the whole population lies. For example, for a numbers needed to treat (NNT) of 10 with a 95% CI of 5 to 15, we would have 95% confidence that the true NNT value lies between 5 and 15.

    b. NNT: The number of patients who need to be treated in order to prevent one additional (successful or poor) outcome.

Section 3: Will the Results Help Me Care for My Patients?

1. Can the results be applied to my patient care? In order for the results of the review to be useful, the results must deal with patients, demographics, and conditions similar to a particular clinical practice or question. If a clinician had a question about the benefit of a particular intervention with his or her geriatric population, a review dealing with a pediatric population may be of limited use. Similarly, there should be no obvious reason (such as poor methodology or indications of potential harm) why the results of this review should not be applied.

2. Were all clinically important outcomes considered? Are the outcomes provided in the review the most appropriate target outcomes for the treatment? For example, if you are interested in the community reintegration of youth after brain injury, a systematic review focused on the outcome of memory would not be an appropriate indicator.

3. Are the likely treatment benefits worth the potential harms and costs? Every treatment is associated with costs and the potential for benefit in relation to harm. It is up to the discretion of individual clinicians (working within potential institutional guidelines) whether

the treatment benefits to clients presented within the review are worth the potential harms and costs associated with that treatment. NNT is often included in reviews. This will help a clinician make that choice.

FINDING SYSTEMATIC REVIEWS

Although systematic reviews are being completed at an increased rate (Duffy, 2005), planning is still involved to find them. Thankfully, a clinician in search of systematic reviews has several options available to them.

First, the American National Library of Medicine offers an electronic text-based search and retrieval system that contains many databases, including PubMed. This site, found at www.ncbi. nlm.nih.gov/sites/gquery, allows you to search full text and abstracts using keywords. As an addition to narrow down your searching, the keyword "systematic reviews" can be added. Although not all articles are full text, this is a good place to begin your searching.

Systematic reviews can also be found while searching databases such as Ovid and MEDLINE. Similar to searching for primary studies and original articles, systematic reviews can be found by entering keywords about the topic for which you are searching. As a strategy to narrow down your search, these databases (and others) allow you to limit your results to only systematic reviews.

Both OTSeeker and the Physiotherapy Evidence Database (PEDro) can be sources of information specific to rehabilitation professionals. OTSeeker, found at www.otseeker.com, is a database that contains abstracts of systematic reviews and randomized controlled trials (RCTs) relevant to occupational therapy. PEDro, found at www.pedro.org.au, offers bibliographic details and abstracts of RCTs, systematic reviews, and evidence-based clinical practice guidelines in physiotherapy. Both of these sites, although not directly linking to full texts, offer an option to select only systematic reviews. Searching these databases provides a method for rehabilitation professionals to see what research has been done in order to have a more specific search strategy in the other databases. Finally, systematic reviews can be accessed through a central location, which will be discussed in more detail.

THE COCHRANE COLLABORATION

What should practitioners do with systematic reviews and meta-analyses once they have been completed? Of course, each reviewer will hold on to completed studies, but that number represents only a handful of reviews potentially completed on the same topic. Could the results of systematic reviews and meta-analyses from around the world somehow be brought together? It was this question that inspired the creation of the Cochrane Collaboration. The Collaboration is named after the British epidemiologist Dr. Archie Cochrane, who strongly advocated for the widespread use of systematic reviews to guide practice. It was Dr. Cochrane's belief that we need to change the way we provide health care because of the outpouring of health care information created each year. To resolve this problem, Dr. Cochrane proposed creating an organization that would conduct systematic reviews in all aspects of health care and would act as a clearinghouse, distributing them worldwide. The creation of the Cochrane Collaboration was also spurred on by the realization that a medical failure can result from the lack of systematic reviews.

As such, the Collaboration itself is based around the following 10 founding principles, which all members attempt to uphold in their work:

1. Collaboration
2. Building on the enthusiasm of individuals

3. Avoiding duplication

4. Minimizing bias

5. Keeping up to date

6. Ensuring relevance

7. Ensuring access

8. Continually improving the quality of its work

9. Continuity

10. Enabling wide participation (Source: www.cochrane.org/about-us/our-principles)

There are a number of tasks that the Cochrane Collaboration undertakes, but the main output of the Cochrane Collaboration is systematic reviews.

The Cochrane Library itself is the mainstay of the Cochrane Collaboration and is composed of a number of parts. First, the Cochrane Controlled Trials Register contains a collection of nearly 300,000 RCTs, which supply high-quality evidence for systematic reviews. A second part of the library is the Cochrane Database of Systematic Reviews, which lists the Cochrane Collaboration's completed reviews and outlines of its reviews in progress. It currently holds approximately 4,500 entries. The Database of Abstracts of Reviews of Effectiveness also lists systematic reviews that were undertaken and published outside of the Cochrane Collaboration. Finally, the Cochrane Review Methodology Database provides information on the procedures, methods, and processes of EBP. The Cochrane Library is available through Wiley Interscience at www.thecochranelibrary.com/view/0/index.html.

To find the Cochrane Centre in your area, consult the list of regional Cochrane Centre Web sites at www.cochrane.org/contact/centres. The Cochrane Collaboration Brochure, from which much of the information about the company was found, is also online at www.cochrane.org. The Cochrane Collaboration represents a vast worldwide effort toward EBP, which will become more and more necessary as the volume of health care information grows while budgets shrink. The Collaboration itself is a first step toward creating a more integrated, evidence-based network for drawing on the vast resources of the entire medical profession to serve clients.

THE CAMPBELL COLLABORATION

A second source for RCT and systematic reviews is the Campbell Collaboration, which is available at www.campbellcollaboration.org. Their objective is to help people make evidence-based decisions regarding interventions through the preparation, maintenance, and dissemination of systematic reviews. The Campbell Collaboration offers researchers, practitioners, and the public access to systematic reviews, titles, and protocols, and can be found at www.campbellcollaboration.org/library.php.

METASYNTHESIS

As discussed previously in the chapter, qualitative research can be reviewed for much the same reasons as quantitative research. In qualitative research, the investigator sets out to "understand the thoughts, feelings, and experiences of individuals, focusing on direct, face-to-face knowledge of patients as human beings coping with their treatment in a given social setting" (Polgar & Thomas, 2000, p. 91). The results from qualitative literature offer a holistic picture of the participants in their natural setting and can be used to provide an in-depth understanding of a particular phenomenon or experience from the participant's point of view (Polgar & Thomas, 2000; Spencer, Ritchie, Lewis, & Dillon, 2003). To the uninitiated reader, qualitative research is very different, because it relies on language-based data rather than the numerical statistics found in quantitative research (Eakin & Mykhalovskiy, 2003).

To date, however, many valuable qualitative research studies have remained isolated from each other, with fewer attempts to put the results together than has been seen in the quantitative world (Sandelowski, Docherty, & Emden, 1997). However, to make these findings more useful and accessible to clinicians, researchers, and policy makers, the pooling together of results has become an increasing need (Finfgeld, 2003). From this need came the metasynthesis (also labeled *meta ethnography*). As Sandelowski and Barroso (2003) said, a metasynthesis is a "study of the processes and results of previous studies in a target domain that moves beyond those studies to situate historically, define for the present, and chart future directions in that domain" (pp. 784–785).

This characteristic is the main difference between the meta-analysis and the metasynthesis; the researcher in the metasynthesis offers an interpretive product as well as an analytic process from the findings of primary authors rather than raw data (Sandelowski & Barroso, 2003). The goal of a metasynthesis is to "produce a new and integrative interpretation of findings that is more substantive than those resulting from individual investigations" (Finfgeld, 2003, p. 893) and can offer clinicians a picture of the meaning or impact a particular phenomenon or intervention can have on their clients (Gewertz, Stergiou-Kita, Shaw, Kirsh, & Rappolt, 2008).

Metasyntheses can also generate new models and theories and determine the existence of different "schools of thought and complement the findings of a systematic review" (Booth, 2001). The completion of metasyntheses, however, is not without controversy. In fact, due to the subjective nature of qualitative research and the potential for different methodological approaches, some authors have suggested that it may not be appropriate to synthesize it at all (Barbour, 1998; Sandelowski, 2006). Despite this controversy, metasyntheses remain an important contribution to health care literature and qualitative research as a whole (Richardson & Lindquist, 2010; Sandelowski & Barroso, 2003).

Finfgeld (2003) has proposed three types of metasynthesis: theory building, theory explication, and descriptive metasynthesis. Theory building sets out to investigate a number of studies in order to move forward with a given theory beyond what is possible in a single study. Syntheses within this category include grounded formal theory and the metastudy. Grounded formal theory uses substantive grounded theory findings to create formal theories. A metastudy brings about three types of formal qualitative analysis to create new theoretical interpretation. Theory explanation examines abstract concepts within the original findings and expands upon them, resulting in a new understanding of that particular phenomenon. Descriptive metasynthesis involves the broad translation of findings across studies dealing with a particular phenomenon. The reader should be aware that other types of metasyntheses may exist, and a single metasynthesis may provide information in more than one category.

Similar to meta-analysis, there is no single accepted method for conducting a metasynthesis. The following graph shows the steps for conducting metasyntheses proposed by Finfgeld (2003), although the reader should be aware that other variations have been proposed (Finfgeld, 2003).

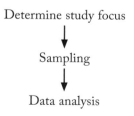

Determine study focus

↓

Sampling

↓

Data analysis

Step 1: Determine Study Focus

Similar to systematic reviews, a metasynthesis must have a clear focus in order to offer more precise results (Mays, Pope, & Popay, 2005). On one hand, the question should be broad enough to encompass all aspects of the phenomenon in question, but it should also be specific enough to be useful for policy makers, readers, and clinicians (Finfgeld, 2003). In setting out to ask a research question, it is important for the investigator to reflect on how the completion of this metasynthesis might be used to "answer existing clinical questions, build theory, [or] inform public policy" (Finfgeld, 2003, p. 898). This may be a more difficult task than first thought, because the investigators must examine their topic of interest and then determine how study findings can be compared. This can be a problem, because it may be difficult to conclude which studies are examining the same phenomenon or aspect of human experience (Sandelowski et al., 1997). For example, within one phenomenon, studies may examine a specific time period, feelings surrounding that experience, or the day-to-day management that the phenomenon entails (Sandelowski et al., 1997).

Step 2: Sampling

Once the question has been proposed, the investigators must begin the process of sampling current research that sets out to answer that question. No consensus exists on the best method for searching; however, many of the same principles that are found in selecting articles for systematic reviews apply for metasyntheses. Setting inclusion criteria is important because this will guide the investigators' choice. Sampling should then occur across disciplines, Internet, conferences, databases, and demographic elements (such as gender and ethnicity) to ensure that no relevant studies have been missed and assist in the generalizability of findings (Booth, 2001; Finfgeld, 2003; Mays et al., 2005). Sandelowski et al. (1997) suggested that studies should not be excluded for reasons of quality because there are many variations within the standards of qualitative research, and valuable information may be missed due to methodological weaknesses. They suggested that although quality should not be a reason for exclusion, it should remain an element within analysis, and it may take a true qualitative artist to distinguish between "surface errors and mistakes fatal enough to discount findings" (Sandelowski et al., 1997).

Searching the databases for qualitative literature can also be challenging because there is no central location for qualitative research similar to the Cochrane Library. Investigators may also come up against poor indexing within databases, as well as variations within indexing terms. For example, CINAHL uses many different indexing terms for qualitative research, whereas MEDLINE does not index qualitative studies at all (Mays et al., 2005). Ensuring that all relevant research has been included may involve explicit strategies other than searching databases (e.g., hand-searching reference lists and contacting researchers in the field of interest; Booth, 2001; Mays et al., 2005).

Questions have been proposed as to how many articles should be included in a metasynthesis. Answers have ranged from 3 articles (Finfgeld, 2003) to no more than 10 articles (Sandelowski et al., 1997) to 292 (Patterson, Thorne, Canam, & Jillings, 2001). These variations may be due to topic breadth or the type of metasynthesis offered (Finfgeld, 2003). It has been cautioned that although no set limit has been accepted, overly large sample sizes may make deep analysis difficult (Sandelowski et al., 1997). If there are too many primary studies to include, the investigator may choose to narrow his or her focus (or question) to produce more manageable results (Dixon-Woods, Agarwal, Jones, Young, & Sutton, 2005).

Step 3: Data Analysis

At this stage, the investigators have a list of primary studies to be included in the metasynthesis. The next step is to determine whether these studies can be compared as well as the similarities and differences between them. Qualitative research offers several methodologies from which to choose (e.g., ethnography, phenomenology, or grounded theory; Creswell, 1998). Investigators must remember, however, that one researcher's grounded theory may be another's ethnography (Sandelowski et al., 1997). Each individual study includes the voice of the initial researcher; as such, it must be detected to assist in the methodological comparability and relationship to the metasynthesis as a whole (Sandelowski et al., 1997). Differences may exist not only between studies but "also among lives-as-lived, lives-as-experienced, and lives-as-told" (Sandelowski & Boshamer, 2006). Once the comparability of original studies has been established, the investigators can begin to identify common or recurring concepts in each of these studies. These concepts are laid out in a table, from which second- and third-order interpretations can be made, leading to larger narratives or general theories derived from all studies (Mays et al., 2005; Sandelowski et al., 1997). The key lies in the investigator's ability to synthesize findings in an understandable way while maintaining the "integrity of individual studies" (Booth, 2001, p. 8).

The following are examples of metasyntheses to further illustrate their construction and use as a clinical tool:

Whalley Hammell, K. (2007). Experience of rehabilitation following spinal cord injury: A meta-synthesis of qualitative findings. *Spinal Cord, 45*(4), 260–274.

Duggan, F., & Banwell, L. (2004). Constructing a model of effective information dissemination in a crisis. *Information Research, 9*(3). Retrieved from http://InformationR.net/ir/9-3/paper178.html

Critically Appraising Metasyntheses

The conduct of metasyntheses is still in its early stages, so there is no agreed-upon method to critically review these works. In general, readers should pay close attention to the following characteristics:

- Did the reviewers ask a clear question that is relevant to your clinical practice?
- What was the rigor of the included studies?
- Were the reviewers clear about their methods for analyzing data?
- Was there a clear description of the similarities and differences between the primary studies?
- Did the reviewer synthesize the studies in an understandable way?

CONCLUSION

The need to critically evaluate the evidence available constitutes an integral aspect of EBP. Through an understanding of the details of different types of studies and the corresponding factors, one can better address the search for evidence to incorporate into practice. Although different methodologies exist for both the completion and appraisal of systematic reviews and metasyntheses, the production of these will allow a clinician to build a better EBP. The efficient finding and use of systematically reviewed qualitative and quantitative evidence can be a valuable tool in a busy clinician's toolbox, one that can contribute to quality client care.

TAKE-HOME MESSAGES

Systematic Reviews

✓ Use scientific strategies to incorporate clinical trials done by different researchers on the same topic.

✓ There are various methodologies for preparing systematic reviews.

✓ Analyze RCTs with respect to methodological quality, precision, and external validity.

✓ All RCTs within the study will have some small error, but those studies with significant error should be rejected.

✓ CONSORT statement consists of checklists and flowcharts to help standardize the researcher-reported RCTs and to guard against methodological error.

✓ Even without positive results, systematic reviews should still be published.

Meta-Analysis

✓ Analysis of analyses; integrate findings from a large variety of individual studies to achieve a systematic review.

✓ Results portrayed in a forest plot with a diagram using confidence intervals.

✓ Meta-analysis often critiqued for publication bias and missing data.

Cochrane Collaboration

✓ Database of systematic reviews and meta-analyses from around the world.

✓ Main output is systematic reviews; groups and databases to address different practice areas.

✓ Represents an integrated evidence-based network

LEARNING AND EXPLORATION ACTIVITIES

The purpose of this chapter was to introduce students to different methods for systematically reviewing the evidence as well as demonstrating some of the appropriate tools with which to perform these evaluations.

1. Systematic Reviews

    a. Read through the systematic review methodologies listed and explore them until you feel that you have a good sense of the commonalities between all of them. Now, write a simple methodology in your own words. Compare this with those your fellow students have prepared. Where do they differ? Where are they similar? If possible, attempt as a group to merge all of your individual methodologies by consensus and produce a methodological statement that is distinctly your own. This will be helpful for understanding why reviews are structured as they are.

    b. Look briefly at the CONSORT statement. What are the important factors that an RCT must have? What makes a good RCT? What makes a poor RCT? Write a short paragraph answering these questions. Now, search for RCTs on a topic of interest (your best bet is to use MEDLINE) and find two or more. Examine each and assess its strengths and weaknesses. Which of the two is better? Why? Justify your answer.

2. Meta-Analysis: Search on MEDLINE for meta-analyses on a topic of your choice. Attempt to find more than one and compare the results. Did they both reach the same conclusion? Why? Why not? What does this say about meta-analysis?

3. The Cochrane Collaboration: Go online and find your local Cochrane Centre. Browse through the page and become familiar with its layout. Go to your local Health Sciences library and find out how to log onto the Cochrane Library from their computers. Search for systematic reviews on a topic of interest and find out how to retrieve them. Continue working until you understand how the software functions and you are comfortable with its features.

4. Review of Evidence: Compare and contrast the methods of qualitative and quantitative reviews. What is each trying to discover? In what instances can one be considered of more use than the other?

WEB LINKS

The following Web sites appear in this chapter:
- Centre for Evidence-Based Medicine: www.cebm.net
- Centre for Evidence-Based Medicine in the University of Alberta: www.ebm.med.ualberta.ca
- University of Toronto's Center for Evidence-Based Medicine: http://ktclearinghouse.ca/cebm
- American National Library of Medicine: www.ncbi.nlm.nih.gov/sites/gquery
- OTSeeker: www.otseeker.com
- PEDro: www.pedro.org.au
- Cochrane Collaboration: www.cochrane.org
- The Campbell Collaboration: www.campbellcollaboration.org/library.php

REFERENCES

Akobeng, A. (2005). Understanding systematic reviews and meta-analysis. *Archives of Disability and Childhood, 90*, 845–848.

Arskey, H., & O'Malley, L. (2005). Scoping studies: Towards a methodological framework. *International Journal of Social Research Methodology: Theory & Practice, 8*(1), 19–32.

Barbour, S. (1998). Mixing qualitative methods: Quality assurance or qualitative quagmire? *Qualitative Health Research, 8*(3), 352–361.

Booth, A. (2001). *Cochrane or cock-eyed? How should we conduct systematic reviews of qualitative research?* Paper presented at the Qualitative Evidence-Based Practice Conference, Taking a Critical Stance, Coventry University, Coventry, England.

Canadian Institutes of Health Research. (n.d.). *A guide to knowledge synthesis.* Retrieved from www.cihr-irsc.gc.ca/e/41382.html

Cochrane Collaboration. (n.d.). Guide to the format of a Cochrane review. Retrieved from www.cochrane-handbook.org/

Counsell, C. (1997). Formulating questions and locating primary studies for inclusion in systematic reviews. *Annals of Internal Medicine, 127*(5), 380–387.

Creswell, J. (1998). *Qualitative inquiry and research design: Choosing among five traditions.* Thousand Oaks, CA: Sage.

Dixon-Woods, M., Agarwal, S., Jones, D., Young, B., & Sutton, A. (2005). Synthesizing qualitative and quantitative evidence: A review of possible methods. *Journal of Health Services Research & Policy, 10*(1), 45–53b.

Duffy, M. (2005). Systematic reviews: Their role and contribution to evidence-based practice. *Clinical Nurse Specialist, 19*(1), 15–17.

Eakin, J., & Mykhalovskiy, E. (2003). Reframing the evaluation of qualitative health research: Reflections on a review of appraisal guidelines in the health sciences. *Journal of Evaluation in Clinical Practice, 9*(2), 187–194.

Finfgeld, D. (2003). Metasynthesis: The state of the art—So far. *Qualitative Health Research, 13*(7), 893–904.

Gewurtz, R., Stergiou-Kita, M., Shaw, L., Kirsh, B., & Rappolt, S. (2008). Qualitative meta-synthesis: Reflections on the utility and challenges in occupational therapy. *Canadian Journal of Occupational Therapy, 75*(5), 301–308.

Greenhalgh, T. (1997). Assessing the methodological quality of published papers. *British Medical Journal, 315*(7013), 305–308.

Klassen, T., Jadad, A., & Moher, D. (1998). Guides for reading and interpreting systematic reviews. *Archives of Pediatric and Adolescent Medicine, 152*, 700–704.

Lapier, T. (2003). Methods for finding systematic reviews relevant to physical therapy: Bridging research and clinical practice. *Cardiopulmonary Physical Therapy Journal, 14*(1), 9–12.

Levac, D., Colquhoun, H., & O'Brien, K. (2010). Scoping studies: Advancing the methodology. *Implementation Science, 5*(69), 1–9.

Mays, N., Pope, C., & Popay, J. (2005). Systematically reviewing qualitative and quantitative evidence to inform management and policy making in the health field. *Journal of Health Services Research & Policy, 10*(1), 6–20.

Moher, D., Jadad, A., & Klassen, T. (1998). Guides for reading and interpreting systematic reviews. *Archives of Pediatric and Adolescent Medicine, 152*, 915–920.

Mulrow, C., & Cook, D. (1997). Formulating questions and locating primary studies for inclusion in systematic reviews. *Annals of Internal Medicine, 127*(5), 380–387.

Oxman, A., & Guyatt, G. (1991). Validation of an index of the quality of review articles. *Journal of Clinical Epidemiology, 44*, 1271–1278.

Patterson, B., Thorne, S., Canam, C., & Jillings, C. (2001). *Meta-study of qualitative health research.* Thousand Oaks, CA: Sage.

Peach, H. (2002). Reading systematic reviews. *Australian Family Physician, 31*(8), 1–5.

Polgar, S., & Thomas, S. (Eds.). (2000). Qualitative field research. In *Introduction to research in the health sciences* (4th ed., pp. 91–103). Toronto, ON: Churchill Livingstone.

Richardson, B., & Lindquist, I. (2010). Metasynthesis of qualitative inquiry research studies in physiotherapy. *Physiotherapy Research International, 15*(2), 111–117.

Rumrill, P., Fitzgerald, S., & Merchant, W. (2010). Using scoping reviews as a means of understanding and interpreting existing literature. *Work, 35*, 399–404.

Sandelowski, M. (2006). "Meta-jeopardy": The crisis of representation in qualitative metasynthesis. *Nursing Outlook, 54*(1), 10–16.

Sandelowski, M., & Barroso, J. (2003). Writing the proposal for a qualitative research methodology project. *Qualitative Health Research, 13*(6), 781–790.

Sandelowski, M., & Boshamer, C. C. (2006). Divide and conquer: Avoiding duplication in the reporting of qualitative research. *Research in Nursing & Health, 29*(5), 371–373.

Sandelowski, M., Docherty, S., & Emden, C. (1997). Qualitative metasynthesis: Issues and techniques. *Research in Nursing & Health, 20*, 365–371.

Shea, B. J., Grimshaw, J. M., Wells, G. A., Boers, M., Andersson, N., Hamel, C., …, Bouter, L. M. (2007). Development of AMSTAR: A measurement tool to assess the methodological quality of systematic reviews. *BMC Medical Research Methodology, 7*(10), 1–7.

Spencer, L., Ritchie, J., Lewis, J., & Dillon, L. (2003). *Quality in qualitative evaluation: A framework for assessing research evidence.* London, England: Government Chief Social Researcher's Office, Cabinet Office.

Whitney, J. (2004). Reading and using systematic reviews. *The Journal of Wound, Ostomy and Continence Nursing, 31*(1), 14–17.

Suggested Reading

Cook, M. D., Mulrow, C. D., & Haynes, R. B. (1997). Systematic reviews: Synthesis of best evidence for clinical decisions. Annals of Internal Medicine, 126(5), 376–380.

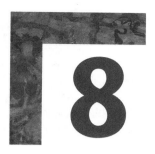

EVALUATING THE EVIDENCE
Economic Evaluations

Mary Law, PhD, OT Reg (Ont), FCAHS; Michael Law, PhD;
and Diane Watson, PhD

LEARNING OBJECTIVES

After reading this chapter, the student/practitioner will be able to:

- Recognize the importance of assessing the value of an intervention to ensure that it offers the most efficient treatment.

- Identify the different types of economic evaluations and determine when they are appropriate for use.

- Search for economic analysis research related to a clinical question including the development of the appropriate question and the use of various electronic databases.

- Critically appraise and communicate this research to his or her clients and managers.

Over the past few years, evidence has increased regarding the effectiveness of rehabilitation interventions in enabling clients to attain specific, desirable outcomes. As a result, practitioners in rehabilitation increasingly search for and utilize evidence-based interventions when making treatment recommendations (Cameron & Ballantyne, 2005; Jette et al., 2003). However, along with examining the effectiveness of an intervention, rehabilitation professionals should also assess the value of these interventions. For example, if two interventions produce identical outcomes but one costs substantially less, both the patient and health system would be better served by using the lower cost alternative. By incorporating knowledge about clinical effectiveness and cost into their treatment decisions, practitioners can ensure that they offer the most efficient means of attaining good outcomes for each patient. Further, if both effectiveness and efficiency information is available, clients, practitioners, and managers can evaluate the costs and outcomes associated with different types of rehabilitation services (Watson, 2000). In the context of shrinking service budgets, these decisions about what services to offer have become increasingly important.

Clients participate in rehabilitation services to attain desirable outcomes at minimal cost to themselves and minimal risk. Services and programs also have to consider relative cost when implementing rehabilitation interventions and making choices between service offerings. We often assume that all health and rehabilitation services are beneficial, but there is substantial evidence

Law M., & MacDermid, J. C.
Evidence-Based Rehabilitation: A Guide
to Practice, Third Edition (pp 175–186).
© 2014 SLACK Incorporated.

from medicine more generally that indicates some interventions can be harmful to one's physical and financial health. For example, it has been estimated that adults receive about 54% of recommended care (McGlynn et al., 2003). In addition, between 45,000 to 195,000 individuals die each year as a result of medical errors (Kohn, Corrigan, & Donaldson, 1999; Leape 2004), and medical bills contributed to up to 62% of bankruptcies in the United States in 2009 (Himmelstein, Thorne, & Woolhandler, 2011). These recent statistics draw attention to the importance of balancing our understanding of potential benefits with insights regarding costs and risks.

In addition to harm, there is research evidence that demonstrates the inappropriate use of many health services and, some research suggests, some rehabilitation services. For example, a review found that most Medicare patients in skilled nursing facilities who received occupational and physical therapy were appropriate candidates and benefited from intervention, but 10% of billed therapy was for services that were "not medically necessary" (Office of the Inspector General, 1999, p. 13). It was also determined that patients who had similar diagnoses, goals, plans, and outcomes varied in the frequency and duration of the therapy services they received from different facilities. These variations suggest that there is either an over- or underprovision of services in different facilities. Evaluations such as this draw attention to the importance of understanding the cost-effectiveness of rehabilitation services and when intervention is excessive.

This chapter provides students, practitioners, and managers with a basic understanding of the research methods that have been used to appraise the costs and outcomes of health services. More extensive information regarding the application of these methods to assess the value of rehabilitation services is published elsewhere (Watson, 2000). Readers can use the knowledge gained in this chapter to search for, critically appraise, and communicate evidence derived from the literature. Other sections in this book highlight the process of seeking evidence regarding the effectiveness of specific services and incorporating this evidence into practice. By comparison, this chapter summarizes how research is conducted in order to evaluate the value of rehabilitation services and describes how practitioners can obtain and appraise this evidence.

ASSESSING THE VALUE OF REHABILITATION SERVICES FOR CLIENTS: ECONOMIC EVALUATION

There has been a long-standing development of research methods in health economics to appraise, describe, and compare the relative value of health and rehabilitation services. These methods have been called *cost-effectiveness analyses* (Russell, Gold, Siegel, Daniels, & Weinstein, 1996) and/or *economic evaluations* (Drummond, Sculpher, Torrance, O'Brien, & Stoddart, 2003). This research is different from clinical evaluations in that it focuses on costs as well as outcomes. The effectiveness and appropriateness of a clinical intervention, however, needs to be established before being combined with an assessment of costs; it would be wasteful to calculate the cost of providing ineffective services (Drummond et al., 2003).

Whereas effectiveness research focuses on the impact of interventions on outcomes such as participation in daily activities and quality of life, economic evaluations focus on the relative value of health services. Within the health care context, the term *value* refers to the relative worth, utility, or importance of a service in meeting the health needs of a defined clientele. For a service to be valuable, clients should receive a fair return (i.e., improvement in health status) for something exchanged (i.e., finances and time invested).

To be informed about the relative value of specific health and rehabilitation services for defined clientele, we must (a) conduct evaluations to determine whether specific interventions are effective at attaining desirable outcomes; (b) evaluate effective interventions to ensure that they offer the most efficient means of attaining specific outcomes; and (c) effectively communicate these results.

Historically, the number of evaluations that have been conducted to assess the relative value of rehabilitation services is smaller than the number of effectiveness studies.

The intent and purpose of economic evaluations are to provide policy makers, managers, clinicians, and patients with information regarding the relative value of particular services in order to inform their decisions. Therefore, these evaluations require that two or more services be compared to assess relative value. One of the comparisons, however, can be a no service alternative, which is equivalent to a control group in experimental research. In this context, a comparison would be made between the cost and benefit of receiving versus not receiving a particular rehabilitation service. For example, Meyer, Wegscheider, Kersten, and Mühlhauser (2005) conducted an economic evaluation when they compared the cost and outcomes of providing versus not providing education and hip protectors for nurses to reduce the number of hip fractures for nursing home patients.

Types of Economic Evaluations

Five different types of economic evaluations have been defined in the literature: cost–consequence, cost minimization, cost-effectiveness, cost utility, and cost–benefit analyses (Drummond et al., 2003). Table 8-1 illustrates how these different research methods might be applied to evaluate the relative worth of a rehabilitation service. Table 8-2 provides examples of economic evaluations that have been published in the literature and highlights the fact that investigators may conduct different types of economic evaluations when assessing the relative value of a health or rehabilitation service.

Cost-Consequence Analysis

A cost–consequence analysis is used to describe a health service or compare two or more health interventions. This type of analysis requires that investigators provide a descriptive profile of the costs (e.g., hospital costs, out-of-pocket expenses) and outcomes (e.g., impact on health and economic circumstances) of one or more interventions. These figures are simply detailed and not further aggregated into ratios. For example, Patel, Knapp, Evans, et al. (2004) described the costs and outcomes of providing caregiver training during rehabilitation of stroke patients.

Cost Minimization Analysis

A cost minimization analysis is conducted to identify the least costly alternative when two or more services produce equivalent outcomes. Evidence that each service produces comparable outcomes must be demonstrated using evidence from the literature or tested as part of the analysis. For example, in a study that determined that there was no significant difference in outcomes for patients who received hospital at home versus hospital inpatient care, a cost minimization analysis was conducted to identify the least costly alternative (Jones et al., 1999).

Cost-Effectiveness Analysis

A cost-effectiveness analysis is conducted when an investigator is interested in describing and comparing the relative costs and outcomes of two or more services. This type of evaluation requires that the services being compared produce the same type of outcome (e.g., both reduce hip fracture rates). For example, Cochrane, Davey, and Edwards (2005) compared the costs and outcomes of individuals who have lower limb osteoarthritis and receive water-based exercise or regular care. A cost-effectiveness analysis was used to study the value of each service option because the goal of each service was to achieve the same type of outcome (i.e., reduce upper extremity impairment and improve health status). The different interventions are always compared using the outcomes they produce, such as the dollar cost per unit of change in upper extremity movement improvement.

Table 8-1

Applying Economic Evaluation Methods to Rehabilitation Services

Consider the following clinical scenario and the contribution of economic evaluation methods to the decision-making process.

Assume that an individual who had a stroke 10 days ago was given the choice to receive rehabilitation services using a number of different approaches to care, and suppose that you have been given the responsibility to be a decision maker regarding the health care services received by this person. You have decided that their decision will primarily be based on the relative value—that is, the relative costs and outcomes—of each alternative.

You have determined that the hospital offers post-stroke rehabilitation services on a general unit or a specialized unit and that home-based rehabilitation services are available. Therefore, the following options are available: (a) hospital-based services on a general unit; (b) hospital-based services on a specialized unit; (c) early discharge from the hospital and home-based rehabilitation; or (d) early discharge and no rehabilitation services.

You have reviewed the literature to determine the relative value of institution-based versus home-based post-stroke rehabilitation versus no intervention. A cost–consequences analysis would provide a descriptive profile of the costs and outcomes of each alternative and any evidence regarding significant differences between these alternatives. Assuming that the goals and objectives of the inpatient post-stroke rehabilitation services were identical and therefore the types of outcomes expected of participants were similar, a cost-effectiveness analysis would provide insight regarding the relative value of the alternatives. Relative value would be measured by determining the cost per unit of health effect (e.g., cost per unit of change in functional status) derived from participation in each service delivery model in comparison to the no service alternative.

Assume that the goals and objectives of the hospital-based programs were to increase independence in activities of daily living and the goals of the home-based programs were to enhance participation of individuals who have experienced a stroke in community-based activities and support programs. In this context, it would be appropriate to conduct a cost utility and/or cost–benefit analysis to compare the relative value of service alternatives that are directed toward different outcomes (i.e., independence in activities of daily living versus enhance community participation). Both outcomes, however, impact health-related quality of life. Therefore, a cost utility analysis would require a comparison of the costs and health-related quality of life of these two service alternatives. Alternatively, a cost–benefit analysis could be conducted to compare the costs, monetary outcomes, and net financial impact of participating in either of these two service alternatives.

Cost Utility and Cost-Benefit Analysis

In contrast, cost utility and cost–benefit analyses are conducted to compare the relative costs and outcomes of two or more services that produce different types of outcomes. Cost utility analyses consider both health status and the value of that status to the client when evaluating outcomes, whereas cost–benefit analyses assess the monetary value of outcomes. Here is an example. A rehabilitation program cannot obtain additional funding to increase staff and the current demand for services exceeds that which is available. The challenge becomes one of trying to determine which clients should receive rehabilitation. For example, should you offer services to individuals who have had an acute back injury or those whose injury has not improved after a specific period of time? Consider making this decision on the basis of which alternative would maximize outcomes for the amount of cost (e.g., money and time) invested. One way to compare outcomes for services that

Table 8-2

Examples of Economic Evaluations in the Rehabilitation Literature

TYPE OF EVALUATION	HEALTH SERVICE AREA	EXAMPLE EVALUATION
Cost–consequence	• Community-based geriatric case management program for frail older patients • Training versus no training for caregivers of stroke patients	Duke (2005) Patel, Knapp, Perez, et al. (2004)
Cost minimization	• Stroke rehabilitation: home or hospital • Use of hip protectors in the prevention of hip fractures in frail institutionalized older patients	Anderson et al. (2000) Jones et al. (1999) van Schoor et al. (2004)
Cost-effectiveness	• Tele-rehabilitation program for older adults in the community • Occupational therapy to promote well-being of older adults living in the community • Use of hip protectors in nursing homes • Home exercise program or no intervention for knee pain • High-intensity exercise program or conventional physical therapy for individuals with rheumatoid arthritis	Bendixen, Levy, Olive, Kobb, and Mann (2009) Clark et al. (2011) Meyer et al. (2005) Thomas et al. (2005) van den Hout et al. (2005)
Cost utility	• Hospital-based rehabilitation or conventional care after an acute coronary event • Home or group-based rehabilitation programs for women with breast cancer • Early discharge of older persons • Stroke unit, stroke team, or domiciliary stroke care • Cardiac rehabilitation prevention program versus conventional therapy	Briffa et al. (2005) Gordon et al. (2005) Miller et al. (2005) Patel, Knapp, Perez, et al. (2004) Yu et al. (2004)
Cost–benefit	• Individual placement and support versus regular employment placement service for mental health patients • Needle exchange program to prevent HIV transmission • Home- versus institution-based psychiatric services	Chalamat, Mihalopoulos, Carter, and Vos (2005) Gold, Gafni, Nelligan, and Millson (1997) Margolis and Petti (1994)

produce different types of outcomes is to measure change in health status on a comparable scale (i.e., cost utility analysis). Commonly the outcomes in cost utility analyses are expressed in terms of quality-adjusted life years (QALYs). A QALY is equivalent to 1 year in perfect health and is decremented for reductions in health status. In other words, measure whether changes in the health status of clients with acute injuries are more, less, or the same as those with more chronic injuries. Another way to compare outcomes is to measure outcomes in financial terms (i.e., cost–benefit analysis). See Tables 8-1 and 8-2 for more examples of economic evaluations.

Conducting Economic Evaluations

Economic evaluations are typically conducted using a multistep process (Drummond et al., 2003). A research question is initially posed to define the purpose and scope of the assessment. The question should describe a service or identify interventions being described or compared, outline the perspective and time horizon of the analysis, specify the scope of the intervention, and detail the costs and outcomes considered. Economic evaluations can be descriptive, comparative, or both. Descriptive evaluations simply describe the goals and objectives of the service, the population for whom the program was provided, the type of intervention offered, the costs of providing and/or consuming the intervention service, and the outcomes or effects of the service. Comparative assessments compare an intervention with appropriate alternative interventions or no intervention.

The perspective of the analysis is important to consider and identify prospectively, because evaluations that are conducted from the same viewpoint as the "user" of the assessment tend to be more relevant and useful (Drummond et al., 2003). Evaluations can be conducted from the perspective of society, payers (e.g., an insurance program), providers (e.g., a hospital), and/or consumers. The perspective will dictate what costs are included. For example, a societal perspective would include the cost of lost work time resulting from foregoing a treatment, whereas the perspective of an insurance program would not. The outcomes to be included should be prespecified. These elements can be identified through a process that considers the goals, objectives, and activities of the rehabilitation service; the needs of the target population and service recipients; and the preference of the audience for whom the evaluation report is intended. The most relevant and important costs and outcomes to include are those that are valued by all stakeholders.

It is important to conduct a literature review during the initial planning stages of an evaluation to enhance understanding of the particular issue and to learn about previous research that is relevant. Evidence regarding the costs and/or the effectiveness of the services being described and/or compared is compiled and evaluated. The process by which evidence can be located in the literature and critically appraised is profiled in Chapters 5 and 6. Economic evaluations should employ rigorous methodologies to determine the efficacy and effectiveness of an intervention and estimate the true costs of intervention as closely as possible.

Good evaluations should include an assessment regarding the robustness of the findings. These assessments—termed *sensitivity analyses*—are required, because investigators must make a number of judgments or assumptions throughout the course of the analysis. A sensitivity analysis presents the range of possible values resulting from variations of a critical judgment (Drummond et al., 2003). For example, the previous studies may have variation in the estimated health outcomes, so sensitivity analysis would investigate whether the conclusions of the study would vary if different assumptions were used. Evaluators also need to make judgments regarding the internal and external validity of their assessments. Sources of bias, contamination, and noncompliance must be described and documented. All studies have limitations, but a final report that includes a description of these will help decision makers to weigh the merits of the evaluation and, thereby, make judgments based on the evidence.

Critically Reviewing Economic Evaluations

The characteristics that describe rigorous economic evaluation projects are those that can be used to critically appraise those articles summarizing the findings of one of these evaluative efforts. Table 8-3 provides a listing of questions that can be used when evaluating evidence in the literature regarding the relative value of health service interventions. This list was developed after reviewing formats that have been used by others to appraise the quality of economic evaluation evidence (Drummond et al., 2003).

Table 8-3

Critically Appraising the Internal and External Validity of Economic Evaluations

INTERNAL VALIDITY

1. Did the research question clearly and accurately define the options compared?
2. Was the perspective of the analysis defined?
3. Were the important and relevant costs and outcomes identified?
4. Were the costs and outcomes properly measured and valued?
5. How rigorous was the methodology that was used to establish costs?
6. How rigorous was the methodology that was used to establish the effectiveness of the service alternatives?
7. Were the differences in costs and outcomes between the options analyzed and compared?
8. Was appropriate allowance made for uncertainties in the evaluation by including a sensitivity analysis incorporating clinically sensitive variations in important variables?

EXTERNAL VALIDITY

1. Are the outcomes worth the costs?
2. Could my patients expect similar health outcomes?
3. Could I expect similar costs?

The National Health Service Research and Development Centre for Evidence-Based Medicine (CEBM) in Oxford, England, was established in 1995 to promote the teaching and practice of evidence-based health care. The CEBM has published guidelines for ranking the level of evidence of effectiveness studies and economic evaluations, and this document is available on the Web at www.cebm.net/index.aspx?o=1421.

Locating Economic Evaluations in the Literature

Economic evaluations that have been published in the literature can be found using traditional health research databases. The National Library of Medicine provides free Internet access through PubMed to enable people to search online databases such as MEDLINE and HealthSTAR. These resources can be accessed by going to www.nlm.nih.gov. MEDLINE is considered to be a premier bibliographic database that contains references and abstracts for journal articles in life sciences with a concentration on biomedicine and the clinical sciences. HealthSTAR is the bibliographic database that provides access to the published literature of health services technology, administration, and research. The National Information Centre on Health Services Research and Health Care Technology provides free Internet access to enable people to search their online databases. This resource can be accessed by going to www.ncbi.nlm.nih.gov/books/NBK16710/.

There are two databases that provide abstracts and critical appraisals of economic evaluations. The National Health Service Centre for Reviews and Dissemination at the University of York in the United Kingdom offers free Internet access to their Economic Evaluation Database. This valuable resource can be accessed by going to http://www.crd.york.ac.uk/crdweb/AboutNHSEED.asp. This database contains structured abstracts and critical appraisals of economic evaluations from 1994 onward. The Office of Health Economics and the International Federation of Pharmaceutical Manufacturers Association offers access to their Health Economic Evaluations Database (HEED) on a subscription basis. This database contains abstracts and structured reviews of economic evaluations, cost analyses, and cost of illness studies from 1967 on. HEED is available in CD format or via the Internet and can be accessed at most university libraries.

CONCLUSION

The number of evaluations that have been conducted to evaluate the effectiveness of rehabilitation interventions and programs has grown rapidly in recent years. By comparison, the number of evaluations that have been conducted to assess the relative value of these services is much smaller. This is not unexpected, because it is important to establish clinical effectiveness before calculating costs. However, economic considerations are increasingly becoming important for health system policy makers and managers, which will only increase the demand for economic evaluations of rehabilitation services.

Research methods have been established to appraise the costs and outcomes of health services to provide clients, consumers, practitioners, and managers with information regarding relative value. It is hoped that these insights will inform their decisions. There are five types of economic evaluations, but these methodological approaches simply differ in how they measure and/or quantify outcomes. A number of good evaluations have been published in the literature, and Table 8-2 provides examples of studies in rehabilitation. Information has been provided to enable the reader to locate and appraise this literature, with the hope that this exercise will inform clinical practice and stimulate enthusiasm among those who wish to conduct this type of research. The challenge for the rehabilitation is clear. We must continue to assess the value of effective interventions to ensure that they offer the most efficient means of attaining specific outcomes and effectively communicate these findings to our clients.

TAKE-HOME MESSAGES

✓ Rehabilitation practitioners must assess the value of effective interventions so that clients and consumers can evaluate costs and outcomes when deciding to participate and so that they can offer the most efficient types of interventions.

✓ We cannot always assume that the potential benefits from receiving a service outweigh the costs and risks.

✓ When making a decision about which service to offer or which intervention to receive, practitioners, managers, and clients must consider the costs, risks, and outcomes of each alternative.

Economic Evaluation

✓ Focus on appraising, describing, and comparing the relative value of specific interventions in order to inform decision making.

✓ Value is the relative worth, utility, or importance of a service in meeting the health needs of a defined clientele.

✓ The following are three aspects of an economic evaluation:
- Evaluate whether specific interventions are effective at attaining outcomes.
- Evaluate effective interventions to ensure they offer the most efficient means.
- Effectively communicate these results.

Types of Economic Evaluations

✓ Cost–consequence: Descriptive profile of the costs and outcomes of one or more interventions.

✓ Cost minimization: Identifies the least costly alternative for services that result in equivalent outcomes.

✓ Cost-effectiveness: Describes and compares the relative costs and outcomes of two or more interventions that result in the same type of outcome.

✓ Cost utility: Describes and compares the relative costs and outcomes of two or more interventions in which the outcomes of interest include health status and the value of the status to the individual.

✓ Cost–benefit: Describes and compares the relative costs and outcomes of two or more interventions in which both the costs and outcomes can be measured in monetary values.

Conducting Economic Evaluations

✓ Research question defines the purpose and scope of assessment.

✓ Descriptive analysis or comparative assessment.

✓ Important to consider the perspective of the analysis (i.e., from society, payers, providers, and/or consumers).

✓ Evaluators of economic analyses should make judgments regarding the internal and external validity of their assessments including source of bias, contamination, and noncompliance.

✓ When critically analyzing economic analyses, it is important to look at both internal and external factors.

Locating Economic Evaluations in the Literature

✓ Research can be found with traditional databases such as MEDLINE and HealthSTAR.

✓ The National Health Service Centre for Reviews and Dissemination (University of York, UK) contains structured abstracts and critical appraisals of economic evaluations from 1994 on.

✓ Economic evaluation
www.rapid-diagnostics.org/app-cost.htm
Outline of economic evaluation for health outcomes of rapid diagnostic tests

✓ Interactive online module regarding health economics
www.nlm.nih.gov/nichsr/edu/healthecon/index.html
Published by the U.S. National Library of Medicine–National Institutes of Health

LEARNING AND EXPLORATION ACTIVITIES

The purpose of this chapter was to provide a basic understanding and appreciation of the research methods that have been used to appraise the costs and outcomes of health services. Upon completion of this chapter, students should be aware of the role that economic evaluations currently play and could potentially play in evidence-based practice.

1. You are the manager for a program providing home-based rehabilitation services for older adults discharged after total hip replacement surgery. It is important to conduct economic evaluations of this program. For each type of economic analysis, describe the purpose of the evaluation and what specific information would be collected to complete such an evaluative study.

    a. Cost–consequences

    b. Cost minimization

    c. Cost-effectiveness

    d. Cost utility

    e. Cost–benefit

2. Select one of the economic evaluation studies listed in Table 8-2. Using the questions in Table 8-3, complete a critical appraisal of this article. What are the implications of the findings for rehabilitation practice?

3. Snoezelen rooms, originating from the Dutch words "to sniff" and "to doze" (Chung & Lei, 2005), have been created as multisensory environments that provide participants with visual, auditory, olfactory, and tactile stimuli (Baker, Doling, Wareing, Dawson, & Assey, 1997). Adults with dementia have become the newest population to use Snoezelen rooms as therapy (Chung & Lei, 2005). Snoezelen rooms may be effective for increasing positive behaviours (i.e., interaction) and decreasing negative behaviours (i.e., aggression and depressed mood) in the short term when used as a form of therapy (Baker et al., 2003; Baillon et al., 2004; Chung & Lei, 2005). However, there is often a hefty price tag that comes with this very technological equipment, and the effects may not generalize or extend to the longer term (Baker et al., 2004; Chung & Lei, 2005). A clinician is left wondering: do the positive effects of Snoezelen rooms warrant the expenses associated with them? How can this clinical question be answered using the five different types of economical evaluation? What research question would address each type of economic evaluation regarding the use of Snoezelen rooms with adults with dementia?

REFERENCES

Anderson, C., Mhurchu, C. N., Rubenach, S., Clark, M., Spencer, C., & Winsor, A. (2000). Home or hospital for stroke rehabilitation? Results of a randomized controlled trial. II: Cost minimization analysis at 6 months. *Stroke, 31*, 1032.

Baker, R., Dowling, Z., Wareing, L., Dawson, J., & Assey, J. (1997). Snoezelen: Its long term and short term effects on older people with dementia. *British Journal of Occupational Therapy, 60*(5), 213-218.

Baker, R., Holloway, J., Holtkamp, C., Larsson, A., Hartman, L., Pearce, R., et al. (2003). Effects of multi-sensory stimulation for people with dementia. *Issues and Innovations in Nursing Practice, 43*(5), 465-477.

Baillon S., Van Diepen, E., Prettyman, R., Redman, J., Rooke, N., & Campbell, R. (2004). A comparison of the effects of Snoezelen and reminiscence therapy on the agitated behaviour of patients with dementia. *International Journal of Geriatric Psychiatry, 19*(11), 1047-1052

Bendixen, R. M., Levy, C. E., Olive, E. S., Kobb, R. F., & Mann, W. C. (2009). Cost effectiveness of a telerehabilitation program to support chronically ill and disabled elders in their homes. *Telemedicine and e-Health, 15*(1), 31–38. doi:10.1089/tmj.2008.0046

Briffa, T. G., Eckerman, S. D., Griffiths, A. D., Harris, P. J., Heath, M. R., Freedman, S. B., ..., Keech, A. C. (2005). Cost-effectiveness of rehabilitation after an acute coronary event: A randomized controlled trial. *Medical Journal of Australia, 183*, 450–455.

Cameron, K. A. V., & Ballantyne, S. (2005). Utilization of evidence-based practice by registered occupational therapists. *Occupational Therapy International, 12*(3), 123–136.

Chalamat, M., Mihalopoulos, C., Carter, R., & Vos, T. (2005). Assessing cost-effectiveness in mental health: Vocational rehabilitation for schizophrenia and related conditions. *Australian and New Zealand Journal of Psychiatry, 39*, 693–700.

Chung, J.C., & Lai, C.K. (2005). Snoezelen for dementia. The Cochrane Database of Systematic Reviews, (3).

Chung, J.C., Lai, C.K., Chung, P.M., French, H.P. (2002). Snoezelen for dementia. The Cochrane Database of Systematic Reviews, (4):CD003152.

Clark, F., Jackson, J., Carlson, M., Chou, C.-P., Cherry, B. J., Jordan-Marsh, M., ..., Azen, S. P. (2011). Effectiveness of a lifestyle intervention in promoting the well-being of independently living older people: Results of the Well Elderly 2 Randomised Controlled Trial. *Journal of Epidemiology and Community Health.* doi:10.1136/jech.2009.099754

Cochrane, T., Davey, R. C., & Edwards, S. M. M. (2005). Randomised controlled trial of the cost-effectiveness of water-based therapy for lower limb osteoarthritis. *Health Technology Assessment, 9*(31), 1–114.

Drummond, M. F., Sculpher, M. J., Torrance, G. W., O'Brien, B. J., & Stoddart, G. L. (2003). *Methods for the Economic Evaluation of Health Care Programmes* (3rd ed). Oxford, England: Oxford University Press.

Duke, C. (2005). The Frail Elderly Community-Based Case Management Project. *Geriatric Nursing, 26*, 122–127.

Gold, M., Gafni, A., Nelligan, P., & Millson, P. (1997). Needle exchange programs: An economic evaluation of a local experience. *Canadian Medical Association Journal, 157*, 255–262.

Gordon, L. G., Scuffham, P., Battistutta, D., Graves, N., Tweeddale, M., & Newman, B. (2005). A cost-effectiveness analysis of two rehabilitation support services for women with breast cancer. *Breast Cancer Research and Treatment, 94*, 123–133.

Himmelstein, D. U., Thorne, D., & Woolhandler, S. (2011). Medical bankruptcy in Massachusetts: Has health reform made a difference? *American Journal of Medicine, 124*(3), 224–228.

Jette, D. U., Bacon, K., Batty, C., Carlson, M., Ferland, A. & Hemingway, R. D. (2003). Evidence-based practice: Beliefs, attitudes, knowledge, and behaviors of physical therapists. *Physical Therapy, 83*(9), 786–805.

Jones, J., Wilson, A., Parker, H., Wynn, A., Jagger, C., Spiers, N., et al. (1999). Economic evaluation of hospital at home versus hospital care: Cost minimization analysis of data from randomized controlled trial. *British Medical Journal, 319*, 1547–1550.

Kohn, L., Corrigan, J., & Donaldson, M. (1999). *To err is human: Building a safer health system.* Washington, DC: National Academy Press.

Leape, L. (2004). 195,000 Annual deaths linked to in-hospital errors, study says. *The Quality Letter for Healthcare Leaders, 16*(9), 10–11.

Margolis, L. H., & Petti, R. D. (1994). An analysis of the costs and benefits of two strategies to decrease length in children's psychiatric hospitals. *Health Services Research, 29*, 155–167.

McGlynn, E. A., Asch, S. M., Adams, J., Keesey, J., Hicks, J., DeCristofaro, A., & Kerr, E. A. (2003). The quality of health care delivered to adults in the United States. *New England Journal of Medicine, 348*(26), 2635–2645.

Meyer, G., Wegscheider, K., Kersten, J. F., Icks, A., & Mühlhauser, I. (2005). Increased use of hip protectors in nursing homes: Economic analysis of a cluster randomized, controlled trial. *Journal of the American Geriatrics Society, 53*, 2153–2158.

Miller, P., Gladman, J. R. F., Cunliffe, A. L., Husbands, S. L., Dewey, M. E., & Harwood, R. H. (2005). Economic analysis of an early discharge rehabilitation service for older people. *Age and Ageing, 34*, 274–280.

Office of Inspector General. (1999). *Physical and occupational therapy in nursing homes: Medical necessity and quality of care.* Washington, DC: Department of Health and Human Services.

Patel, A., Knapp, M., Evans, A., Perez, I., & Kalra, L. (2004). Training care givers of stroke patients: economic evaluation. *British Medical Journal, 328*, 1102–1107.

Patel, A., Knapp, A., Perez, I., Evans, A., & Kalra, L. (2004). Alternative strategies for stroke sare. Cost-effectiveness and cost-utility analyses from a prospective randomized controlled trial. *Stroke, 35*, 196–203.

Russell, L. B., Gold, M., Siegel, J. E., Daniels, N., & Weinstein, M. C. (1996). The role of cost-effectiveness analysis in health and medicine. *Journal of the American Medical Association, 276*, 1172–1177.

Thomas, K. S., Miller, P., Doherty, M., Muir, K. R., Jones, A. C., & O'Reilly, S. C. (2005). Cost effectiveness of a two-year home exercise program for the treatment of knee pain. *Arthritis & Rheumatism, 53*, 388–394.

van den Hout, W. B., de Jong, Z., Munneke, M., Hazes, J. M. W., Breedveld, F. C., & Vliet Vlieland, T. P. M. (2005). Cost-utility and cost-effectiveness analyses of a long-term, high-intensity exercise program compared with conventional physical therapy in patients with rheumatoid arthritis. *Arthritis & Rheumatism, 53*, 39–47.

van Schoor, N. M., de Bruyne, M. C., van der Roer, N., Lommerse, E., van Tulder, M. W., Bouter, L. M., & Lips, P. (2004). Cost-effectiveness of hip protectors in frail institutionalized elderly. *Osteoporosis International, 15*, 964–969.

Watson, D. E. (2000). *Evaluating costs and outcomes: Demonstrating the value of rehabilitation services.* Bethesda, MD: American Occupational Therapy Association.

Yu, C., Lau, C., Chau, J., McGhee, S., Kong, S., Cheung, B. M., & Li, L. S. (2004). A short course of cardiac rehabilitation program is highly cost effective in improving long-term quality of life in patients with recent myocardial infarction or percutaneous coronary intervention. *Archives of Physical Medicine and Rehabilitation, 85*, 1915–1922.

Suggested Readings

Drummond, M. F., Richardson, W. S., O'Brien, B. J., Levine, M., & Heyland, D. (1997). Users' guide to the medical literature. How to use an article on economic analysis of clinical practice: Are the results of the study valid? *Journal of the American Medical Association, 277*, 1552–1557.

Gottlieb, S. (2000). Medical bills account for 40% of bankruptcies. *British Medical Journal, 320*(7245), 1295.

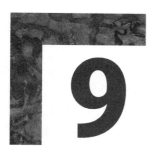

KNOWLEDGE TRANSLATION

Mary Law, PhD, OT Reg (Ont), FCAHS and
Joy C. MacDermid, PhD, PT Reg (Ont), FCAHS

LEARNING OBJECTIVES

After reading this chapter, the student/practitioner will be able to:

- Define knowledge exchange and translation (KET) and distinguish between the various models of knowledge translation (KT).
- Identify effective KET models.
- Recognize the differences between knowledge-driven models and problem-driven models of evidence-based policy.
- Characterize the roles and challenges of evidence-based policy within evidence-based practice (EBP).

Transferring research into practice and policy seems to be the very reason for the existence of EBP, and it would be reasonable to assume that it is something at which evidence-based practitioners would be skilled. Despite the need for research transfer, however, the best methods for doing it are still being developed and evaluated. Traditionally, transfers of health care information took place through either the undiscriminating distribution of print media (such as a bulletin or a journal article) or through large-group continuing education seminars. For a long time, this was thought to be enough; however, practitioners have recently realized that these methods are inadequate. The problems were substantial—either the information was not reaching those who needed it, it was not convenient for the practitioners who wanted to learn, or the format of the material alienated the participants. In the past decade, there have been major efforts made to create strategies that will ensure effective research transfer.

Let us start by looking at the term *knowledge translation*. This term has been defined by the Canadian Institutes of Health Research (CIHR) as:

> The exchange, synthesis and ethically-sound application of knowledge—within a complex system of interactions among researchers and users—to accelerate the capture of the benefits of research for Canadians through improved health, more effective services and products, and a strengthened health care system. (CIHR, 2008, p. 5)

Law M., & MacDermid, J. C.
*Evidence-Based Rehabilitation: A Guide
to Practice, Third Edition* (pp 187–203).
© 2014 SLACK Incorporated.

Figure 9-1. Knowledge to action model. (From "Lost in Knowledge Translation: Time for a Map," by I. D. Graham, et al., 2006, *Journal of Continuing Education in the Health Professions,* 26(1). Reprinted with permission from John Wiley & Sons, Inc.)

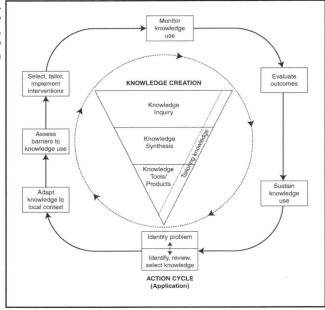

Since this time, other terms such as *knowledge exchange and translation*, *research dissemination*, and *knowledge mobilization* have also been used to describe a similar process.

Knowledge development is a complex process, and transfer of knowledge is equally complex. There are many more considerations than just the fact that the research has been done correctly. We must also examine the characteristics of the different pieces in the KET process. What are the characteristics of the scientific evidence used? Who are the decision makers who will be examining it? In what organizational context do we expect this research information to be used? There are a rich variety of variables that must be considered, and their interplay is discussed in the chapter on evidence-based policy. Effective research transfer can sometimes be more of an art than a science.

MODELS OF KNOWLEDGE EXCHANGE AND TRANSLATION

Let us begin by examining models about how research/knowledge transfer works in health care and other fields. Some research theories about how to transfer knowledge into practice have centered on changing the behavior of individual practitioners, whereas others have centered more on changing the organizations in which practitioners work.

One of the most widely used models of KT is the knowledge-to-action framework developed by Graham et al. (2006). As can be seen in Figure 9-1, the knowledge-to-action framework depicts both the process for creating knowledge and the action cycle through which knowledge is applied to specific identified issues or problems. In the center of the framework, Graham et al. (2006) illustrated how research and inquiry builds knowledge, which is then synthesized and developed into tools or products for translation and dissemination. These tools or products can be used as part of the action cycle to transfer research information into practice and policy. In the action cycle, all stakeholders are involved in identification of the issues, adaptation of knowledge to fit local context, and selections of methods by which to complete the KT. During the action cycle, it is important to address potential barriers to knowledge use, monitor the impact of dissemination, and evaluate outcomes. The knowledge-to-action framework is dynamic in nature and acknowledges the complexity of the KT process. Because of this, the framework can be useful to guide practitioners and policy makers throughout the process of KT.

The knowledge-to-action framework has been used to discuss how evidence regarding falls research can be implemented into practice and policy (Tetroe, Graham, & Scott, 2011). For specific examples of how the knowledge-to-action framework has been used, see Chapter 13 in this book.

The readiness-to-change model (the transtheoretical model) by Prochaska and DiClemente is an example of a model that looks specifically at the individual. It incorporates features of a variety of behavior models and suggests that change in behavior is modulated by a person's readiness to make changes at the time the information is provided (Dalton & Gottlieb, 2003; Kerns & Habib, 2004). This model is useful to understand how clinicians respond to KT. The stages of change in this model, as outlined by Sherman and Carothers (2005), are as follows:

- Precontemplation (no awareness of or intention of taking action toward an idea)

- Contemplation (awareness of an idea and consideration of changing)

- Preparation (making plans to change behavior)

- Action (engaging in a new behavior)

- Maintenance (continuing the behavior and making it part of a routine)

There are also processes of change, which are as follows (Prochaska, Norcross, & DiClemente, 1995, p. 33, as cited in Sherman & Carothers, 2005):

- Consciousness-raising ("increasing information about self and problem")

- Emotional arousal ("experiencing and expressing feelings about one's problems and solutions")

- Commitment ("choosing and committing to act, or belief in ability to change")

- Reward ("rewarding self, or being rewarded by others, for making change")

- Environmental reevaluation ("assessing how one's problem affects the physical environment" Prochaska et al., 1992, p. 1108, as cited in Sherman & Carothers, 2005)

KT strategies can be tailored using this information about how people respond to change. For example, providing information that increases conscious thoughts about an intervention is more effective for those at the consciousness raising or emotional arousal stages, whereas behavioral interventions such as rewards are more effective for the action and maintenance stages (Sherman & Carothers, 2005).

Some research has shown that interventions influencing individuals have not had a large impact on KT (Davies & Nutley, 2002). Researchers such as Rogers (1995) have taken a more combined or "diffusion of innovations" approach—one that focuses on both the individual and the organization. Rogers (1995) proposed a model called the *innovation decision process model*. He defined diffusion as "the process by which an innovation is communicated through certain channels over time among the members of a social system." In short, his model looks at how individuals and organizations change over time, how they become familiar with new research information, how they use this information, and the types of information that are most effective within a given stage of the process. This model has been used in health research and in other disciplines and other models have built upon it. The five stages of the model are as follows:

1. Knowledge (learning about a new idea)

2. Persuasion (forming an opinion about the idea)

3. Decision (deciding whether to use the idea or not)

4. Implementation (trying out the new idea)

5. Confirmation (evaluating the implementation of the idea to determine if it is producing the desired outcome—continuing to seek out information along the way). It is important to note that these stages may not always occur in the order presented.

Rogers (1995) also discussed a two-pronged strategy for communication and KT. He referred to two types of communication channels within the innovation decision process model: mass media channels and interpersonal channels. In other words, he suggested that the way information is delivered should differ depending on the stage of the model the individual or organization is working through. The use of mass media channels such as TV, radio, peer-reviewed journals, and teleconferences is most effective during the knowledge and awareness phase. For an example of the use of mass communication for persons with disabilities, see Kurtovich et al. (2010). Alternatively, interpersonal channels (face-to-face communications) such as interactions between colleagues, small-group discussions, and knowledge brokering work best within the persuasion and decision stages.

Another model for research transfer comes from researchers Dobbins, Ciliska, Cockerill, Barnsley, and DiCenso (2002). Researchers broke the research transfer process into the same five key stages as Rogers (1995; knowledge, persuasion, decision, implementation, and confirmation) but built on the model by applying it to health care research. Dobbins et al.'s (2002) model extends to evidence-based policy, as do many larger models of research transfer activities, because the two (research transfer and policy making) interact. Each of Dobbins et al.'s (2002) five phases has a specific purpose. The knowledge stage begins when research is complete and attempts to identify the best ways for presenting that knowledge to others (discussed later in this chapter). The persuasion stage is twofold—it includes persuading other practitioners and policy makers of the merits of one's research. Third, the decision stage leads to evidence-based decision making on whether or not this innovation will be put to use. The fourth and fifth stages, implementation and confirmation, deal more specifically with evidence-based policy.

KT cannot be a passive endeavor. Agencies will distribute clinical guidelines and evidence-based policy; however, it is up to individuals to assimilate much of the knowledge on their own. The strategy of teaching practitioners the process and having them perform short, self-directed inquiries into subjects is better than distributing information that will not be used. More important, perhaps, than even the content of the evidence being transferred is the method of transfer. Choosing a research transfer flow that accords practitioners respect for their experience and makes them enthusiastic about using their own critical appraisal skills—while simultaneously encouraging researchers when they see that the fruits of their labor put to good use—is the ultimate goal.

Early in a KT process, the emphasis is on preparing practitioners to gather and assimilate new knowledge. When the research transfer process starts, it begins with a topic that is a current clinical problem in the practitioner's everyday setting. The surest way to alienate practitioners new to EBP is to make them work on esoteric, theoretical cases because they will soon lose interest and respect for the evidence-based process. If practitioners are set to work on improving care in an area that is known to be a clinical problem, however, they will respond much more positively and will see it as a chance to test themselves against real clinical challenges. One must ensure that practitioners feel supported and capable of working with the evidence they have gathered and, if not, that they have access to experienced help.

KNOWLEDGE TRANSFER NEEDS THE INVOLVEMENT OF ALL STAKEHOLDERS

Ho, Bloch, et al. (2004) described a push-down and pull-up system (KT cycle) in which all stakeholders work together. They described three key groups in the health care system that possess different types of valuable information and therefore must work together as a system to pass knowledge along:

1. Knowledge producers (the community of researchers)
2. Knowledge consumers (the community of practice—clinicians)
3. Knowledge beneficiaries (the community of patients)

Although research can inform practice, the reverse is also very important, whereby patients inform research about the most relevant issues. Practitioners are in the middle, linking the two ends together. KT strategies need to keep in mind the needs of patients at all times (Ho, Bloch, et al., 2004).

Factors influencing the process of KT can be conceptualized in a matrix model. KT is initiated either by knowledge producers or the system in a push configuration or by knowledge consumers and beneficiaries in a pull operation. In the former case, practitioners remain in a passive role as information receivers. In the latter case, the practitioner is actively seeking specific information.

SPECIFIC RESEARCH TRANSFER STRATEGIES

As was mentioned previously, when a practitioner is undertaking a research transfer project, he or she will need to be able to teach others what he or she found when finished. It was also stated that conventional speech and print methods were found to be inadequate for effective, long-lasting research transfer. Research transfer dissemination strategies, which are more effective, are those that conform to the personal learning needs of the researcher and utilize two or more different approaches simultaneously.

Evidence from randomized controlled trials and systematic reviews, which examined practitioners' habits, indicates that there is no one optimal way to disseminate knowledge to other practitioners. In their powerful article, "No Magic Bullets: A Systematic Review of 102 Trials of Interventions to Improve Professional Practice," Oxman, Thomson, Davis, and Haynes (1995) concluded that "there are no 'magic bullets' for improving the quality of health care, but there are a wide range of interventions available that, if used appropriately, could lead to important improvements in professional practice and patient outcomes" (p. 142). These interventions can include provision of educational materials through conferences, visits, or mail; use of local opinion leaders; audit and feedback; electronic reminders; provision of materials directly to patients; and many forms of direct marketing.

Specific combinations of KT strategies must be made to suit the content being disseminated. Strategies such as using local opinion leaders, audit and feedback, and reminders are discussed in this chapter as well as later articles by Oxman and coworkers and show that research transfer works well when personalized to individuals practitioners' needs (Jamtvedt, Young, Kristoffersen, O'Brien, & Oxman, 2006; O'Brien et al., 1999; Oxman et al., 1995). A recent Cochrane Collaboration review indicated that audit and feedback work best (changes ranging from –10% to 70%) when the baseline adherence to procedures or intervention protocols is low and when the feedback is provided more intensively (Jamtvedt et al., 2006). Continuing education can lead to small changes in practice, particularly if sessions use mixed interactive and didactic learning strategies and focus on outcomes that are considered relevant and serious by the attendees (Forsetlund et al., 2009).

The Provincial Centre of Excellence for Child and Youth Mental Health at the Children's Hospital of Eastern Ontario, Canada has published a toolkit for knowledge transfer entitled "Doing More With What You Know: A Toolkit on Knowledge Exchange." This toolkit is an excellent source of knowledge and includes frameworks for KT, checklists to follow, scenarios, and several suggested vehicles for KT. The overall message of the toolkit is that KT "takes innovative and creating thinking." Five key strategies for KT that can all include the production of lay summaries, introducing online forums, inviting media, and linking researchers with patients/clinicians are as follows:

1. Cultural approach: Using artifacts or symbols to get information across. For example, storytelling and socializing can be a great way to affect tacit knowledge.

2. Multisector partnerships: Bring different organizations/strengths together.

3. Conferences/conference leverage: Good place to push out and pull in knowledge.

4. Research summaries: Specific to a wide range of stakeholders.

5. Supportive infrastructures within organizations.

The article also summarizes necessary processes that effect KT. Working together in partnerships, building capacity, writing in plain language, and evaluating KT approaches are highlighted.

Specific types of interpersonal channels that have shown some positive effects on knowledge uptake in practice settings are as follows:

*   Two-way communications (e.g., interactive workshops) where clinicians are actively involved as opposed to one-way sessions (which have not shown positive change).

*   Information presented by local opinion leaders.

*   Educational outreach visits by trained people to clinicians.

*   Problem-based learning groups (clinicians work together to solve problems).

A further application of research transfer dissemination strategies is through organizations known as journal clubs. Long popular with physicians, journal clubs are a group of practitioners who split up the literature to be read, with each person focusing on one particular article, journal, or group of journals. When the journal club convenes, practitioners summarize and present what they have garnered from their reading to the other participants, thereby cutting down the amount of slogging through the medical literature that must be done by each practitioner. Jaan Siderov (1995) wrote an article in which he meta-analyzed the habits of 131 journal clubs for medical residents. His main conclusions were that the crucial elements that make a good journal club include mandatory attendance from participants, meetings with the provision of food, fewer full staff attending (thus giving students the feeling of greater freedom to debate and discuss without being evaluated), and a modest size to preclude feelings of exclusion.

Finally, technology-enabled knowledge translation (TEKT) or information and communication technology has been shown to be an effective method of pushing out evidence (Davis et al., 2003; Ho, Bloch, et al., 2004; Ho, Lauscher, et al., 2004). Examples are handheld PDAs that give physicians immediate access to knowledge and technologies that provide summaries of evidence. Ho, Lauscher, et al. (2004) stated that the use of technology as a vehicle for KT may be extremely useful because technology can do the following:

*   Assist practitioners with access and uptake of information.

*   Improve the uptake of research in policy making because it speeds up the KT process.

*   Facilitate the transfer of public data (e.g., national health surveys) to policy makers more quickly.

*   Can support communities of practice where groups share knowledge and information regarding specific topic(s) of interest.

In their article "Technology-Enabled Knowledge Translation: Frameworks to Promote Research and Practice," Ho, Bloch, et al. (2004) discussed a framework for implementing TEKT as well as evaluation and dissemination methodologies. The framework focuses on measuring the effectiveness of KT across several dimensions—structural, subjective, cognitive, behavioral, and systemic use. Although the importance of TEKT has been recognized and will likely be the way of the future, few innovative technologies have been developed in general and none have been developed for rehabilitation.

Information from a conference organized by the Canadian Research Transfer Network (2001) is useful in helping therapists and researchers focus the most effective strategies for KT. These strategies, as outlined in the following sections, center on engaging the audience, constructing a clear message, and ensuring effective delivery. In terms of the audience, it is important to focus on the information they want or need, tailor messages according to the group you are trying to reach and according to the values that are important to that group, and speak in terms of what you think they "need to know" rather than what they "ought to know." A good way to achieve these goals is to involve members of the audience in each step of the KT process. The message also needs to be valuable to the audience. It should be tangible, compelling, and clear. It is wise to spread the message to different groups so that word of mouth will continue to pass the information along to people or areas you may not have considered. When delivering the message, a fellow stakeholder who is trusted is the best type of messenger. The messenger should speak the same language as the audience (do not use too much jargon or technical wording) and listen to the audience. It is important to go at their pace and remember that creating new policies takes time.

EVIDENCE-BASED POLICY

Evidence-based policy is a relatively new field of study in the realm of EBP. Evidence-based medicine (EBM) and the work of Dr. Archie Cochrane were the inspirations for the movement; however, all of the evidence gathered and analyzed for EBM was concentrated on better patient care. The idea that evidence could be used on policy successes and failures could be gathered in the same way did not initially pique the same outpouring of interest and work, but it is becoming increasingly important. Hanney, Gonzalez, Block, Buxton, and Kogan (2003) stated, "Policy-making can be viewed as involving the 'authoritative allocation of values,' and when interpreted broadly can include people making the policy as government ministers and officials, as local health service managers, or as representatives of a professional body" (p. 3). Nutley, Davies, and Walter (2002) noted that "policy making is always inherently political" (p. 1).

Bowen and Zwi (2005), in an article entitled "Evidence-Informed Policy and Practice Pathway," discussed the place of evidence in the policy-making process. Figure 9-2 details the framework used for the various political and rapidly changing factors that go into the decision-making process.

There are reasons why evidence-based policy has been slow to catch on. The material we have covered in EBP up to this point has been primarily logical, rational processes. This makes sense, because EBP is an attempt to introduce a more systematic approach to the use of health care knowledge. When entering into the realm of evidence-based policy, however, logic cannot always be trusted. The creation of policy from research findings is a fundamentally different exercise than the careful synthesis and analysis of academic data. EBP, as a process, is based on individual or small-group consideration of knowledge and research information. In contrast, evidence-based policy is based on the consideration of health care research by large groups that must come to a consensus and by those who may not be experts in the field; namely, managers and policy makers. As such, processes that worked in EBP cannot necessarily be completely replicated in the creation of policy.

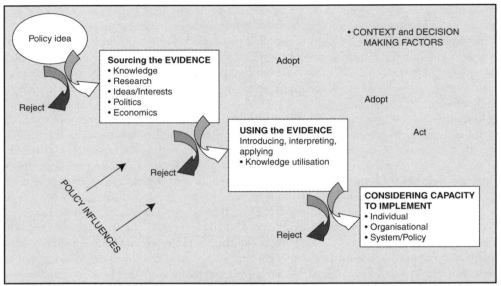

Figure 9-2. The evidence-informed policy and practice pathway. (From "Pathways to 'Evidence-Informed' Policy and Practice: A Framework for Action" by S. Bowen, A. B. Zwi, 2005, *PLoS Med 2*(7): e166. doi:10.1371/journal. pmed.0020166. Reprinted with permission.)

MODELS OF KNOWLEDGE TRANSFER INTO POLICY

One of the major obstacles to policy being made along evidence-based lines is the fact that the two contributors to policy—scientists and managers—perceive and value research differently. A good example of this problem was given by Dr. Francois Champagne, a researcher at Quebec's Université de Montréal. Presenting at a 1999 conference in Toronto, Dr. Champagne discussed the differences by proposing that evidence-based policy making can be perceived through two fundamentally different models (Champagne, 1999).

The first, which Champagne calls the *knowledge-driven model*, is one that makes sense in a rationally determined environment. It follows five steps:

1. Research (basic, then applied)
2. Technological development
3. Use (adoption of technology)
4. Quality of implemented actions
5. Outcome

This model is the view most commonly held by scientists who work primarily in the first steps of the model, doing research that could be directed toward certain ends. This model is built on several inherent assumptions. The knowledge-driven model assumes that once new knowledge exists, it will naturally be pressed toward use. In evidence-based policy making, however, this is not necessarily the case. "Perfect knowledge" would be required for policy making to work in this way.

Perfect knowledge implies that all evidence is applied in exactly the most beneficial way. This rests on the idea that policy makers and scientists are able to omnisciently see exactly where basic and applied research could be put to use. Furthermore, it assumes that all relevant knowledge will be adopted in its field without impediments. Unfortunately, however, there are many factors standing in the way of research being used in this manner. Basic and applied research is distributed in health care journals, which grow in number and size each month. Scientists and policy makers are not able to sort through all of the new knowledge or see how it could be applied to their work; thus, new findings sometimes go unused. Even when evidence and research findings are identified as important, the process of implementing them into policy is often a long and difficult one. Even the best evidence can be doomed by hasty decision making, poor presentation, or political reasons. There are often reasons other than evidence that support implementation of specific policies. This leads to an important truth of evidence-based policy making: management, or the creation of new policies from research, is inherently based in its context. The environment in which policy is made has a strong hand in shaping its eventual outcome.

A second model of evidence-based policy making, known as the *problem-driven model*, takes an alternative approach to the process and avoids some of the idealism of the knowledge-based model (Champagne, 1999). Realizing the contextual nature of health care policy, this model does not begin with research but rather with a problem or question.

This model, a view more commonly held by managers, suggests that evidence-based policy is made according to the following logic:

- Definition of problem
- Identification of missing knowledge
- Acquisition of knowledge through various possible channels
- Interpretation for the problem situation
- Use (adoption of technology)

In the problem-driven model, once a problem or information need has been understood, policy makers decide which evidence they will require and use various channels to obtain it. Furthermore, both of the channels by which the model suggests that research knowledge is obtained take note of realities. In the problem-driven model, research findings will generally come from either a pool of knowledge already available to policy makers or through commissioned research into a specific problem. This understanding of the realities of how research findings come to practice acknowledges the fact that evidence distribution is not always perfect and that policy makers do tend to draw upon knowledge already available to them. Once policy makers have the research they require, they will interpret it for the situation at hand and finally use it.

The problem-driven model approximates the "real" processes of policy making better than the knowledge-driven model, but why is that? Why do scientists tend to believe that evidence will be used in a different way than managers do? Investigation into this problem has shown that different groups perceive how research should be used in different ways. In a 1981 article, Weiss and Weiss posed the question, "What is meant by using research for policy making?" (p. 846). Though seemingly simple, this question is central to the issue, because it highlights the differences of opinion between groups (researchers and policy makers) and reasons why misunderstandings do occur.

What Weiss and Weiss (1981) found is that researchers see the use of evidence in policy as a fundamentally rational, linear process. When new evidence is published, they feel that it should, and will be, expediently put to use in the most applicable field. Decision makers, on the other hand, see a greater and more varied number of ways to use research and are less willing to act on specific pieces of research alone. Much more is required than just top-notch research for policy makers to implement evidence into policy. They see evidence-based policy making as a holistic, multifaceted, nonlinear process. Champagne (1999) summarized that "researchers and decision makers belong to separate communities with different values and different ideologies and [thus] these differences impede utilization."

Decision making in complex situations is not necessarily a rational process; decision makers and managers draw in a great deal of evidence and assess it in a holistic manner. Instead of affording

Table 9-1		
Contextual/Systematic Differences for Researchers, Clinical Practitioners, and Administrative and Legislative Decision Makers		
CONTEXT/SETTING	**TYPES OF EVIDENCE PREFERRED**	**COMMUNICATION FORMATS USED**
Research		
Universities; private sector; discipline oriented; long-term time frames	Original research; peer reviewed; scientific > qualitative; basic > applied research	Academic journals; academic meeting; Internet
Clinical		
Community practice; clinical management; patient oriented; short-term time frames	Practical summaries; clinical application; patient preferences; applied > basic research	Colleagues/conferences; summaries/reviews; audit/feedback; professional journals
Administrative		
Public agencies; program oriented; population oriented; varying time frames	Practical summaries; program evaluations; cost effectiveness; applied > basic research	Summaries/reviews; personal contacts; conferences/meeting; Internet, journals, media
Legislative		
Elected fora; problem oriented; responsive to crises; varying time frames	Problem summaries; policy solution; cost effectiveness; anecdotal > scientific	Staff briefings; personals contacts; polls; constituents; media

Reprinted with permission from "So Much Research Evidence, So Little Dissemination and Uptake: Mixing the Useful With the Pleasing," by C. Waddell. (2002). *Evidence Based Nursing*, 5(38), p. 39.

evidence weight based purely on its methodology and scientific rigor, policy makers are much more apt to take in and consider a great deal of evidence simultaneously, sometimes placing more emphasis on proximate sources, the opinions of local experts, etc. They also generalize the results of many studies together, working with this accumulated evidence. Finally, managers may not always use research purely for the purposes of making the best policy. As Champagne (1999) said, they may use knowledge "deliberately, politically, tactically, and conceptually" to manipulate or work within the context of their policy environment.

Table 9-1, from Charlotte Waddell's (2002) article, shows the differences in the types of evidence that the various decision-making groups prefer. Table 9-2 lists the different types of evidence that policy makers use.

CHALLENGES OF MOVING EVIDENCE INTO POLICY

Does the complexity of the policy-making process mean that EBP fundamentally breaks down during its final stage? Not necessarily. Although evidence-based policy making is not necessarily a linear exercise, it can still yield valid and useful conclusions. Therefore, is there anything that health care professionals can do to influence policy makers to use our high-quality evidence?

Table 9-2

Types of Evidence and How They Are Used in Policy Making

TYPES OF EVIDENCE	INFORMATION AND INFLUENCE ON DECISION MAKING
Research	• Empirical evidence from randomized control and other trials • Analytic studies such as cohort or case control studies • Time series analyses • Observations, experiences, and case reports • Qualitative studies • Before and after studies
Knowledge and information	• Results of consultation processes with networks/group • Internet • Published documents/reports (including policy evaluation and statistical analyses)
Ideas and interests	• Opinion and view—"expert knowledge" of individuals, groups, networks (shaped by past personals and professional experiences, beliefs, values, skills)
Politics	• Information relevant to the agenda of government • Political risk assessment and saleability • Opportunity • Crises
Economics	• Finance and resource implication • Cost effectiveness or other forms of economic evaluation • Opportunity cost

Reprinted with permission from "Pathways to 'Evidence-Informed' Policy and Practice: A Framework for Action" by Bowen S., & Zwi A.B. (2005). *PLoS Med 2*(7): e166. doi:10.1371/journal.pmed.0020166.

Dobbins et al. (2002) suggested that "tailoring" evidence to fit the needs and desires of policy makers is a good way to get evidence heard. They looked specifically at systematic overviews of research and how to get decision makers to agree to them. Decision makers, it must be remembered, have specific needs for the evidence they use. Among these, as Champagne (1999) said, is the need for data to be available, accessible, and valid. Without these characteristics, even the most methodically rigorous study is liable to be given less importance than it may deserve.

> Even when the evidence about outcomes and effectiveness is clear, local circumstances dictate how that evidence is translated into practice. Opportunities have recently emerged to share evidence globally about the outcomes and effectiveness of health care (globalization) and then translate that evidence into improved heath care at the local level (localization). To succeed in globalizing the evidence, policy makers must realize that opportunities to do so will be tempered by three competing core values: choice, efficiency, and equity. (Elsenberg, 2002, p. 166)

Chunharas (2006) discussed the complexity of the knowledge chain and stated that KT for policy works best if a learning organization is built within the health services and policy field. His definition of a learning organization is an environment "structured in such as way as to facilitate learning as well as the sharing of knowledge among members or employees" (p. 652). Characteristics of a learning organization include the regular sharing of information among colleagues, ensuring that the environment of the organization is considered in the transfer of knowledge and a focus on developing a problem-solving cycle as the best means to use knowledge for management and policy decisions.

The author reported the following types of knowledge that are used by health services decision makers:

- Information from their own organization via policies and guidelines about how to deal with and decide upon certain issues.

- Information from their own personal experience, knowledge, or discipline.

- Information from research evidence. (According to Chunharas [2006], this type of information is relied upon least often by decision makers. Reasons for this are similar to the reasons clinicians find it difficult to use EBP.)

Nuyens and Lansang (2006, p. 590) wrote an editorial that summarizes lessons from knowledge translation initiatives at the national level. The five lessons that they referred to are as follows:

1. The systems context is extremely important.

2. Continuity between past, current, and future research is important.

3. "Complexity should be considered"—KT messages need to be modified for the intended recipient.

4. The various stakeholders should be involved in the KT process (knowledge brokers can be used to aid this process).

5. KT efforts need to pay more attention to increasing the skills and competencies needed to transfer the information ("capacity strengthening") and not just pay attention to the information itself.

In addition to macrolevel work on evidence-based policy which attempts to understand the entire system, there are also smaller steps that have been taken toward moving research into policy. By examining the literature on evidence-based policy, common trends of the field can be understood. The first article to consider appeared in the journal *Health Policy* and discussed practice guidelines. The authors (Lohr, Eleazer, & Mauskopf, 1998) contended that practice guidelines are the main format of evidence-based policy today. A practice guideline consists of a series of clinical recommendations or dictates on an issue assembled from the best possible evidence. Practice guidelines are distributed by national clearinghouses to avoid conflict between them and to allow care to be standardized to one high standard. Guidelines are discussed in detail in Chapter 10.

The five steps for KT into policy are as follows (Tugwell, Robinson, Grimshaw, & Santesso, 2006, p. 645):

1. Barriers and facilitators. Assess values, awareness, resources (e.g., skills, financial, human) for the following six *P*s by socioeconomic status (SES): public, patient, press, practitioner, policy maker, and private sector.

2. Prioritize modifiable barriers across six *P*s by SES.

3. Choose KT interventions to address key barriers. adapt evidence-based actionable messages, tailored for relevant audiences by SES.

4. Knowledge transfer effectiveness. Evaluate both process and health outcomes using appropriate study designs by SES.

5. Knowledge management and sharing. Dissemination, diffusion, and application to other clinical conditions for six *P*s.

Birch (1997) has discussed whether there are characteristics of organizations themselves that can make them more open to considering new policies. Champagne (1999) has worked on the question and suggested that there are. Organizations that have an informal atmosphere, specialize in a particular field of knowledge, and participate in interorganizational networks of knowledge sharing are most likely to adopt new innovations and recommendations with greater ease. In conventional institutions, problems with adopting new ideas may arise such as the resistance of established health care professionals to new ideas due to their familiarity with the old. In more informal and less hierarchical systems, however, practitioners are more apt to feel as if they have a stake in shaping the use of a policy for their institution; therefore, they may be more willing to follow it.

A comprehensive discussion of EBP guidelines can be found in Gray, Haynes, Sackett, Cook, and Guyatt's (1997) article, "Transferring Evidence From Research Into Practice." Evidence-based policy and clinical guidelines, however, will be most apparent when examined on a case-by-case basis in which the blend of research and politics is evident. A good rule of thumb for all evidence-based policy making is that policies must apply to a wide range of people, be adaptable to the needs of local practitioners, and keep the best evidence at hand while spurring on toward future research.

TAKE-HOME MESSAGES

Research Transfer Into Practice

✓ New innovations to replace usual transfer of research using widespread print media and large conferences.

✓ Research transfer can be achieved through preparing practitioners to gather and assimilate new information, interpret this knowledge so that it can be used, and reflect on its actual use.

✓ Effective research transfer dissemination strategies conform to the personal learning needs of the researcher and utilize at least two different strategies simultaneously.

Evidence-Based Policy

✓ Not always a logical process but based on the considerations of health care policy research and the consensus of a group who may not always be experts.

✓ Knowledge-driven model: Requires perfect knowledge and assumes that knowledge will be adopted without impediment; unrealistic.

✓ Problem-driven model: Alternative approach; begins with a problem rather than research; acknowledges that evidence distribution is not always perfect and that policy makers tend to draw upon currently available information.

✓ Practice guidelines: Consist of series of clinical recommendations that have been assembled from the best possible evidence.

✓ Researchers see evidence in policy as a fundamentally linear and rational process; decision makers see more variety and are less likely to act on a single piece of evidence.

WEB LINKS

What Is a Critically Appraised Topic?

http://www.cebm.net/index.aspx?o=1216

This page at the CEBM is a great overview on critically appraised topics, including how they work and how they are put together.

United States Agency for Health Care Policy and Research

www.ahcpr.gov

This site has a great deal of information on health care policy as well as a list of practice guidelines that can be downloaded and examined.

Canadian Health Services Research Foundation

www.chsrf.ca

Contains information on KT as well as research summary information and ways to access research-based evidence.

The Provincial Centre of Excellence for Child and Youth Mental Health at the Children's Hospital of Eastern Ontario

www.onthepoint.ca

Toolkit to support KT as well as online forum.

LEARNING AND EXPLORATION ACTIVITIES

The purpose of this chapter is to build upon the previous methods of organizing evidence in order to demonstrate the methods for transferring that evidence into practice and policy. These exercises highlight various sections of the chapter through leading the student through exercises both as an individual and as a group, which allow opportunities to utilize this understanding of the different types of evidence.

1. Research Transfer Into Practice

   a. What methods work best when transferring research findings? Oxman et al.'s (1995) chart suggests a number of ways of transferring research. Can you think of any more? Why would some be better than others? Which kind of learners are they primarily aimed at? Is there a way to make research transfer strategies that speak equally well to many different learning styles?

   b. Try out your own research transfer. Choose a field and find a piece of previously (to your knowledge) unapplied research. Through careful examination of the research conclusions, determine which parts of the research can be transferred into practice, and develop ways to do this (again, Oxman et al.'s [1995] methodologies will help here). If working in a group, each participant may attempt this exercise, and all can take turns at teaching others what they have found. Whose research transfer strategy worked the best (was memorable for the most people)? Why is this?

2. Evidence-Based Policy

   a. This exercise will take some preparation and is best attempted in a group. Choose a topic of clinical interest and find a current clinical policy related to it. In the reference list of the policy should be a list of articles and academic sources used in its creation. Find two or three of the articles on this list and assign one to each group member. Have each person read both the policy and their assigned article and then convene together as a group. How was each person's article reflected in the policy? Which articles received more or less weight? Why might this have been? Does this policy make good use of current knowledge?

   b. Attempt the same exercise in reverse: Find a number of articles on a subject and convene a policy conference around them. You will probably want to assign one article to each person and have him or her argue for it in the conference, as well as designating some nonaligned administrators and decision makers. Even more complex (and interesting) would be if every member of the group was given a specific interest that he or she was to support during the meeting but that he or she could not directly reveal to others. After you have finished the exercise, evaluate your performance. How did you interact in the conference? What forms of discussion worked best? Were everyone's needs met to their satisfaction? Who "won"?

REFERENCES

Birch, S. (1997). As a matter of fact—Evidence-based decision making unplugged. *Health Economics, 6,* 547–559.

Bowen, S., & Zwi, A. B. (2005). Pathways to evidence informed policy and practice: A framework for action. *PLos Medicine, 2*(7), e166.

Canadian Institutes of Health Research. (2008). *Knowledge translation strategy 2004–2009.* Retrieved from www.cihr-irsc.gc.ca/e/26574.html#defining

Canadian Research Transfer Network. (2001). Knowledge transfer: Looking beyond health. Retrieved from www.chsrf.ca/knowledge_transfer/resources_e.php

Champagne, F. (1999). *The use of scientific evidence and knowledge by managers: Closing the loop.* Paper presented at the Third International Conference, Toronto, ON.

Chunharas, S. (2006). An interactive and integrative approach to translating knowledge and building a "learning organization" in health services management. *Bulletin of the World Health Organization, 84*(8), 652–657.

Dalton, C. C., & Gottlieb, L. N. (2003). The concept of readiness to change. *Journal of Advanced Nursing, 42*(2), 108–117.

Davies, H. T. O., & Nutley, S. M. (2002). *Evidence-based policy and practice: Moving from rhetoric to reality* (Discussion Paper 2). St Andrews, Scotland: Research Unit for Research Utilisation, University of St. Andrews.

Davis, D., Evans, M., Jadad, A., Perrier, L., Rath, D., Ryan, D., et al. (2003). The case for knowledge translation: Shortening the journey from evidence to effect. *British Medical Journal, 327*(7405), 33–35.

Dobbins, M., Ciliska, D., Cockerill, R., Barnsley, J., & DiCenso, A. (2002). A framework for the dissemination and utilization of research for health care policy and practice. *Online Journal of Knowledge Synthesis for Nursing, 9*(7).

Elsenberg, J. M. (2002). Globalize the evidence, localize the decision: Evidence-based medicine and international diversity. *Health Affairs, 21*(5), 166–168.

Forsetlund, L., Bjørndal, A., Rashidian, A., Jamtvedt, G., O'Brien, M.A., Wolf, F., …, Oxman, A. D. (2009). Continuing education meetings and workshops: effects on professional practice and health care outcomes. *Cochrane Database of Systematic Reviews, 2,* CD003030. doi:10.1002/14651858.CD003030.pub2

Graham, I. D., Logan, J., Harrison, M. B., Straus, S. E., Tetroe, J., Caswell, W., & Robinson, N. (2006). Lost in knowledge translation: Time for a map. *Journal of Continuing Education in the Health Professions, 26*(1), 13–24.

Gray, J. A., Haynes, R. B., Sackett, D. L., Cook, D. J., & Guyatt, G. H. (1997). Transferring evidence from research into practice: 3. Developing evidence-based clinical policy. *Evidence-Based Medicine, 2*(2), 36–38.

Hanney, S. R., Gonzalez-Block, M. A., Buxton, M. J., & Kogan, M. (2003). The utilization of health research in policy-making: Concepts, examples and methods of assessment. *Health Research and Policy Systems, 1*(2). Retrieved from http://www.ncbi.nlm.nih.gov/pmc/articles/PMC151555/

Ho, K., Bloch, R., Gondocz, T., Laprise, R., Perrier, L., Ryan, D., et al. (2004). Technology enabled-knowledge translation: Frameworks to promote research and practice. *Journal of Continuing Education in the Health Professions, 24*(2), 90–99.

Ho, K., Lauscher, H. N., Best, A., Jervis-Selinger, S., Fedeles, M., & Chockalingam, A. (2004). Dissecting technology-enabled knowledge translation: Essential challenges, unprecedented opportunities. *Clinical and Investigative Medicine, 27*(2), 70–78.

Jamtvedt, G., Young, J. M., Kristoffersen, D. T., O'Brien, M. A., & Oxman, A. D. (2006). Audit and feedback: Effects on professional practice and health care outcomes. *Cochrane Database of Systematic Reviews, 2,* CD000259. doi:10.1002/14651858.CD000259.pub2

Kerns, R. D., & Habib, S. (2004). A critical review of the pain readiness to change model. *Journal of Pain, 5*(7), 357–367.

Kurtovich, E., Ivey, S. L., Neuhauser, L., Graham, C., Constantine, W., & Barkan, H. (2010). A multilingual mass communication intervention for seniors and people with disabilities on Medicaid: A randomized controlled trial. *Health Services Research, 45*(2), 397–417.

Lohr, K. N., Eleazer, K., & Mauskopf, J. (1998). Health policy issues and applications for evidence-based medicine and clinical practice guidelines. *Health Policy, 46*, 1–19.

Nutley, S., Davies, H., & Walter, I. (2002). *Evidence based policy and practice: Cross sector lessons from the UK* (Working Paper 9). St. Andrews, Scotland: Research Unit for Research Utilisation Department of Management, University of St. Andrews.

Nuyens, Y., & Lansang, M. A. D. (2006). Knowledge translation: Linking the past to the future. *Bulletin of the World Health Organization, 84*(8), 590–591.

O'Brien, M. A., Oxman, A. D., Haynes, R. B., Davis, D. A., Freemantle, N., & Harvey, E. L. (1999). Local opinion leaders: Effects on professional practice and health care outcomes. *Cochrane Database of Systematic Reviews, 1,* CD000125. doi:10.1002/14651858.CD000125

Oxman, A. D., Thomson, M. A., Davis, D. A., & Haynes, R. B. (1995). No magic bullets: A systematic review of 102 trials of interventions to improve professional practice. *Canadian Medical Association Journal, 153*(10), 1423–1431.

The Provincial Centre of Excellence for Child and Youth Mental Health at the Children's Hospital of Eastern Ontario. (2006). *Doing more with what you know: A toolkit on knowledge exchange.* Retrieved from www.onthepoint.ca

Rogers, E. M. (1995). *Diffusion of innovations* (4th ed.). New York, NY: The Free Press.

Sherman, M. D., & Carothers, R. A. (2005). Applying the readiness to change model to implementation of family intervention for serious mental illness. *Community Mental Health Journal, 41*(2), 115–127.

Siderov, J. (1995). How are internal medicine residency journal clubs organized and what makes them successful? *Archives of Internal Medicine, 155*, 1193–1197.

Tetroe, J. M., Graham, I. D., & Scott, V. (2011). What does it mean to transform knowledge into action in falls prevention research? Perspectives from the Canadian Institutes of Health Research. *Journal of Safety Research, 42*(6), 423–426.

Tugwell, P., Robinson, V., Grimshaw, J., & Santesso, N. (2006). Systematic reviews and knowledge translation. *Bulletin of the World Health Organization, 84*(8), 643–651.

Waddell, C. (2002). So much research evidence, so little dissemination and uptake: Mixing the useful with the pleasing. *Evidence Based Nursing, 5*(38), 38–40.

Weiss, C. H., & Weiss, J. A. (1981). Social scientists and decision makers look at the usefulness of mental health research. *American Psychologist, 36*(8), 837–847.

Suggested Reading

Teplicky, R. (2005). *Facilitating the use of family-centred service in a children's rehabilitation centre.* Hamilton, ON: McMaster University.

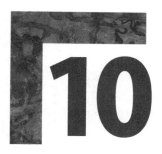

10

STRATEGIES TO BUILD EVIDENCE INTO PRACTICE

Mary Law, PhD, OT Reg (Ont), FCAHS and
Joy C. MacDermid, PhD, PT Reg (Ont), FCAHS

LEARNING OBJECTIVES

After reading this chapter, the student/practitioner will be able to:

- Develop an understanding of building evidence for practice of how to incorporate evidence into clinical practice.

- Apply strategies to limit the influence of potential barriers to the implementation of evidence-based practice (EBP).

- Understand the different tools available to enhance EBP such as critically appraised topics (CATs), critically appraised papers (CAPs), EBP resource sites, "push" e-mail programs, and other technologies (e.g., literature-searching services).

- Identify the essential components and different types of CATs.

- Understand and explain the use of CATs in EBP.

Using EBP as an occupational therapist or a physical therapist means processing and organizing a lot of information from the research literature. This task can seem quite challenging in a busy practice setting (Law, Pollock, & Stewart, 2004). Each time you use your evidence evaluation skills (i.e., identifying new clinical questions, searching for relevant studies in the literature, and integrating your findings into practice), you will be exposed to vast amounts of information which can seem overwhelming. Instead of inundating yourself with evidence about the many interventions that could be used, it is vital that you implement strategies to quickly locate the evidence you require. Remember that EBP is not only about using research evidence, but about using it in partnership with excellent clinical reasoning and paying close attention to the client's stated goals, needs, and values.

Law M., & MacDermid, J. C.
Evidence-Based Rehabilitation: A Guide
to Practice, Third Edition (pp 205–231).
© 2014 SLACK Incorporated.

IMPLEMENTATION MODELS

Researchers have proposed models or strategies to help therapists implement EBP more efficiently and effectively. Some of these models have been outlined in this section.

In describing evidence-based medicine, the originators described a five-step process (Sackett, 1997; Sackett, Straus, Richardson, Rosenberg, & Haynes, 2000):

1. Convert your information needs into answerable questions.

2. Track down, with maximum efficiency, the best evidence with which to answer them.

3. Critically appraise that evidence for its validity and usefulness.

4. Integrate this appraisal with your clinical expertise and apply it in practice.

5. Evaluate your performance.

A similar step-by-step model for therapists to follow has been suggested by several researchers (Corcoran, 2006; Law et al., 2004; Tickle-Degnan, 2000). Once a clinical problem or issue is identified, the therapist can carry out the following steps:

1. Write a clinical question/formulate a relevant practice question.

2. Search for evidence related to the question.

3. Evaluate/critically appraise evidence to determine the evidence that best informs the clinical question.

4. Speak with the client and his or her family and decide in partnership with them whether to act upon the evidence.

5. Evaluate the outcomes of these actions.

6. Save the evidence-based information you have acquired for future reference for you and your colleagues; post this information on a Web site (e.g., www.otevidence.info).

When formulating the practice question (Step 1), it is helpful to break it down into components (Bennett & Bennett, 2000). For example, think about the primary client; the rehabilitation and health issues; the desired outcome; and whether the focus of the practice encounter is assessment, intervention, or both (Law et al., 2004). The various components can help you formulate different search words to use in the literature search (Bennett & Bennett, 2000). A strategy that can be used to define clinical questions is the P.I.C.O. approach, where P = the patient (type), I = intervention of interest, C = the comparison choice/intervention, and O = the outcome of interest. Differentiating these can help define specific clinical research questions.

When searching for evidence (Step 2), it may be necessary to search multiple databases, redesign your search for each database, and use thesaurus terms and text searches. Refer back to Chapter 5 for detailed search strategies. When determining whether to act upon the evidence (Step 4), clinicians should determine whether the evidence "fits" with the features of the client's context (personal skills/values/preferences, living environment, and daily activities/demands). Factors such as the environment in which the client lives as well as his or her cultural beliefs, priorities, and values ultimately determine the usefulness of research evidence for informing clinical practice. Consideration is also given to the practice setting, clinical expertise, and resources available to the therapist.

In 1999, Rosswurm and Larrabee proposed a model for EBP that guided practitioners through the process, from determining the clinical question to integrating the new protocol into practice. Their proposed process is composed of the following steps (Figure 10-1):

1. Assess: The practitioner's assessment of the need for change is the first step in the process. The impetus for change can arise from questions that arise during patient interactions or from patient dissatisfaction, new research findings, or quality improvement data.

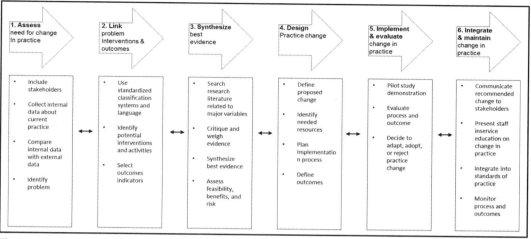

Figure 10-1. A model for evidence-based practice. (From "A Model for Change to Evidence-Based Practice," by M. A. Rosswurm, & J. H. Larrabee, 1999, *Journal of Nursing Scholarship, 31*(4), pp. 317-322. Reprinted with permission.)

2. Link: Practitioners need to use a common language to define their clinical issue in order to provide common language to link with other disciplines and identify potential interventions.

3. Synthesis: The next step in the process involves searching for, critiquing, and synthesizing the best available evidence in combination with clinical judgment to determine the best options to consider.

4. Design practice change: Once the best intervention option is chosen, the practitioner must determine the resources available, plan the pilot implementation, and propose outcome measures to evaluate the change.

5. Implementation and evaluation: As the change is implemented, it is important to evaluate both the process and the outcome to determine whether the practice change has had the desired effect.

6. Integration and maintenance: If the change has been successful, it is important to involve relevant stakeholders to incorporate it into daily clinical practice. Continuing education and staff in-service are useful tools to help reinforce and maintain the new evidence-based change.

Corcoran (2006) included a step-by-step model *within* her concept about what busy practitioners need to do to incorporate evidence into practice. She said that "making positive changes requires attitude, knowledge and skills" (p. 127). In terms of attitude, Corcoran (2006) urged clinicians to consider the importance of staying current with and implementing literature to provide clients with the best possible treatments. Such practices also encompass a professional and ethical obligation toward continuous learning. In terms of knowledge, practitioners can learn about evidence and how to apply it. This is where the step-by-step model fits best. Finally, she stated that "you will need to develop skills that make using evidence a vital part of everyday clinical reasoning" (Corcoran, 2006, p. 128). To do this one should do the following:

- Familiarize yourself with the EBP resources that are available via the Internet.
- Bookmark the sites that will help you quickly obtain the best information.
- Learn how to use keywords.
- Look for services that find information for you (these will be discussed later in this chapter).

Gillespie and Gillespie (2003) outlined a similar approach regarding where and how to find useful information. They suggested that clinicians can perfect the art of searching by moving through three stages of questioning:

1. Patient-focused questioning to ascertain specific functional problems

2. Primary research questioning

3. Secondary research questioning

They then suggested that clinicians become familiar with search terms, exploding/focusing terms, and combining terms and that they should learn to use search databases such as the Physiotherapy Evidence Database (PEDro) and the Cochrane Libraries. See Chapter 5 of this book for information on searching for evidence. Clinicians may find it useful to use the tutorials available on PubMed or from journal clubs to facilitate this learning.

Bennett and Bennett's (2000) model is based on the notion that EBP is a process that involves clinical expertise, relevant research, colleague support, and family and client choice. To integrate EBP into practice, clinicians must do the following:

- Ask a clinical question classified into diagnosis, treatment prevention, or prognosis.

- Formulate the question into P.I.C.O. (patient/disease, intervention, comparative intervention, outcome) and search the literature using that information. Hierarchies of evidence relevant to each question are presented. They cautioned users to focus on peer-reviewed journals.

- Critically appraise the evidence that you find by deciding whether the information is valid and clinically significant (see Chapter 6). This can be accomplished by asking four questions:

  ○ Do the results apply to my client?

  ○ Does the treatment fit into my client's values and preferences?

  ○ Do I have the resources to implement this treatment?

  ○ Do I have the training or skill necessary to implement these interventions?

McCluskey and Cusick (2002) believe that managers are extremely important to the implementation of EBP and may need to lead and support the change within an organization. Managers can facilitate the use of evidence in practice by championing its use and ensuring that EBP is a core value for their service. Support to therapists by managers promotes positive attitudes toward EBP and confirms that the use of evidence is valued by the organization. Managers can also work closely with therapists to identify real and potential barriers to implementation. Through strategic planning and the use of strengths, weaknesses, opportunities, and threats (SWOT) analyses, managers and therapists together can plan opportunities and strategies most suitable to the organization in order to facilitate EBP. In Chapter 3, extensive information about becoming an evidence-based practitioner is provided.

Remember, change takes time. According to Drake, Torrey, and McHugo (2003), there are three stages to implementing EBP:

1. Motivational or educational interventions to prepare for change.

2. Enabling or skill building interventions to enact a new practice.

3. Reinforcing, structuring, or financing interventions to sustain change.

As Drake et al. (2003) stated:

> Multifaceted changes that involve all stakeholders, rearrange daily workflow to support new practices and are reinforced by financing and regulatory strategies are more likely to succeed than those focusing exclusively on changing practitioners' behaviour. … Program implementation is most likely to be successful when it matches the values, needs and concerns of practitioners.

Factors within the change itself (e.g., quality, complexity, and clarity), the practitioner (e.g., experience, perceptions, and beliefs), the patient (e.g., expectations and preferences), and the practice context (e.g., resource availability, organizational culture, and opinion leaders) can all affect implementation success (Stergiou-Kita, 2010).

Specific information about what all stakeholders can do to help implement EBP will be discussed in this chapter. The taxonomy for strategies that can be used to characterize knowledge translation strategies can also be used to develop a strategy for implementing evidence in practice (see Appendix H).

EVIDENCE-BASED PRACTICE: BARRIERS AND SOLUTIONS

Bennett et al. (2003) studied the attitudes regarding EBP in a group of occupational therapists and found that though most participants felt that EBP was important and helpful in improving client care, they most frequently made decisions based on their clinical experience. Therefore, it is important to look at many of the common barriers to practicing EBP that people describe as well as effective solutions that have been put in place. Several research studies have found that the barriers and solutions that clinicians note to implementing EBP include the following.

Barriers

- Difficulty finding the time to search for evidence and then appraise and implement it (Bartlet et al., 2011; Bennett et al., 2003; Grimmer-Sommers, Lekkas, Nyland, Young, & Kumar, 2007; Iles & Davidson, 2006; Koehn & Lehman, 2008; Law et al., 2004; Nail-Chiwetalu & Bernstein Ratner, 2007; Schrieber, Stern, Marchetti, & Provident, 2009; Solomons & Spross, 2011; Upton & Upton, 2006).
- Limited quantity of evidence in specific practice areas (Bennett et al., 2003).
- Lack of resources such as staff shortages and money (Curtin & Jaramazovic, 2001; Upton & Upton, 2006).
- Insufficient quality of evidence (Herbert, Sherrtington, Maher, & Moseley, 2001).
- Lack of access to computers and journal articles that are needed to carry out EBP (Bennett et al., 2003; Curtin & Jaramazovic, 2001).
- Lack of training about EBP and how to carry it out (Curtin & Jaramazovic, 2001).
- The influence of personal factors (those who are self-motivated, have a personal interest in EBP, and are willing to work EBP into their work and personal time are more likely to actively use EBP; Curtin & Jaramazovic, 2001).
- Research does not provide certainty since findings cannot be applied to individual patients (Herbert et al., 2001).
- Clinical research does not tell of client's experiences (Herbert et al., 2001).
- Lack of clinical confidence in how to search for, interpret, and implement evidence (Brown, Tseng, Casey, McDonald, & Lyons, 2009; Grimmer-Somers et al., 2007; Iles & Davidson, 2006; Koehn & Lehman, 2008; Lyons, Brown, Tseng, Casey, & McDonald, 2011; Nail-Chiwetalu & Bernstein Ratner, 2007; Salbach et al., 2007).
- Lack of useful research summaries (Iles & Davidson, 2006).
- Lack of organizational support (Brown et al., 2009; Lyons et al., 2010; Salbach et al., 2007).

Solutions

- Support from managers (Curtin & Jaramazovic, 2001).
- Access to and effective distribution of relevant resources (Curtin & Jaramazovic, 2001).
- Personal factors (self-motivated, personal interest; Curtin & Jaramazovic, 2001).
- Postgraduate education was linked to greater use of current research literature (Bennett et al., 2003).
- The use of alerting services or technological services that push out evidence.
- Databases of preappraised evidence such as PEDro and OTSeeker.
- Availability of clinical trials and synthesized evidence such as systematic reviews, meta-analyses, practice guidelines. The role of clinical trials is to provide information about the size of treatment effects, not to tell whether something will or will not definitely work in every situation. Clinical trials cannot tell how an individual client will react to a therapy; however, they do give an idea of a likely result based on certain criteria.

In order to deal with these problems, clinicians need the support of mangers and to be given access to necessary resources such as computers, journals, and ongoing training (Curtin & Jaramazovic, 2001). Haynes (1998) suggested that managers and organizations should do the following:

- Produce policies for how to develop evidence-based clinical guidelines.
- Use information systems that integrate evidence and guidelines with patient care.
- Develop facilities and incentives to encourage effective care and better disease-management systems.
- Improve effectiveness of educational and quality improvement programs for practitioners.
- Implement technology designed for practice (Phillippi & Buxton, 2010).
- Point of care evidence summaries (Banzi, Liberati, Moschetti, Tagliabue, & Moja, 2010).

Therapists, in turn, need to make EBP a priority for themselves. They can be self-motivated and willing to spend some personal time learning to use EBP (Curtin & Jaramazovic, 2001) because the more time is spent searching, appraising, and applying evidence, the easier and therefore less time consuming it will become (Herbert et al., 2001). We also recognize that although time is reported as a common barrier, this is a surrogate for the priority given to EBP. When therapists see EBP as a strategy to provide effective and efficient care, time is less of a barrier.

Specific instructions for clinicians on how to overcome EBP barriers were given by Bennett and Bennett (2000, p. 178):

- Seek out continuing education opportunities.
- Make use of EBP resources such as Web sites and journal clubs.
- Participate in research evaluating interventions within your discipline.
- Participate in or establish a journal club.
- Seek out or contribute to evidence-based clinical practice guidelines.
- Negotiate work time to search and appraise research.

ISSUES RELATED TO SKILL LEVEL

A major problem reported by clinicians was a lack of skill level in finding, appraising, and applying research evidence. Clinicians do not always know how to determine the quality of the evidence or how it should be applied to their own practice. Bennett et al. (2003) found that most occupational therapists were confident in finding literature (60.8%) and determining the clinical significance of results (49.6%). They were less sure of how to determine study design (37%) and validity (37%) and using Cochrane databases (15%).

In addition to utilizing the implementation strategies discussed at the beginning of this chapter and looking for continuing education opportunities as discussed previously, therapists should familiarize themselves with the numerous EBP resources that are available. For example, the Internet contains EBP directories that provide access to articles and instructions on how to carry out EBP and free Web sites that give access to electronic databases and systematic reviews. There are also methods that help organize your search and that discover, summarize, evaluate, and even rank methodology and study implications for you (Bennett et al., 2003; Corcoran, 2006; Herbert et al., 2001). These and other methods for enhancing EBP will be discussed in detail later in this chapter.

ISSUES RELATED TO THE
QUANTITY AND QUALITY OF RESEARCH EVIDENCE

Within the research literature, there are areas where there is so much evidence that it can be overwhelming for clinicians because of both the amount and complexity of the research (Haynes, 1998). The amount of evidence available to therapists is growing daily. Therefore, it is very difficult for therapists to keep up with the research literature in their area of practice. There are also topic areas in which it is difficult to find any relevant research literature (Bennett & Bennett, 2003; Herbert et al., 2001). Finally, it has been found that clinicians feel that the quality of evidence is not always good enough (Herbert et al., 2001).

Again, in cases where there is too much information or complicated information or when you are unsure of the quality of the study methodology, make use of resources such as those that abstract, synthesize, and evaluate the information for you (Haynes, 1998). Keep practicing your EBP skills and continue to look for educational opportunities about research methods. In addition, it may be helpful to know that search databases, such as PEDro, have increased randomized controlled trials (RCTs) scores (from 3 to 5) in an attempt to weed out inferior studies (Herbert et al., 2001).

USING TECHNOLOGY TO SUPPORT EVIDENCE-BASED PRACTICE

Recent innovations in technology and the use of push-out services are changing this situation. New evidence-based services (such as electronic databases, systematic reviews, and journals that summarize evidence) are now being developed and will make accessing current best evidence feasible and easy in clinical settings.

PEDro (www.pedro.org.au) and OTSeeker (www.otseeker.com) are Web sites that contain abstracts and appraised information about systematic review and RCTs relevant to physical therapy and occupational therapy. By searching these sites, therapists can access information easily and be assured that it has been rated using a standard quality rating system. Therapists can use the information on these two databases to judge whether a particular intervention is appropriate for specific clients. Both of these databases are growing rapidly. For example, as of 2012, PEDro listed over 24,000 RCTs and OTSeeker listed 6,500 RCTs relevant to physical therapy or occupational therapy, respectively.

An example of an innovative use of push-out technology is McMaster Premium Literature Service (PLUS). McMaster PLUS was originally developed for physicians with funding from the Ontario Ministry of Health and Long-Term Care in Canada and provides an innovative solution to these problems by "pushing-out" valuable current evidence. Specifically, MacPLUS (a) identifies the clinical interest of individual practitioners; (b) rates the scientific merit, clinical relevance, and newsworthiness of new evidence; (c) alerts practitioners about new high-quality research findings in their area; and (d) provides a cumulative database so that practitioners can look up information when needed. The service does not duplicate library services but enhances their functionality. Currently, there is a rehabilitation version of MacPLUS in development (see http://hiru.mcmaster.ca/hiru/ for more information).

Therapists can also access information to support EBP from Web resource sites on the Internet. Web portal sites, with links to many EBP resources, are also beginning to be developed. An example recently completed for occupational therapy is at www.otevidence.info. The American Physical Therapy Association has "Hooked on Evidence" that allows members to access and contribute to a database of article extractions, view Web sites and resources that support EBP, and access tutorials on using the *Guide to Physical Therapist Practice* at www.hookedonevidence.com. Other sites are listed at the end of this chapter. Therapists can also sign up for e-mail alert services. For example, the Gerontological Society of America will alert users to publication of articles that match key words or authors previously identified by the user, as does PubMed. Many journals offer sign-up services that push out their tables of content with links, and these can be very useful to find evidence in your speciality. PubMed allows the user to create custom searches and have then run at set intervals. These can be sent through e-mail under "My NCBI." Finding the strategies that reduce the burden of finding evidence can make EBP more time efficient.

WHAT TO DO WHEN THERE IS LITTLE EVIDENCE

There are likely to be clinical areas where there is little research evidence. Dealing with weak or conflicting evidence can reduce confidence in EBP. In clinical areas where there appears to be little or no research evidence available, the problem may be that the clinician is unaware of the research that is available or that can be useful. Many practitioners indicate that they are concerned about a lack of evidence in their practice area, which limits their ability to become evidence-based practitioners. Lack of evidence, however, is not as clear a concept as one may think. Evidence lacking in one field may, in fact, be plentiful in other disciplines. In addition, search terms used in the databases can be quite specific and therefore provide narrow results, making it seem that there is no evidence. Using plurals or synonyms of terms will often reveal far more evidence than first thought. In some cases, however, there is little evidence and a combination of clinical judgement, client outcome, and peer input must be used (Bennett et al., 2003).

Some forms of evidence may never have Level 1 evidence. Some problems are so rare or diverse that clinical trials are not possible; for example, congenital malformations. In other cases the interventions are complex and customized, so the trials can provide little guidance on how the intervention should be provided to individual patients. For example, though many trials suggest that patient education is important in rehabilitation, the specific information that patients need (e.g., how to set goals, etc.) is not usually explicitly defined, nor can its best format be easily evaluated by the RCT design. It is unlikely that this or other similar topics will be studied in this way. Therefore, the specific information that is necessary to implement best practice may not be readily available. Using alternative forms of evidence such as expert panels, Delphi consensus processes, and qualitative studies may enrich our understanding of these issues.

After all searches have been completed, there may be clinical questions for which little evidence exists. In such cases it may be necessary to draw on lower levels of evidence, including observations made on small numbers of patients in case series or even theoretical foundations, physiologic principles, or lab-based research. In such situations, practitioners can help generate evaluative data through consistently tracking outcomes in their practice or implementing small, single-case studies.

The best way to begin tracking outcomes or doing small studies is often through a research partnership with a rehabilitation faculty member in a university.

BARRIERS AND SOLUTIONS REQUIRING HELP FROM ALL STAKEHOLDERS

Some of the barriers associated with EBP are difficult for rehabilitation practitioners to deal with on their own. These barriers include current health policies, organizational barriers, and biases within the research evidence (Maher, Sherrington, Elkins, Herbert, & Moseley, 2004). Maher et al. (2004) suggested that clinicians and researchers need to work together and do the following:

- Publish all RCTs, regardless of outcome.
- Petition MEDLINE and CINAHL for complete coverage in rehabilitation journals.
- Expand free access to databases.
- Expand access to free text.
- Include translations of non-English research.
- Use relevant research to predict the treatment effect and adjust that prediction based on clinical experience.

Other suggestions on how to narrow the gap between research and practice are for research professionals to demand or "emphasise the timely transfer of research and theoretical knowledge into practice" (Law et al., 2004) and to create linkages and partnerships between researchers and practice participants (Forsyth, Summerfield-Mann, & Kielhofner, 2005; Hayes, 2000). A model proposed and tested by Forsyth et al. (2005) drew the following conclusions:

- In order to create an EBP, there must be a research alliance with all key stakeholders (i.e., researchers, students, administration, and clinicians).
- These stakeholders can join to form a community of practice, or community of practice scholars.
- In order to successfully close the gap between theory and practice, three factors should be considered:
  - Those who use knowledge should be involved in helping to generate and refine it.
  - A scholarship of practice should be developed to create new educational and research opportunities.
  - Models developed should show clear links between theoretical concepts and the everyday work of therapists.
- A centralized agency should oversee the transfer of knowledge between all practice scholars.

Burns (2003) suggested that research studies should be carried out in the field to involve practitioners to begin with and ensure that studies are relevant to current practice. Burns proposed a clinic/community intervention development model as follows (p. 964):

- Develop the research question in the setting where it is to be treated
- Initial efficacy trial under controlled conditions to determine potential benefit
- Single case applications in a clinical setting
- Initial effectiveness trial in a clinic
- Full test of effectiveness under everyday practice conditions
- Effectiveness of treatment variations

- Assessment of goodness of fit with host organization, practice setting, or community

- Dissemination of information to other organizations

Recent trends have included recognition of the need for practice-based evidence, effectiveness research, and other forms of clinical research as important evidence to inform practice (Fritz, MacDermid, & Snyder-Mackler, 2011).

HOW TO ENHANCE EVIDENCE-BASED PRACTICE

There are specific strategies that therapists can use to enhance their use of evidence in practice. The CAT is an excellent method for organizing your thoughts and keeping your evidence straight.

Critically Appraised Topics

CATs are the preferred categorization format for quick studies in EBP. The CAT was originally developed at McMaster University (Sauve et al., 1995), but several CAT formats have evolved since then. Simply put, a CAT is a one- or two-page "summary of a search and critical appraisal of the literature related to a focused clinical question, which should be kept in an easily accessible place so that it can be used to help make clinical decisions" (Center for Evidence-Based Emergency Medicine, n.d.-a). The most essential characteristics of CATs are that they be simultaneously brief, informative, and useful.

To give a more general understanding of the basis for CATs, it is important to be able to place them in the complete EBP process. The University of Oxford's Center for Evidence-Based Medicine (n.d.) breaks up the evidence-based information search process into five parts. They suggest that once you have realized that you have an information need, you should do the following:

- Translate these needs into answerable questions.

- Track down the best evidence to answer them.

- Appraise that evidence for its validity and applicability.

- Integrate that evidence with clinical expertise and apply it in practice.

- Evaluate the performance of the intervention.

This definition meshes with that of the Centre for Evidence-Based Emergency Medicine's (n.d.-b) definition of a CAT, which states, "A CAT is a one- or two-page summary of all of the preceding steps involved in your evidence-based approach to the literature. It provides immediate access to your method and results."

CATs have a hand in all of the steps of the evidence-based process. They require that one have a focused question, categorize the evidence found, allow for the evaluation of that evidence, and produce a clinical bottom line that will be developed into practice. Finally, CATs can be reviewed on a regular basis and their successes passed on for further analysis and use.

Different Types of Critically Appraised Topics

There are five major types of CATs:

1. Diagnosis/screening

2. Prognosis

3. Evaluating risk and harm in a case-control study

4. Evaluating risk and harm in a cohort study

5. Intervention studies (treatment, prevention, and screening)

Figure 10-2. Table used for diagnostic calculations. (Reprinted with permission from the Centre for Evidence-Based Medicine.)

	Disease Positive	Disease Negative
Test Positive	a	b
Test Negative	c	d

Diagnosis/Screening

CATs for diagnosis are one of the easiest to understand. This type of CAT involves finding relevant studies that identify disease symptoms and assessing the diagnostic accuracy of those symptoms. If the symptom in question is present, how likely is it that the patient has the disease or condition? Diagnostic CATs compare new diagnoses with the gold standard, or the most highly accurate diagnostic test that currently exists. The CAT for diagnosis has a two-by-two table for entering the evidence numbers (Figure 10-2) and a formula for calculating the likelihood ratios for the new diagnosis or how likely it is that a person has the disease if he or she shows the symptom.

A likelihood ratio is a simple calculation of the probability that a client has a certain condition given the results of a test. There are two equal and opposite types of results to consider when examining the results of clinical tests—sensitivity and specificity. These two factors interplay with each other to produce results. The sensitivity of a diagnostic test is the proportion of people who actually have the disease or problem in question who come up with a positive test. The specificity of a test is the equal and opposite result—the proportion of people who do not have the disease who come up (rightfully) with a negative test. From the pictured graphic the following can be determined:

$$\text{Sensitivity} = \frac{a}{(a + c)}$$

$$\text{Specificity} = \frac{d}{(b + d)}$$

Thus, the likelihood ratio is the sensitivity of the test (the chance that it will rightly include clients with the condition) divided by the opposite of the specificity (1 – specificity, or the chance that it will wrongly exclude clients with the condition). A likelihood ratio (LR) is thus:

$$LR = \frac{\text{sensitivity}}{(1 - \text{specificity})}$$

$$LR = \frac{\frac{a}{(a + c)}}{\frac{d}{(b + d)}}$$

If this is still unclear, we suggest that you consult a medical statistics textbook or online resource such as the Centre for Evidence-Based Medicine's Glossary, which is located at www.cebm.net/index.aspx?o=1116. Likelihood ratios are most often used by physicians for medical diagnostic questions, but they are also used in rehabilitation for screening issues (e.g., the identification of a developmental delay).

Prognosis

A CAT for prognosis will assess the ability of a symptom to forecast probable outcomes. The difference between a diagnosis CAT and a prognosis CAT is that diagnosis CATs attempt to establish whether or not persons have a condition, whereas prognosis CATs try to predict the future of a condition for one person. An example in rehabilitation is the predictive validity of screening tests, such as the Motor Assessment of Infants.

Evaluating Risk and Harm in a Case-Control Study

Risk is very simply defined as the probability that an event will occur, and the two types of CATs discussed attempt to find the risk for patients with a certain condition in two different ways. A case-control study is "a study that starts with identification of people with the disease or outcome of interest (cases) and a suitable control group without the disease or outcome" (Cochrane Reviewer's Handbook Glossary version 4.1.6, 2003).

The case-control CAT, therefore, analyzes information on the presence of risk factors using a statistical technique called an *odds ratio* (OR). An OR is simply the odds of a patient in the experimental group suffering an adverse event relative to the odds of a patient in the control group suffering the same event. There are two numbers to consider when calculating an OR: the experimental event odds (EEO) and the control event odds (CEO). The OR is the following:

OR = EEO

1 – EEO

CEO

1 – CEO

Once again, if this is not clear, consult a text or the Centre for Evidence-Based Medicine (NHS Research and Development, n.d.-b).

Evaluating Risk and Harm in a Cohort Study

Cohort studies differ from case-controlled studies in that the two types of studies approach populations differently. Cohort studies are studies in which subsets of a defined population are identified. These groups may or may not be exposed to factors hypothesized to influence the probability of the occurrence of a particular outcome. The cohorts are then followed forward in time to determine differential outcomes based on exposure or no exposure. In cohort studies, it is necessary to calculate the relative risk of the experimental and control groups.

A relative risk is simply the number of people exposed to a risk factor who developed the unwanted outcome taken as a percentage of the whole. The relative risk will differ for groups that are categorized differently, because the population considered is different. An easy analogy that illustrates this concept is the example of taxation. Each year, a percentage of citizens in a country who file tax returns are randomly chosen and are subjected to an in-depth audit. The number of citizens audited taken as a percentage of the total number of citizens who file tax returns is the relative risk of an audit. For those who are not legally required to file tax returns (e.g., children), the relative risk of an audit is different; for those who decide to illegally refrain from filing a tax return, the relative risk of an audit is different again. It is crucial to understand that though each subgroup has its own relative risk, the complete sample (the entire population of the country) has its own relative risk as well (which would be a weighted average of the relative risks of its subgroups).

Intervention Studies (Treatment, Prevention, and Screening)

CATs in this category typically use evidence from RCTs but can include other evaluative studies as well. This type of CAT distills information from an article on a treatment into a final conclusion on the number needed to treat (NNT).

The NNT, as defined by the NHS Research and Development Centre (n.d.-a), is as follows:

> The NNT is the number of persons you need to treat to prevent one additional bad outcome (stroke, poor function, etc.). … An NNT of 5 … means you have to treat 5 people with the intervention to prevent one additional bad outcome or create one good outcome.

ELEMENTS PRESENT IN RELIABLE CRITICALLY APPRAISED TOPICS

There are elements present in all reliable CATs, regardless of the type of CAT used (i.e., general form or specific CAT for each situation). Those elements—and a discussion of their purpose in the CAT—are provided in the following sections.

The Date of Completion

Although this seems straightforward, all CATs require that a date of completion be prominently displayed. As will be discussed, CATs are inherently transitory creations, with a "shelf life" hovering between a few months and a few years (depending on the advance of knowledge in the field). When you are reviewing your CATs, or if others are examining them for use with their clients, it is imperative that they know when you completed your evidence-based analysis of the literature and whether or not they should do their own search to find out whether any advances in knowledge have been made in the interim.

The Question

At the heart of the CAT is your clinical question. Care should be taken in preparing and wording this question because its structure will dictate the course of your research. It has been suggested (Richardson, Wilson, Nishikawa, & Hayward, 1995) that a question's "anatomy" should consist of these four parts:

1. The person or problem being addressed (P)
2. The intervention or exposure being considered (I)
3. The comparison intervention or exposure, when relevant (C)
4. The outcomes of interest (O)

If a question encompasses all four aspects (P.I.C.O.), it will be usable in a literature search and will likely yield results that will be helpful. A sample question could be phrased as follows: For persons with condition A, will treatment X be more effective than treatment Y in leading to outcome P or increasing function in outcome P? If a question cannot be made to fit these criteria, more work needs to be done in defining it.

The Clinical Bottom Line

The clinical bottom line is where you summarize your findings for yourself and others to have readily available. After your examination of the evidence, your final evaluation and the actions you will take based on that evidence are briefly summarized here. The clinical bottom line is more than the results of the article you read. Rather, you should report your critical evaluation of the evidence you have reviewed and your clinical judgment on how those results could be generalized to apply to your client.

The Evidence

Because this is EBP, there is room on the CAT to list the evidence that you have found that pertains to the question. It is a good idea to summarize the evidence you are using to make your case. The CAT is your clinical lifeline—it is the backup you have for your decision on a person's treatment. If required, you can refer back to the CATs and explain them as the basis for your clinical judgment. It is important to cite the article's source on the CAT and, if your institution uses paper CATs, advisable to attach the article and proof that you found to the final document. The information (or critical review) written up in the CATs also includes the numerical and statistical bases of the evidence.

The Gold Standard

On CATs that specifically have to do with diagnosis or screening (e.g., asking whether test A can accurately diagnose condition B), there is room to describe the current gold standard test. The gold standard will be a known, valid diagnostic or screening tool. Your diagnostic tool (based on the evidence you have found) should be offered up for comparison to the gold standard in its likelihood ratios. You can also input information gleaned from journal articles to calculate LRs (discussed previously). Other types of CATs, such as those for evaluating risk and harm, do not have a gold standard treatment with which to be compared, but they should be measured against other existing treatments for the specific condition in question.

Notes

This section, sometimes titled "comments" or "additional information," is where information goes that does not fit into any of the other categories but that you feel should be added to the CAT. It is a good idea to note any important issues that came up in the critical appraisal or any other costs or consequences of a proposed clinical bottom line that were not mentioned before. This section could also be used to record your personal reflections on the evidence you have found and its application. This section will be especially helpful if your CAT is used by others in the field because it provides a human dimension to the making of the CAT.

Sample Critically Appraised Topics Format

The sample CAT format (Figure 10-3) was developed by Dr. Annie McCluskey for the OT CATs Web site and is available from www.otcats.com/template/index.html. This template is shown as Figure 10-3.

Students should look at the following sample CATs:

- www.otcats.com
  - This Web site is a resource for CATs and CAPs. Many of the CATs and CAPs on the site have been completed by practitioners.
  - The CATs on this site are reviewed by an academic faculty member prior to posting them on the site.
- http://qspace.library.queensu.ca/handle/1974/213
  - This Web site contains CATs completed by graduate students in rehabilitation at Queen's University, Canada.

Finally, the Centre for Evidence-Based Medicine has developed a software program called the CATmaker, which assists in the creation of computerized CATs. A demonstration version of the software is available for download at www.cebm.net/index.aspx?o=1216.

CRITICALLY APPRAISED TOPIC

TITLE

Notes on the Title

> ➤ The title may or may not be declarative (ie, one that declares the findings of the appraisal). If a series of studies are being appraised and synthesised into a CAT, it may be better to use a more descriptive title (eg, "Effectiveness of X or Y for children with autism")
>
> ➤ For previous examples, see CAPs in Australian Occupational Therapy Journal and previous CATs on the OT – CATS website.
>
> ➤ It is suggested that authors do NOT include the level (eg, 1b) in the title since the difference countries/organisations use different hierarchies, and the terms can have different meanings for studies of therapy effectiveness vs prognostic/diagnostic studies

AUTHOR

Prepared by		Date	
Email address			
Review date	[Usually 2 years later]		

CLINIAL SCENARIO

FOCUSSED CLINICAL QUESTION

SUMMARY OF SEARCH
[Best evidence appraised and key findings]

CLINICAL BOTTOM LINE

Important note on the limitation of this CAT

This critically appraised paper (or topic) has /has not been peer-reviewed by one other independent person/lecturer

Please AIM to FIT AS MUCH OF THE ABOVE INFORMATION ONTO THE FIRST PAGE OF YOUR CAT/CAP

Figure 10-3. Sample CAT format. (Reprinted with permission from Annie McCluskey, PhD, MA, DipCOT.)

SEARCH STRATEGY

Terms used to guide the search strategy

- **P**atient/Client Group:
- **I**ntervention (or Assessment):
- **C**omparison:
- **O**utcome(s):

Databases and Sites Searched	Search Terms	Limits Used

INCLUSION and EXCLUSION CRITERIA

Inclusion Criteria

Exclusion Criteria

RESULTS OF SEARCH

Figure 10-3 (continued). Sample CAT format. (Reprinted with permission from Annie McCluskey, PhD, MA, DipCOT.)

A total of ____ *(insert number)* relevant studies were located and categorised as shown in Table 1 (based on Levels of Evidence, Centre for Evidence Based Medicine, 2011)

Table 1: Summary of Study Designs of Articles Retrieved

Study Design/Methodology of Articles Retrieved	Level	Number Located	Author (Year)

Note

If you search for and locate evidence-based clinical guidelines, note this at the end of your table, and include in your reference list. The level of evidence should be recorded as Not Applicable (NA) for qualitative studies, and a footnote added to identify levels for non- intervention studies (i.e. prognostic or diagnostic).

BEST EVIDENCE

Figure 10-3 (continued). Sample CAT format. (Reprinted with permission from Annie McCluskey, PhD, MA, DipCOT.)

The following study/paper was identified as the 'best' evidence and selected for critical appraisal. Reasons for selecting this study were:

➢

➢

➢

SUMMARY OF BEST EVIDENCE

Table 2: Description and appraisal of (name study design) by (authors, Year)

Aim/Objective of the Study/Systematic Review:

Study Design
[eg, systematic review, cohort, randomised controlled trial, qualitative study, grounded theory. Includes information about study characteristics such as blinding and allocation concealment. When were outcomes measured, if relevant] Note: For systematic review, use headings 'search strategy', 'selection criteria', 'methods' etc. For qualitative studies, identify data collection/analyses methods

Setting
[eg, locations such as hospital, community; rural; metropolitan; country]

Participants
[N, diagnosis, eligibility criteria, how recruited, type of sample (eg, purposive, random), key demographics such as mean age, gender, duration of illness/disease, and if groups in an RCT were comparable at baseline on key demographic variables; number of dropouts if relevant, number available for follow-up]

Figure 10-3 (continued). Sample CAT format. (Reprinted with permission from Annie McCluskey, PhD, MA, DipCOT.)

Intervention Investigated

[Provide details of methods, who provided treatment, when and where, how many hours of treatment provided]

Control

Experimental

Outcome Measures (Primary and Secondary)

Give details of each measure, maximum score for each measure and range, administered by whom, where

Main Findings

[Insert table of mean scores/mean differences/treatment effect, 95% confidence intervals and p-values etc where provided – if you need to calculate these data yourself put calculations here and add interpretation later, under 'critical appraisal' on next page]

Original Authors' Conclusions

[paraphrase as required. If providing a direct quote, add page number]

Figure 10-3 (continued). Sample CAT format. (Reprinted with permission from Annie McCluskey, PhD, MA, DipCOT.)

Critical Appraisal

Validity

[Methodology, rigour, selection, bias, provide PEDro score/PEDro partitioned score and sub-test items 1-10 for RCTs; other study designs, follow headings used in critical appraisal checklist forms.

Comment on missing information in original paper.

Interpretation of Results

[Favourable or unfavourable, specific outcomes of interest, size of treatment effect, statistical and clinical significance, minimal clinically important difference – some of which you may have calculated yourself.

Email original authors for information needed such as additional data needed to calculate confidence intervals.

Summary/Conclusion

Repeat the above table as needed for additional studies included in the CAT.

If more than one paper is included, an additional table that provides a comparative summary of each paper may be added.

Figure 10-3 (continued). Sample CAT format. (Reprinted with permission from Annie McCluskey, PhD, MA, DipCOT.)

Table [x]: Characteristics of included studies

	Study 1 [Author and Year]	Study 2 [Author and Year]	Study 3 [Author and Year]
Intervention investigated			
Comparison intervention			
Outcomes used			
Findings			

IMPLICATIONS FOR PRACTICE, EDUCATION and FUTURE RESEARCH

Notes

- *This section synthesises your comments from appraisal section, and may mention other related research, both quantitative and qualitative.*
- *Comment on whether the intervention is used in practice in your region/country, cost of that treatment, need for education of local therapists/undergraduates about this intervention and/or outcome measures used in the study).*
- *Students may wish/need to discuss implications with clinicians for suggestions*
- *Read recent CATs from the OT-CATS website and CAPS in Australian Occupational Therapy Journal for ideas to include in this section.*

REFERENCES
[List references in alphabetical order using APA style and format]

- *AIM TO SUMMARISE YOUR CAT IN 8-12 PAGES IF ONLY APPRAISING ONE KEY STUDY (CAP= Critically Appraised Paper).*
- *A LONGER DOCUMENT IS ACCEPTABLE IF YOU ARE APPRAISING AND SYNTHESISING SEVERAL STUDIES (CAT = Critically Appraised Topic).*

Figure 10-3 (continued). Sample CAT format. (Reprinted with permission from Annie McCluskey, PhD, MA, DipCOT.)

Using Critically Appraised Topics

As was stated at the beginning of this chapter, CATs are used to summarize and organize evidence for specific clinical situations in practice. However, they are even more useful if they are available to a network of health care professionals. Some health care centers have set up collections of CATs called CATbanks, which contain all of the CATs their staff have put together. This way, each practitioner's evidence-based work is made available to the entire unit. Several good examples of CATbanks are the following:

- The University of Washington EBM Page

   www.mebi.washington.edu/ebm-uwsom/indexbody.html

- University of North Carolina CATs

   www.med.unc.edu/medicine/edursrc/!catlist.htm

- University of Michigan CATs

   www.med.umich.edu/pediatrics/ebm/cat.htm

- University of Western Sydney

   www.otcats.com

Drawbacks of Critically Appraised Topics

Despite their usefulness as a tool in EBP, CATs have their drawbacks. Each CAT is the product of either one individual or a small group of individuals and, as such, is subject to error, bias, and other limitations that are inherent to non-peer-reviewed material. CATs are designed to be dated as well and are only used as short-term or interim guides until more conclusive evidence in the form of RCTs or systematic reviews can provide more conclusive evidence on the topic in question. Sauve et al. (1995) suggested that "when others research and reappraise the same clinical problem the next time a client presents it, the old CAT may be used as the starting point rather than the last word."

Summary of Critically Appraised Topics

CATs are quick, easy, and intuitive organizational tools for using EBP. They can be created around a variety of topics and methods of looking at evidence. Despite some differences in format, they consist of several basic categories that must be completed. CATs are useful in that they can be collected and can serve as a pool of the EBP knowledge created by a specific unit; however, CATs can be flawed because of the inherent speed of their creation. CATs represent an advance in the organization and dissemination of research transfer knowledge and should be integrated into the repertoire of the evidence-based practitioner.

Critically Appraised Papers

A CAP is very useful in helping practitioners quickly figure out the quality of a newly published research study and how to apply it. CAPs are similar to CATs but specific to individual papers. Their characteristics include the following:

- They are "succinct appraisal of a single research study ... comprised of a declarative title, a structured abstract, and a commentary" (Canadian Association of Occupational Therapists, n.d.).

- They are written by a clinician or methodologist who describes the strengths and weaknesses of a study, "places the study in the context of other research, and discusses implications for practice, education, and future research" (Canadian Association of Occupational Therapists, n.d.).

The *Australian Journal of Occupational Therapy* regularly publishes CAPs that are peer reviewed. The Canadian Association of Occupational Therapists (n.d.) has developed a Web resource for CAPs that are free to members or can be purchased by e-mail. The CAPS on this site are peer reviewed. Queen's University, Canada, has a Web site for CATs in rehabilitation science that have been completed by students in their programs (see http://qspace.library.queensu.ca/handle/1974/213).

CAPs are useful because they cover many different types of evidence including RCTs, qualitative studies, systematic reviews, and metasyntheses of qualitative research. They are easy to share among colleagues or at meetings (www.otcats.com).

CAPs also have limitations. Many CAPs have more of a medical than a rehabilitation focus. Not all CAPs have been peer reviewed, so it is important to take note of this. CAPs are meant to provide a guide because they are based on someone else's interpretation of the methods, results, and statistics of a paper. These interpretations may not always be accurate and the suggestions on implications for practice might not apply to your own situation, setting, or specific client.

Sample Critically Appraised Papers and How to Use Them

Information on how to use CAPs and sample CAPs can be accessed at the following Web sites:
- www.otcats.com (see description in CATs section)
- The Canadian Association of Occupational Therapists

  www.caot.ca/default.asp?pageid=1295:

  - The CAPs on this site are free to members or can be purchased by e-mailing the following address: publications@caot.ca.

  - Online discussion forums also exist on this site so that therapists can speak with each other about how to apply findings.

  - The CAPs on this site are peer reviewed.

- Many other CAP samples are available on the Internet and can be found by typing "critically appraised paper" into your Web browser. Examples include the New South Wales, Speech Pathology Evidence-Based Practice Interest Group in Australia. A sample CAP can be found at http://www.nswspeechpathologyebp.com.au/critically-appraised-papers-and-topics.

WEB-BASED RESOURCE SITES

Numerous sites exist to teach therapists about EBP and how to search for, appraise, evaluate, and apply evidence. These sites often contain links to other sites on the topic. One of the most comprehensive of these sites is the new Evidence-Based Occupational Therapy Web Portal. This site is a one-stop destination containing most of the information that therapists need for finding out about and using evidence. The Web site includes up-to-date articles on EBP as well as lists of search databases and systematic reviews. The site is located at www.otevidence.info

Searchable databases are very useful in supporting EBP. Therapy specific sites include the following:

OTSeeker

Contains abstracts of systematic reviews and RCTs "that have been critically appraised and rated to assist you to evaluate their validity and interpretability. These ratings will help you to judge the quality and usefulness of trials for informing clinical interventions" (www.otseeker.com).

As previously mentioned, OTseeker (www.otseeker.com) listed 6,500 randomized controlled trials in 2012 relevant to occupational therapy.

RehabTrials.org

www.kesslerfoundation.org

This site provides links to research publications on topics such as spinal cord injury, traumatic brain injury, and strokes.

Physiotherapy Evidence Database

www.pedro.org.au

Physiotherapy evidence database provides free access to many RCTs, systematic reviews, and clinical practice guidelines.

CLINICAL GUIDELINES

Clinical Guidelines

www.guidelines.gov

A public resource of compiled clinical guidelines; tools on this site provide additional information from experts and allows one to conduct a side-by-side comparison of two guidelines.

Exter Health Library

http://services.exeter.ac.uk/eml/ehlguidelinespage.html

A list of additional useful Web sites compiled by the Exter Health Library.

The Ottawa Hospital Library Service

www.ottawahospital.on.ca/wps/portal/Base/TheHospital/EducationAndLearning/TOHMedicalLibraryServices

Orthopaedic Web Links

www.orthopaedicweblinks.com

A comprehensive assembly of Web links regarding orthopedics.

SUM Search

http://sumsearch.org

SUM search is a metasearch engine (simultaneously conducting a search through multiple Web sites).

TRIP Database

www.tripdatabase.com

A search engine that classifies results with a hierarchy of evidence to allow for a search restricted to a certain level of evidence.

Evidence-Based Medicine Guidelines

http://onlinelibrary.wiley.com/book/10.1002/0470057203

A database of evidence-based clinical guidelines; subscription is required for access.

Sources of systematic reviews and trials include the following:

The Cochrane Library

www.cochrane.org/cochrane-reviews

Cochrane Reviews are internationally recognized systematic reviews; plain-language summaries with a link to the full review are available for public access.

National Health Service Center for Reviews and Dissemination

www.york.ac.uk/inst/crd/

Clinical Evidence

www.clinicalevidence.com

This site provides systematic reviews for common clinical interventions.

Getting Hooked on Evidence

www.apta.org (The more specific URL is www.hookedonevidence.org/search.cfm)

A database with articles regarding evidence for physical therapy interventions by the American Physical Therapy Association; subscription is required for access.

TAKE-HOME MESSAGES

EBP is not only about using research evidence but about using it in partnership with excellent clinical reasoning and paying close attention to the client's stated goals, needs, and values. Use of a step-by-step model to gather and use evidence will improve the process of building evidence for your practice.

Critically Appraised Topics

✓ A CAT is a one- or two-page summary of a search and critical appraisal of the literature related to a focused clinical question.

✓ CATs are brief, informative, and useful.

✓ The five types of CATs are the following: diagnosis/screening; prognosis; evaluating risk/harm in a case controlled study; evaluating risk/harm in a cohort study; treatment, prevention, and screening.

✓ Necessary elements of CATs are date of completion, question, clinical bottom line, evidence, gold standard, and notes.

✓ CATs are a quick, easy, and intuitive tool but are also subject to error or bias.

✓ Should be seen as a starting point in a decision-making process rather than a final word.

Learning and Exploration Activities

The purpose of this chapter is to introduce the definition and uses of CATs to students. The following exercises allow students to practice developing and using CATs so that they become an effective tool of EBP.

1. Compare the different CAT templates suggested in this chapter. Which one makes the most sense to you? Which information do you think is the most crucial in a CAT? Which is the least important? Why? Using the CAT templates given as examples, create your own CAT template that incorporates the information that you feel is essential.

2. Choose a topic in rehabilitation and make a CAT about it. This can be something you have been studying in class or a topic of personal interest. Do this exercise along with a number of your classmates and when you have finished, exchange CATs and discuss their strengths and weaknesses. If you are really energetic, the class may want to create a paper or electronic CATbank of your collected CATs, which can be expanded as you collectively continue your studies in EBP.

REFERENCES

Banzi, R., Liberati, A., Moschetti, I., Tagliabue, L., & Moja, L. (2010). A review of online evidence-based practice point-of-care information summary providers. *Journal of Medical Internet Research, 12*, e26.

Bartlet, T. C., Ziebert, C., Sawin, K. J., Malin, S., Nugent, M., & Simpson, P. (2011). Evidence-based practice: Perceptions, skills, and activities of pediatric health care professionals. *Journal of Pediatric Nursing, 26*(2), 114–121.

Bennett, S., & Bennett, J. (2000). The process of evidence based practice in occupational therapy: Informing clinical decisions. *Australian Journal of Occupational Therapy, 47*, 171–180.

Bennett, S., Tooth, L., McKenna, K., Rodger, S., Strong, J., Ziviani, J., Gibson, L. (2003). Perceptions of evidence based practice: A survey of Australian occupational therapists. *Australian Occupational Therapy Journal, 50*, 13–22.

Brown, T., Tseng, M. H., Casey, J., McDonald, R., & Lyons, C. (2009). Knowledge, attitudes, practices and barriers of pediatric occupational therapists to evidence-based practice and research utilization. *WFOT Bulletin, 60*, 38–48.

Burns, B. (2003). Children and evidence based practice. *Psychiatric Clinics of North America, 26*, 955–970.

Canadian Association of Occupational Therapists. (n.d.). Critically appraised papers: An introduction for readers. Retrieved from www.caot.ca/default.asp?pageid=1295

Center for Evidence-Based Emergency Medicine. (n.d.-a). Critically appraised topics bank. Retrieved from www.cebm.net.

Center for Evidence-Based Emergency Medicine. (n.d.-b). Formulating a critically appraised topic. Retrieved from www.cebm.net.

Corcoran, M. (2006). A busy practitioner's approach to evidence-based practice. *The American Journal of Occupational Therapy, 60*(2), 127–128.

Curtin, M., & Jaramazovic, E. (2001). Occupational therapists views and perceptions of evidence based practice. *British Journal of Occupational Therapy, 64*(5), 214–221.

Drake, R. E., Torrey, W. C., & McHugo, G. J. (2003). Strategies for implementing evidence-based practices in routine mental health settings. *Evidence-Based Mental Health, 6*, 6–7.

Forsyth, K., Summerfield-Mann, L., & Kielhofner, G. (2005). Scholarship of practice: Making occupation-focused, theory-driven evidence-based practice a reality. *British Journal of Occupational Therapy, 68*(6), 260–268.

Fritz, J. M., MacDermid, J. C., & Snyder-Mackler, L. (2011). Counting what counts. *Journal of Orthopaedic & Sports Physical Therapy, 41*, 907–908.

Gillespie, L., & Gillespie, W. (2003). Finding current evidence: Search strategies and common databases. *Clinical Orthopaedics and Related Research, 413*, 133–145.

Grimmer-Somers, K., Lekkas, P., Nyland, L., Young, A., & Kumar, S. (2007). Perspectives on research evidence and clinical practice: A survey of Australian physiotherapists. *Physiotherapy Research International, 12*(3), 147–161.

Hayes, R. L. (2000). Viewpoint: Evidence-based occupational therapy needs strategically-targeted quality research now. *Australian Occupational Therapy Journal, 47*(4), 186–190.

Haynes, B. (1998). Barriers and bridges to evidence based clinical practice. *BMJ, 317*, 273–276.

Herbert, R., Sherrtington, C., Maher, C., & Moseley, A. (2001). Evidence based practice: Imperfect but necessary. *Physiotherapy Theory and Practice, 17*, 201–211.

Iles, R., & Davidson, M. (2006). Evidence based practice: A survey of physiotherapists' current practice. *Physiotherapy Research International, 11*(2), 93–103.

Koehn, M. L., & Lehman, K. (2008). Nurses' perceptions of evidence-based nursing practice. *Journal of Advanced Nursing, 62*(2), 209–215.

Law, M., Pollock, N., & Stewart, D. (2004). Evidence-based occupational therapy: Concepts and strategies. *New Zealand Journal of Occupational Therapy, 51*(1), 14–22.

Lyons, C., Brown, T., Tseng, M.-H., Casey, J., & McDonald, R. (2011). Evidence-based practice and research utilisation: Perceived research knowledge, attitudes, practices and barriers among Australian paediatric occupational therapists. *Australian Occupational Therapy Journal, 58*(3), 178–186.

Maher, C., Sherrington, C., Elkins, M., Herbert, R., & Moseley, A. (2004). Challenges for evidence-based physical therapy: Accessing and interpreting high quality evidence on therapy. *Physical Therapy, 84*(7), 644–654.

McCluskey, A., & Cusick, A. (2002). Strategies for introducing evidence-based practice and changing clinician behaviour: A managers toolbox. *Australian Occupational Therapy Journal, 49*(2), 63–70.

Nail-Chiwetalu, B., & Bernstein Ratner, N. (2007). An assessment of the information-seeking abilities and needs of practicing speech-language pathologists. *Journal of the Medical Library Association, 95*(2), 182–188, e56–e57.

NHS Research and Development Centre for Evidence-Based Medicine. (n.d.-a). NNT. Retrieved from http://www.cebm.net/?o=1044

NHS Research and Development Centre for Evidence-Based Medicine. (n.d.-b). Odds ratios. Retrieved http://www.cebm.net/index.aspx?o=1160

Phillippi, J. C., & Buxton, M. (2010). Web 2.0: Easy tools for busy clinicians. *Journal of Midwifery & Womens Health, 55*, 472–476.

Richardson, W., Wilson, M., Nishikawa, J., & Hayward, R. (1995). The well-built clinical question: A key to evidence-based decisions. *ACP Journal Club, 123*, A12–A13.

Sackett, D. L. (1997). Evidence-based medicine. *Seminars in Perinatology, 21*, 3–5.

Sackett, D. L., Straus, S. E., Richardson, W. S., Rosenberg, W., & Haynes, R. B. (2000). *Evidence-based medicine. How to practice and teach EBM* (2nd ed.). Toronto, ON: Churchill Livingstone.

Salbach, N. M., Jaglal, S. B., Korner-Bitensky, N., Rappolt, S., Davis, D., & Duncan, P. W. (2007). Practitioner and organizational barriers to evidence-based practice of physical therapists for people with stroke. *Physical Therapy, 87*(10), 1284–1305.

Sauve, S., Lee, H. N., Meade, M. O., Lang, J. B., Faroukh, M., Cook, D. J., et al. (1995). The critically appraised topic: A practical approach to learning critical appraisal. *Annals of the Royal College of Physicians and Surgeons of Canada, 28*(7), 396–398.

Schreiber, J., Stern, P., Marchetti, G., &Provident, I. (2009). Strategies to promote evidence-based practice in pediatric physical therapy: A formative evaluation pilot project. *Physical Therapy, 89*(9), 918–933.

Solomons, N. M., & Spross, J. A. (2011). Evidence-based practice barriers and facilitators from a continuous quality improvement perspective: An integrative review. *Journal of Nursing Management, 19*(1), 109–120.

Stergiou-Kita, M. (2010). Implementing clinical practice guidelines in occupational therapy practice: Recommendations from the research evidence. *Australian Occupational Therapy Journal, 57*(2), 76–87.

Tickle-Degnen, L. (2000). Evidence-based practice forum. Communicating with clients, family members, and colleagues about research evidence. *The American Journal of Occupational Therapy, 54*(3), 341–343.

University of Oxford Center for Evidence-Based Medicine. (n.d.). What is a CAT? Retrieved from www.jr2.ox.ac.uk/cebm/docs/cats/catabout.html

Upton, D., & Upton, P. (2006). Knowledge and use of evidence-based practice by allied health and health science professionals in the United Kingdom. *Journal of Allied Health, 35*(3), 127–133.

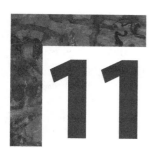

Evidence Synthesis
Practice Tools
Guidelines, Algorithms, Clinical Pathways, Prediction Rules, and Patient Decision Aids

Joy C. MacDermid, PhD, PT Reg (Ont), FCAHS

Learning Objectives

After reading this chapter, the student/practitioner will be able to:

- Identify the role of evidence synthesis products in evidence-based practice.
- Contrast and compare commonly used evidence synthesis tools/products: clinical practice guidelines (CPGs), algorithms, clinical prediction rules (CPRs), clinical pathways (CPs), and patient decision aids (PDAs).
- Identify the steps required to formulate evidence-based practice guidelines.
- Be aware of the variations in how guidelines are developed and the potential implications.
- Be aware of resources for obtaining CPGs and PDAs pertaining to rehabilitation.
- Be able to critically evaluate CPGs using a structured critical appraisal instrument.
- Be able to evaluate the implementability or adaptability of CPGs using a structured tool.
- Be aware of resources to appraise or implement CPs.
- Recognize barriers to evidence synthesis products and be able to formulate an implementation plan.

Background

In the knowledge-to-action cycle (Graham & Tetroe, 2007), the knowledge creation funnel starts with individual research studies and is then distilled down into syntheses of the best quality studies, which are then used to develop evidence-based tools and products. Knowledge syntheses such as

Law M., & MacDermid, J. C.
Evidence-Based Rehabilitation: A Guide
to Practice, Third Edition (pp 233–274).
© 2014 SLACK Incorporated.

systematic reviews and meta-analyses are evidence-based research summaries that can reduce the burden of evidence-based practice on clinicians by taking on the effort of searching in a methodical fashion for the best quality evidence and synthesizing it into summary recommendations. The process for finding, developing, and evaluating these has been reviewed in previous chapters. Systematic reviews and meta-analyses are highly valued by clinicians because they are able to bring together a large body of evidence on a clinical topic and can save a tremendous amount of time that would be involved in independently searching for and evaluating primary studies. However, one of the challenges that evidence-based practitioners have when attempting to use these syntheses is that the recommendations or conclusions may not be sufficiently detailed to facilitate implementation in their practice. The topics covered in this chapter deal with that transition from evidence synthesis to clinical tools and products that may help clinicians move evidence synthesis into action. We will cover the most common of these and attempt to understand how they are developed and evaluated, where to find them, and how to implement them.

A variety of new evidence synthesis products have recently started to proliferate in rehabilitation literature. These can range from comprehensive documents that make clinical recommendations for comprehensive management of the disorder to evidence-based tools that focus on a single decision point. The common feature across these tools is that they are based on taking the best quality evidence and packaging it into a knowledge product or tool that should facilitate implementation in clinical practice. Variants on evidence knowledge products are available for public health/health promotion, public policy, and clinical care. We will focus on the most common ones used in rehabilitation clinical practice which include CPGs, algorithms, CPRs, CPs, and PDAs.

Clinical Practice Guidelines

The Institute of Medicine defines CPG as "systematically developed statements that assist practitioner and patient decisions about appropriate health care for specific clinical circumstances" (Canadian Medical Association, 1994; Field & Lohr, 1992). CPGs have also been referred to as *practice parameters, practice policies, appropriateness criteria,* or *consensus statements,* although these terms are more generic and do not necessarily imply the same rigor of development as a CPG. However, the term *practice guideline* is also sometimes used to refer to clinical protocols or consensus statements that were not developed using an evidence synthesis. Historically, in some areas of health care including rehabilitation practice, protocols were developed based on expert opinion alone. Such documents have little role in evidence-based practice. Therefore, practitioners have to be cautious about understanding how CPGs should be developed and be prepared to use a structured quality appraisal process to filter out lower quality CPGs.

Ideally, CPGs should be based on strong evidence that would provide clear and comprehensive recommendations regarding all of the relevant issues on a particular clinical topic, provide a framework to monitor the process and outcome of implementing the CPG into clinical practice, and incorporate a regular review and updating process. The process of developing and maintaining guidelines is challenging for most guideline development groups because the evidence synthesis process can be costly and requires strong methodological skills. The process for obtaining and sustaining the broad interprofessional partnership and ongoing funding required can be difficult. It can be even more problematic to obtain funds for updating guidelines at regular intervals to ensure that they remain up to date on the latest evidence. Despite these challenges, professional groups and funders are increasingly diverting resources to guideline development as a means to promote better process and outcomes in practice.

The majority of guidelines are developed to assist with specific patient populations and ideally should provide comprehensive recommendations across the range of clinical activities required for persons with that health problem. This should include assessment/diagnosis, prognosis, intervention selection/effectiveness, monitoring for adverse events, and evaluating the outcomes of clinical management. CPGs are often developed based on the existing evidence and evaluated for quality based on the extent to which they follow the correct process, rather than the extent to which they provide comprehensive and useful advice to clinicians. Therefore, practitioners also need to be aware that even when they are successful in locating an evidence-based CPG, some areas of practice may not be delineated in the CPG.

The medical profession has invested heavily in guideline development and the majority of guidelines currently available relate to medical practice. Rehabilitation professions have recognized the potential benefits of CPG and have recently become more engaged in this process. Occupational and physical therapy associations are increasingly focusing on the role of evidence-based CPGs through either position statements or developing guidelines (see Web links). For example, the American Physical Therapy Association has developed CPGs for areas of orthopedic practice and other professional associations have focused on compiling/appraising relevant guidelines. CPGs are increasingly appearing in rehabilitation literature where they have been subject to peer review (Gross et al., 2002; Johnston, Wood, Stason, & Beatty, 2000; McPoil et al., 2008; Rodin, Saliba, & Brummel-Smith, 2006; Scholten-Peeters et al., 2002). As the number of CPGs developed increases, it is increasingly becoming possible to do reviews of practice guidelines to establish scope and quality (Berrigan, Marshall, McCullagh, Velikonja, & Bayley, 2011; Brooks et al., 2005; Hurkmans, Jones, Li, & Vliet Vlieland, 2011; MacDermid, 2004). Brooks and coauthors (2005) published a paper summarizing the quality of 50 CPGs used in physical therapy, demonstrating wide variability in quality. When comparing mean quality scores of CPGs developed prior to 2000 with those developed in 2000 or later, the newer CPGs scored better, suggesting that as the methods for developing and evaluating CPGs evolved, there have been improvements in quality.

There are logical reasons why guideline development may be lagging in rehabilitation practice when compared to some areas of health care such as cancer or cardiovascular medicine, because the funds required to develop evidence-based guidelines may be more difficult to compile. Furthermore, CPGs are best developed where there is a substantial base of high-quality clinical trials upon which to make evidence-based recommendations. Barriers to conducting these trials in rehabilitation practice are well known (Fritz, MacDermid, & Snyder-Mackler, 2011; Goldsmith, Gross, MacDermid, Santaguida, & Miller, 2011) and include the complex nature of rehabilitation practice. In rehabilitation it is common to use a multidimensional assessment to identify multidimensional goals that are tailored to the individual patient and lead to a multimodal treatment plan that is modified over time to optimize outcomes unique to that individual patient. Though this may be very patient centered, it can fall outside the usual research paradigm where variables are very tightly controlled. There are certainly other challenges to conducting trials in rehabilitation. However, in most areas of rehabilitation we lack sufficient randomized controlled trials (RCTs) to answer all of our clinical questions. Rehabilitation may be challenged to ensure that the guideline development process can embrace the nature of rehabilitation practice. Nevertheless, the need to establish guidelines for efficacious and efficient rehabilitation intervention is critical to the success of rehabilitation. Recent guidelines have attempted to incorporate evidence and conceptual frameworks like the *International Classification of Functioning, Disability and Health* (ICF) as a way to manage this complexity.

The methodology to develop, critically appraise, and implement CPGs has only recently emerged as a scientific methodology in its own right. One can look at any element of the guideline development and evaluation process and see a rapidly evolving science about how this work should be conducted and evaluated. CPGs are typically founded on evidence syntheses such as systematic reviews, reviews of reviews (or overviews), metasyntheses, etc. Each of these evidence synthesis processes is an evolving science unto itself. In addition to considering the evidence, some component of expert consensus is often involved in development of CPGs. Techniques for obtaining expert input and consensus are also emerging. Finally, CPGs must have explicitly structured recommendations, and the process for designating these recommendations is also evolving. Current guidelines contain many variations about how recommendations are constructed. We will discuss the exemplar of the Grading of Recommendations Assessment, Development, and Evaluation (GRADE). GRADE is an international consensus-based process for moving from evidence synthesis to specific recommendations (Brozek et al., 2009; Guyatt et al., 2008). Finally, the process by which these recommendations are communicated, disseminated, and implemented also vary (Davis, 2006; Eccles & Grimshaw, 2004; Grimshaw, Eccles, & Tetroe, 2004). In this chapter, we will only deal with some aspects of implementation. The reader is advised to consult with the chapter on knowledge translation and the taxonomy for knowledge translation interventions presented in Appendix H.

We recognize that the following are substantial barriers to the development of CPGs, many of which include comprehensive and clear recommendations:

- The lack of sufficient high-quality research on a number of rehabilitation issues/interventions.
- The lack of standards about reporting the detailed specifications of rehabilitation interventions when reporting clinical research.
- Gaps between the interventions used in practice and those investigated in the clinical literature.
- The complex nature of rehabilitation practice.
- The multidimensional nature of rehabilitation outcomes such as function and quality of life.

Despite these concerns, there is a substantial theoretical rationale supporting the large public and professional investments going into the development of CPGs. CPGs have been shown to provide reduced variations in health care delivery and, in some cases, improved outcomes (Bahtsevani, Uden, & Willman, 2004; Grimshaw & Hutchinson, 1995). For example, increased adherence to CPGs in management of low back pain is associated with fewer functional limitations and fewer treatment visits (Rutten et al., 2010). Similarly, patients with major depression are most likely to see improvements in their symptoms if their routine treatment is guideline compliant, although only 29% of patients in a community-based sample received guideline-compliant treatment (Fortney, Rost, Zhang, & Pyne, 2001). Overall, despite challenges, CPGs have the potential to improve rehabilitation practice and thus there is an onus on the professions to ensure that high-quality, relevant CPGs are developed and implemented.

Ideally, CPGs would incorporate tools, customized for the different end-users, to assist with the implementation of best practices. The types of implementation tools that are most commonly employed by guideline developers are brief summaries of the recommendations that may be written in alternate forms for clinicians, patients, or decision makers. Other implementation tools are less common but can include treatment algorithms, PDAs, electronic decision supports, or implementation guides. The methods of disseminating CPGs can also be an important aspect of the implementation plan. Dissemination can be through peer-reviewed journals, professional Web sites, and guideline databases such as the National Guideline Clearinghouse. When planning or evaluating a strategy for implementation of CPGs, one might use the Taxonomy of Knowledge Translation Interventions in Appendix H.

The Guideline Development Process

Guideline development follows a systematic process. Review Table 11-1 for further key elements of the process. However, there is considerable variation between guideline development teams about how this process is operationalized. Sufficient experience on the process of developing CPGs now exists so that key elements to the process are recognized. CPGs are developed by teams with sufficient breadth of clinical, professional, content, and methodological skills to proceed through the detailed, systematic process required to ensure that relevant high-quality information

Table 11-1

Steps for Developing a Clinical Practice Guideline or Clinical Pathway in Rehabilitation

1. Assemble a development team. The team should contain the following individuals
   - Multidisciplinary representation
   - Clinicians who practice in the area
   - Methodological expertise on appraisal and development of CPG/CP
   - Prior experience in development of guidelines
   - Patients/consumers and/or their representatives
2. Define the clinical question(s) or scope:
   - The clinical population(s) (P)
   - The range of interventions to be addressed
   - The outcomes of interest
   - The disciplines involved
   - The type of evidence to be included
3. Define current clinical practice (to define scope of practice in areas that should be addressed within the guidelines; in some cases it will be necessary to draw on clinical practice patterns where evidence is lacking):
   - Clinical populations treated, important clinical subgroups
   - Range of interventions used (practice–evidence gaps)
   - Clinical and/or patient surveys on values/preferences
   - Data/research on efficacy or treatment mediators
4. Devise and document a strategy to locate the best quality evidence on the clinical question, as defined:
   - Retrieve all relevant systematic reviews
   - Determine search terms and databases to locate primary studies
   - Identify what quality cutoffs will be used in areas where there is a substantial number of primary studies
   - Identify what quality cutoffs will be used where there are few primary studies
   - Identify a strategy to deal with areas where there is no evidence (expert consensus may be useful in this case)
   - Develop a method for collecting expert feedback
   - Identify a strategy to integrate patient opinions and their preferences with evidence
5. Identify a strategy for evaluating quality of the available evidence:
   - Identify an appropriate rating system for summarizing and labeling the quality of the evidence (suggest GRADE approach or definitions)
   - Define effect mediators, values/preferences, and costs/resources issues that might affect how evidence is interpreted or applied
6. Identify a process for documenting specific recommendations:
   - Identify an appropriate rating process including a method for resolving disagreements on ratings (establish a defined consensus process)
   - Identify and document evidence summaries into specific recommendations (suggest GRADE approach or principles)
   - Identify and use a consistent process within the CPG for presenting clinical recommendations and identifying the level of supporting evidence
7. Establish outcome measures that could be used to monitor the impact of the CPG/CP implementation:
   - Recommend standardized, reliable, and valid measures that fit within a rehabilitation framework
   - Consider process and outcomes indicators
   - Consider qualitative and quantitative elements

(continued)

Table 11-1 (continued)

Steps for Developing a Clinical Practice Guideline or Clinical Pathway in Rehabilitation

8. Consider whether a CPG can be used to establish a CP or algorithm:
   - Consider treatment or outcome mediators
   - Consider contraindications
   - Consider the rate of progression and how patients move from one element/stage of the rehabilitation program to the next level
   - Consider where guidelines can be linked to form CPs
9. Identify forms of documentation to be used for dissemination and implementation:
   - Identify the needs of stakeholders in terms of receiving and implementing the guideline
   - Consider the use of clinical tools, executive summaries, primary and secondary publications, research and training presentations, and different vehicles for information exchange
   - Establish the process time line for developing each component
10. Establish a process for external review of the completed guidelines:
    - Include all disciplines involved
    - Include a range of expertise
    - Implement pilot testing where possible
11. Revise based on feedback
12. Devise a schedule and process for updating the guideline (every 3 years is suggested):
    - Updating the literature review and recommendations
    - Reevaluating and revising tools and communications
    - Fixing problems identified
13. Disseminate and participate in ongoing knowledge translation to different stakeholders to facilitate implementation of CPG (see Appendix H):
    - Disseminate to increase awareness
    - Develop tools/guides including operational manuals for interventions if needed
    - Develop decision tools for interventions with variable risk/benefit
    - Consider multiple media/formats

is appropriately synthesized. In most cases, a multidisciplinary approach is preferable because the guideline can help with role definition and coordination of care. Guidelines should also include a patient perspective. This can range from including qualitative information about patients to active leadership of patient participants in the development process. At a minimum, patients and/or their representatives should be included on this team to provide a consumer perspective. Increasingly, guideline developers and clinical researchers are starting to become more aware of the specific skills needed by patient/consumer representatives in order to take an active role. In some areas such as arthritis, the development of the role of a highly qualified consumer has provided a mechanism for more active engagement of patients.

The scope of the CPG is defined by the development team and should include agreement on specific research questions that must be addressed or a definition of the scope of literature that will be reviewed. Making the clinical topic clearer involves defining the specific population and condition to be addressed, the range of interventions to be considered, and the extent and nature of the multidisciplinary team that will be included. CPG developers must develop a strategy to search for/retrieve high-quality evidence. Teams usually have strategies to deal with lower quality evidence because important practice areas may not have sufficient high-quality evidence. Teams may need to develop consensus processes to develop recommendations in areas of practice where published evidence is absent. CPGs most typically involve a strong reliance on published clinical trials, although other forms of evidence should be considered. In some cases, practice pattern reviews or surveys are a useful strategy to identify the scope of interventions used, the perceived efficacy of such interventions, and the gaps between clinical practice and research evidence. These have been used effectively by some developers to support guideline development processes (Bitzer, Klosterhuis, Dorning, & Rose, 2003; Gulich, Engel, Rose, Klosterhuis, & Jackel, 2003).

The strategies for finding and evaluating evidence are key elements of guideline development and were addressed in earlier chapters. Critical appraisal focuses on determining the quality (or level of evidence) of individual studies. Methods for critical appraisal of different types of clinical research studies were covered in previous chapters. During guideline development, the focus is on making recommendations considering the entire body of evidence (all of the good research) available. Although developers may need to cross different types of evidence in order to be comprehensive, it is important that they provide clear guidance about the quality of evidence supporting specific recommendations. For example, a CPG on the management of lymphedema following breast cancer surgery listed some recommendations that were based on high-quality evidence, and another set of recommendations was presented separately and identified as being based solely on recommendations from clinicians and patients (Harris, Hugi, Olivotto, & Levine, 2001). This second set enhanced the patient-centeredness of the guideline by including considerations around patient values and preferences. Development teams must also decide how they will achieve consensus on clinical recommendations and how those recommendations will be formatted in various publications arising from the CPG development process. A formal consensus process can promote efficiency and circumvent group members dominating the process or decisions (Pagliari & Grimshaw, 2002; van der Sanden, Mettes, Plasschaert, Grol, & Verdonschot, 2004).

Different guideline development groups have used different recommendation criteria and terminology. In fact, more than 60 different rating systems have been described. Formats for grading recommendations include letter grades like those used by the Center for Evidence-Based Medicine or the Scottish Intercollegiate Guidelines Network (www.sign.ac.uk/guidelines/fulltext/50/annexb. html). Other groups have used terminology like *platinum* and *bronze*. Recently, Australian guideline developers suggested the use of a framework, the form framework, that consists of five components (evidence base, consistency, clinical impact, generalizability, and applicability), which are used to structure the strength of a recommendation (Hillier et al., 2011). A study of six of the most commonly used guideline recommendation rating systems indicated problems with reliability (Atkins et al., 2004).

Although there is no clear consensus on how to format recommendations, one may be emerging. GRADE is the international consensus-based process. A recent trial compared four different recommendation systems in a single pediatric context and suggested that GRADE was somewhat more understandable to clinicians (Cuello Garcia, Pacheco Alvarado, & Perez, 2011). The GRADE system for making evidence-based recommendations (Brozek et al., 2009, 2011) classifies the quality of evidence in one of four levels—high, moderate, low, and very low (see Table 11-1). One of the favorable aspects of GRADE is that it does not decide on quality on the basis of research design alone but rather takes a more comprehensive view on the likelihood that research evidence is certain and unbiased. Thus, RCTs start off being considered as high-quality evidence but can be downgraded for overriding concerns including study limitations, inconsistency of results across trials, indirectness of evidence, imprecision in the estimates of effect within trials, and reporting bias. Although observational studies—cohort and case-control studies—are initially considered as low quality, their rating can be upgraded if the magnitude of the treatment effect is very large, if there is evidence of a dose–response relationship, or if all plausible biases that could discount the treatment effect have been considered. The process of implementing GRADE requires that guideline developers extract specific information and consider these factors in a structured way. But, ultimately,

Table 11-2

Determinants of Strength of a GRADE Recommendation

FACTOR	INTERPRETATION
Balance between desirable and undesirable effects	The larger the difference between the desirable and undesirable effects, the higher the likelihood that a strong recommendation is warranted. The narrower the gradient, the higher the likelihood that a weak recommendation is warranted.
Quality of evidence	The higher the quality of evidence, the higher the likelihood that a strong recommendation is warranted.
Values and preferences	The more values and preferences vary, or the greater the uncertainty in values and preferences, the higher the likelihood that a weak recommendation is warranted.
Costs (resource allocation)	The higher the costs of an intervention—that is, the greater the resources consumed—the lower the likelihood that a strong recommendation is warranted.

From "Going From Evidence to Recommendations," by G. H. Guyatt, A. D. Oxman, R. Kunz, et al., 2008, *British Medical Journal, 336*(7652), pp. 1049-1051. Reprinted with permission.

the purpose is to determine the overall quality of the evidence, considering the balance of evidence, so that the quality rating will reflect the extent to which we are confident that the research evidence has defined the anticipated outcome of an intervention decision according to the following GRADE definitions:

- High quality—Further research is very unlikely to change our confidence in the estimate of effect.

- Moderate quality—Further research is likely to have an important impact on our confidence in the estimate of effect and may change the estimate.

- Low quality—Further research is very likely to have an important impact on our confidence in the estimate of effect and is likely to change the estimate.

- Very low quality—Any estimate of effect is very uncertain.

Another important aspect of GRADE is that recommendations are not based solely on the quality of evidence but also take into consideration other important factors (Table 11-2). These include the balance between desirable and undesirable effects, the quality of evidence, values and preferences, and costs/use of resources. These are important considerations and allow one to consider that factors other than the evidence might determine when it is appropriate to make a uniform recommendation that should be routinely implemented versus one that acknowledges the need for more latitude and individual decision making to consider a range of potential actions.

This allows guideline developers to make recommendations that would suggest more routine implementation when it is warranted—the evidence is strong, the benefit is clear, the effect is consistent and can reasonably be expected to apply to a broad array of patients, and there are no contentious downsides or adverse effects. Conversely, where the benefit is more marginal in comparison to other alternatives, considerations such as variations in risks, types of adverse events/side effects, costs, or other considerations suggest that a homogeneous approach might not be warranted. These considerations could easily mean that one patient might benefit from one intervention whereas another patient might benefit from a different one. For example, manipulation may provide a small additional benefit in recovery of neck pain in addition to a well-designed specific exercise program (Gross et al., 2007). However, clinicians will vary in their skills and opinions with respect to cervical neck manipulation. Patients are likely to have different opinions about this procedure as well. The relative risks and benefits remain somewhat uncertain. Cost considerations will vary across contexts. For this reason, guideline developers might consider making a weak recommendation about the use of cervical neck manipulation to treat neck pain, even in the presence of strong evidence of a small benefit.

Despite the number of factors considered in making a recommendation, ultimately, GRADE makes a simple binary strength of recommendation. This course was selected by the GRADE working group "in an attempt to provide clearer direction to patients, clinicians, and policy makers." One of the positive aspects of this binary approach is that unless the evidence is clear that a consistent approach is needed, it recognizes that clinical experience and judgment may take a lead role in making decisions. This should provide flexibility for CPG development in rehabilitation, even in areas where the evidence is weak.

The implications of a strong recommendation are as follows:

- For patients—Most people in your situation would want the recommended course of action and only a small proportion would not; request discussion if the intervention is not offered.
- For clinicians—Most patients should receive the recommended course of action.
- For policy makers—The recommendation can be adopted as a policy in most situations.

The implications of a weak recommendation are as follows:

- For patients—Most people in your situation would want the recommended course of action, but many would not.
- For clinicians—You should recognize that different choices will be appropriate for different patients and that you must help each patient to arrive at a management decision consistent with her or his values and preferences.
- For policy makers—Policy making will require substantial debate and involvement of many stakeholders.

Rehabilitation therapists should be aware of how GRADE recommendations (Brozek et al., 2009) are formulated and recognize the intention behind how the recommendations are worded. It is common for well-developed guidelines to be associated with scientific publications and alternate publication formats including detailed reports such as all evidence tables, executive summaries, tailored synopses, and brief reports. GRADE recommendations have relatively straightforward language that could be used consistently across these different formats.

CPGs are intended to be updated on a regular basis to ensure that the recommendations remain consistent with current best evidence. Three years has been suggested as the optimal time frame for this reevaluation. It can be problematic to find groups who have an ongoing commitment to update CPGs, particularly when one considers that it may take 3 years to develop a single evidence-based CPG. For this reason, it is beneficial to have the involvement of professional associations who may support an ongoing commitment. Clinicians should recognize that CPGs older than 3 years may contain outdated recommendations. In such cases, they will need to search the primary research to determine whether recent evidence may provide conflicting or additional findings.

The Guideline Adaptation Process

Given the time and resources required to develop evidence-based CPGs, a potential course of action is to adapt CPGs developed in one context to a different context. This makes further sense because the resources that are available to support evidence-based practice would be better spent on assisting with the implementation of useful guidelines rather than re-creation of new guidelines where marginal differences exist between contexts. The ADAPTE process (Table 11-3) describes a process and provides supporting tools for adaptation of guidelines. (www.g-i-n.net/document-store/adapte-resource-toolkit-guideline-adaptation-version-2). It was developed to be usable by either organizations or individuals so that they could approach the adaptation process with a specific framework but allows sufficient flexibility in the process to be usable across different situations.

The adaptation process consists of three phases: a setup phase, an adaptation phase, and a finalization phase (see Table 11-3). During setup, guideline adapters are required to identify the resources and expertise necessary to complete the process. During the adaptation phase, guideline adapters clarify their clinical questions; locate relevant CPGs; and determine the currency, content, and applicability of the available guidelines. This allows the group to make decisions about adaptation of the guideline and facilitates preparation of a draft adaptive guideline. The group then consults with both the stakeholders who would be using the adaptive guideline and the original guideline developers to verify relevancy and accuracy of the recommendations. The ADAPTE Web site provides a guide, tools that can be used to implement the adaptation process, and an exemplar. An adaptation working (sub) group of the Guideline International Network continues to develop the ideas and resources around guideline adaptation (www.g-i-n.net/activities/adaptation).

Finding Clinical Practice Guidelines

Currently, there are thousands of CPGs available—most on medical issues. Because guidelines are most commonly developed by guideline development organizations or professional associations, they are not always disseminated through peer-reviewed literature. Hence, searching electronic databases of scientific research alone will not identify many of the existing CPGs. Increasingly, guideline developers are recognizing the value of having a scientific publication and, where possible, developers are using peer-reviewed journals as one arm of their dissemination plan. However, not all journals are open to publishing such documents.

Therefore, a three-pronged approach is advisable for therapists seeking to find CPGs in their clinical practice area. One can certainly use a traditional search engine like PubMed. In PubMed, clinical queries filters are automated to help clinicians target the type of evidence they would prefer. The category of systematic reviews in clinical queries actually displays citations for systematic reviews, meta-analyses, reviews of clinical trials, evidence-based medicine, consensus development conferences, and guidelines. Therefore, using clinical queries can be a good strategy to identify published CPGs. Such searches may also identify articles that have synthesized information about guidelines in subspecialty areas of rehabilitation. For example, descriptions of the CPGs that pertain to rehabilitation practice have been described (Brooks et al., 2005; Brosseau et al., 2004; Hurdowar et al., 2007; MacDermid, 2004) and provide lists of rehabilitation CPGs.

A second approach for finding CPGs is to look within professional specialty organizations. Professional organizations are often motivated to develop or share guidelines relevant to their members. For example, the American Physical Therapy Orthopedic Division has developed and disseminated guidelines for rehabilitation of common orthopedic conditions (www.orthopt.org/ICF.php). Other organizations compile lists of relevant CPGs to help their members locate these. In terms of searching for guidelines on professional associations, Google may be a more appropriate search engine.

The third approach to searching for relevant guidelines can be focused on databases or repositories that house guideline information. The National Guidelines Clearinghouse Web site (www.guideline.gov) serves as the database of existing guidelines. It provides open access to some guidelines though others must be obtained from national associations or developers. The National Guidelines Clearinghouse offers a sign-up service so that subscribers can receive regular

Table 11-3

ADAPTE—Steps in Adapting an Existing Guideline

Preparation

1. Check whether adaptation is feasible
2. Establish an organizing committee
3. Select a topic
4. Identify skills and resources needed
5. Complete setup tasks
6. Write protocol

Setup Phase

7. Determine the health questions
8. Search for guidelines and other relevant documentation
9. Screen retrieved guidelines
10. Reduce total number of guidelines if there are more than can be dealt with by the panel

Adaptation Phase

11. Assess guideline quality (AGREE)
12. Assess guideline currency
13. Assess guideline content
14. Assess guideline consistency (search strategies, selection of studies, links between evidence and recommendations)
15. Assess acceptability/applicability of the recommendations
16. Review assessments to aid decision making
17. Select between guidelines and recommendations to create an adapted guideline
18. Prepare a document that respects the needs of the end users and provide a detailed transparent explanation of the process

Finalization Phase

19. External review by target users
20. Consult with relevant endorsement of bodies
21. Consult with developers of source guidelines
22. Acknowledge source documents
23. Plan for aftercare of the adapted guideline
24. Produce high-quality final guideline

From "The ADAPTE Process: Resource Toolkit for Guideline Adaptation, Version 2.0," by the ADAPTE Collaboration (2009). Available at: http://www.g-i-n.net. Reprinted with permission.

e-mail updates about newly developed guidelines. An advantage of using the National Guideline Clearinghouse is that it can quickly provide access to potentially relevant CPGs and indicate how they can be located. Many of them have been appraised. The downside to the repository is the fact that rehabilitation guidelines are the exception rather the rule within the database. The Guideline International Network is a professional organization that attracts guideline developers but also contains a variety of resources useful for clinicians wishing to find or implement CPGs (www.g-i-n.net/).

Evaluating the Quality of Clinical Practice Guidelines

Like other evidence syntheses, practitioners can expect to find multiple versions of CPGs on topics relevant to their clinical practice. The next decision becomes how to choose between multiple evidence syntheses. Quality appraisal is a fundamental issue to consider when choosing between different CPGs. A variety of instruments have been developed to evaluate CPGs (Graham, Calder, Hebert, Carter, & Tetroe, 2000). Although numerous guideline appraisal instruments exist, the most commonly used instrument in current literature is the Appraisal of Guidelines Research and Evaluation (AGREE), located at www.agreetrust.org/. This instrument has evolved based on methodological evaluation. The original instrument was based on a yes/no scale and then evolved into a 4-point Likert scale and most recently has become a 7-point evaluation scale where raters endorse items ranging from *strongly disagree* to *strongly agree* (The AGREE Collaboration, 2001, 2003; Brouwers et al., 2010a, 2010b, 2010c; MacDermid et al., 2005). AGREE has been used both by guideline developers to ensure quality during the development process and by users to help select between different guideline options.

One of the benefits of using AGREE to evaluate the quality of guidelines is that it is a structured process using a well-validated tool. The original validation study (The AGREE Collaboration, 2003) demonstrated a strong foundation for AGREE and this was further substantiated by a similar study that reproduced these findings when physical therapists used AGREE to evaluate CPGs developed for a spectrum of rehabilitation issues (MacDermid et al., 2005). Two barriers commonly encountered by individual clinicians in using AGREE are the amount of time required to complete the evaluation and the fact that there is no cutoff score to indicate whether something should or should not be implemented. These barriers are less critical when a team or organization is undertaking a review of guidelines because the organization often recognizes the need to proceed with caution when implementing new practices that may cost the organization time and resources. Appraisal of guidelines allows an organization to follow a process to ensure the optimal guideline choice is selected.

AGREE II (see Table 11-4 for a list of items) Brouwers et al., 2010a, 2010b, 2010c) is the most current version of the guideline appraisal tool and has a dedicated Web site that contains both online and PDF versions of the tool (available at www.agreetrust.org/resource-centre/agree-ii/). In addition, there are training resources on the Web site to facilitate use of the tool. AGREE II consists of 23 key items organized within six domains followed by two global rating items (overall assessment). Each domain captures a unique dimension of guideline quality. The domains as described by AGREE are as follows:

- Domain 1: Scope and purpose is concerned with the overall aim of the guideline, the specific health questions, and the target population (items 1 to 3).

Table 11-4

Items From the Appraisal of Guidelines Research and Evaluation II Guideline Appraisal Tool

DOMAIN 1. SCOPE AND PURPOSE

1. The overall objective(s) of the guideline is (are) specifically described

2. The health question(s) covered by the guideline is (are) specifically described

3. The population (patients, public, etc.) to whom the guideline is meant to apply is specifically described

DOMAIN 2. STAKEHOLDER INVOLVEMENT

4. The guideline development group includes individuals from all relevant professional groups

5. The views and preferences of the target population (patients, public, etc.) have been sought

6. The target users of the guideline are clearly defined

DOMAIN 3. RIGOR OF DEVELOPMENT

7. Systematic methods were used to search for evidence

8. The criteria for selecting the evidence are clearly described

9. The strengths and limitations of the body of evidence are clearly described

10. The methods for formulating the recommendations are clearly described

11. The health benefits, side effects, and risks have been considered in formulating the recommendations

12. There is an explicit link between the recommendations and the supporting evidence

13. The guideline has been externally reviewed by experts prior to its publication

14. A procedure for updating the guideline is provided

DOMAIN 4. CLARITY OF PRESENTATION

15. The recommendations are specific and unambiguous

16. The different options for management of the condition or health issue are clearly presented

17. Key recommendations are easily identifiable

DOMAIN 5. APPLICABILITY

18. The guideline describes facilitators and barriers to its application

19. The guideline provides advice and/or tools on how the recommendations can be put into practice

20. The potential resource implications of applying the recommendations have been considered

21. The guideline presents monitoring and/or auditing criteria

DOMAIN 6. EDITORIAL INDEPENDENCE

22. The views of the funding body have not influenced the content of the guideline

23. Competing interests of guideline development group members have been recorded and addressed

From "Comparison of Original AGREE and AGREE II Items" by the AGREE Research Trust, 2009, www.agreetrust.org. Adapted with permission.

- Domain 2: Stakeholder involvement focuses on the extent to which the guideline was developed by the appropriate stakeholders and represents the views of its intended users (items 4 to 6).

- Domain 3: Rigor of development relates to the process used to gather and synthesize the evidence and the methods to formulate the recommendations and to update them (items 7 to 14).

- Domain 4: Clarity of presentation deals with the language, structure, and format of the guideline (items 15 to 17).

- Domain 5: Applicability pertains to the likely barriers and facilitators to implementation, strategies to improve uptake, and resource implications of applying the guideline (items 18 to 21).

- Domain 6: Editorial independence is concerned with the formulation of recommendations not being unduly biased with competing interests (items 22 to 23).

- Overall assessment includes the rating of the overall quality of the guideline and whether the guideline would be recommended for use in practice.

The individual items are listed in Table 11-4. Readers should explore the full documentation of AGREE and how it is applied/scored as outlined on the AGREE Web site. A recommended process for combining reader scores is provided on the Web site. Typically, raters perform independent assessments. Ideally, the process of rating CPGs using this tool would typically involve some initial training on the use of the tool either by the organization and/or through use of the online training materials, a calibration review performed jointly with experienced raters, and then a process of independent review followed by either averaging or consensus of the ratings. After appraising the individual items, raters make a global assessment about the overall quality of the guideline and whether they would recommend it (with or without modifications). Clinicians who want to determine whether a CPG is useful for their practice can also use AGREE independently and can use the training resources on the Web site to help clarify the meaning of any of the items.

Barriers to Implementation and Uptake of Clinical Practice Guidelines

Although there are benefits of implementing CPGs, the impact has been unclear. The reasons for this are likely multifactorial and include the challenges to developing rehabilitation guidelines, concerns about the guidelines themselves, and challenges in changing practice.

CPGs can be controversial. Those who fear that evidence-based practice may result in "cookbook medicine" may point to CPGs as an example. That CPGs contain recommendations that might not adequately recognize the importance of clinical expertise is a concern of some practitioners. Clinicians may be uncomfortable with prescriptive statements or concerned that CPG fail to address important elements of their specialty practice (Farquhar, Kofa, & Slutsky, 2002; Garfield & Garfield, 2000). Clinicians may feel that their expertise is insufficiently recognized when CPGs are implemented (Garfield & Garfield, 2000). More specifically, it is sometimes perceived that their ability to be client centered or use their clinical experience to optimize treatment will be impeded by a CPG (Farquhar et al., 2002).

Some suspect that cost reduction, not quality, is the primary motivation for CPG implementation (Browman, 2000). Some practitioners might also be concerned that CPGs might pose a liability issue (Farquhar et al., 2002), because not all clinics/practitioners may be able to provide interventions for which there is supporting evidence. Some worry about the legal implications in cases where the practitioner does not follow the course of action recommended by a guideline even though they may feel that their rationale is justified.

A relatively common concern is that CPGs are not necessarily applicable to complex patients and are unable to deal with the interaction between different comorbid conditions. Practitioners know that patients often present with multiple health problems and can struggle to apply multiple guidelines that treat these conditions as separate entities. This can be exacerbated by the way the clinical research is conducted because recommendations within CPGs often arise from clinical trial evidence where complex patients may have been excluded. Thus, clinicians may find that CPGs contain recommendations that are not appropriate for some patients or that CPG recommendations may be conflicting for different comorbid disorders.

An alternative concern is that guidelines do not provide enough specific information to define how interventions can be implemented. For example, a study of guidelines for physical therapy management of rheumatoid arthritis noted that the guidelines lacked details concerning mode of delivery, intensity, frequency, and duration of treatment (Hurkmans et al., 2011). Vague recommendations cannot be implemented. Furthermore, practitioners reading vague recommendations may feel validated and perceive that their practice is already evidence based in that it appears to be consistent with a CPG recommendation without recognizing that their application method or dosage is not consistent with what was specified in the clinical trials. Thus, when CPGs do not include specific recommendations, they may not accomplish the goal of reducing inappropriate practice variations. In fact, one might argue that these CPGs could be counterproductive.

Another concern is that low-quality CPGs may adversely affect practice (Savoie, Kazanjian, & Bassett, 2000), because they may not be evidence based or provide clear, valid recommendations. This concern is reinforced when clinicians observe different CPGs that make different recommendations or contradict each other. Fortunately, CPGs developed more recently tend to be of higher quality (Brooks et al., 2005).

Practical barriers to the implementation of guidelines also exist. For example, guidelines may contain many recommendations and implementing all would be impossible. Therefore, individuals or organizations may struggle with where to start. The process of change in practice is difficult (see chapters dealing with knowledge translation). Many guidelines do not indicate how one can monitor the impact of implementation to help individuals or organizations be more confident that they are achieving improved outcomes. Finally, CPG may recommend a course of action but not provide sufficient detail on the exact nature of how that recommendation should be implemented, leaving a substantial adaptation and implementation burden on the user. This is particularly true in rehabilitation where complex interventions are implemented and the information on skill development/requirements, dosing, combining, and progression is poorly articulated in primary trials.

Facilitating Implementation of Clinical Practice Guidelines

Despite the broad public investment, uptake of guidelines has been more modest than hoped for across most areas of health care where CPGs are available. This has been demonstrated in both simple recommendations such as the use of antibiotics or ordering of diagnostic imaging as well as multimodal interventions. For example, despite intensive guideline development and promotion within The Netherlands, a cross-sectional survey of 1,500 private practice physiotherapists that measured guideline adherence through the use of validated clinical vignettes found an average guideline adherence rate of 50% (Rutten, Kremers, Rutten, & Harting, 2009). Only 38% of the physiotherapists had realistic perceptions of their personal performance.

Factors that mediate rehabilitation guideline uptake have to do with the nature of the guideline itself (e.g., quality, complexity, and clarity); factor within the practitioner and users (e.g., experience, perceptions, and beliefs); the patient target audience (e.g., expectations and preferences); and the practice context (e.g., resource availability, organizational culture, and opinion leaders; Stergiou-Kita, 2010). An extensive study of the evidence documenting barriers for physician adherence to CPGs reviewed 76 published studies addressing perceived barriers and identified 293 potential barriers to physician guideline adherence. Most commonly addressed included awareness/familiarity with the guideline, agreement with guideline recommendations, self-efficacy issues around use of guidelines, difficulties in changing practice, external barriers, and outcome expectancy (Cabana et al., 1999). In rehabilitation, adherence has been linked to the perceived relative advantages and awareness of adherence to the perceived social norm (Rutten et al., 2009).

Strategies for Successful Implementation

We have discussed challenges specific to implementing CPGs. The reader is referred to the knowledge translation chapter for more generic information about the theoretical basis and evidence for changing practice behaviors. There is a considerable body of evidence around guideline implementation and related knowledge translation. A systematic review of 714 primary studies involving 22,512 clinicians evaluated CPG implementation strategies found that studies were highly variable and difficult to compare. Effective implementation strategies include multifaceted interventions, interactive education, and clinical reminder systems. The review also concluded that didactic education and passive dissemination strategies were ineffective. The active involvement of clinicians throughout the process was also identified as a facilitator of successful implementation (Prior, Guerin, & Grimmer-Somers, 2008). Effective CPG implementation strategies will require development of a clear implementation plan and an ongoing commitment to these more time-consuming and resource-intensive interventions (Moulding, Silagy, & Weller, 1999).

Typically, when an organization or individual decides that they might improve their practice through the use of CPGs, they are faced with finding an appropriate guideline and potentially choosing between different guidelines that address the same topic. One aspect of choosing between guidelines is evaluation of their quality. Other considerations include the implementability of the guideline or its recommendations. Finally, it may be necessary to adapt an existing guideline or recommendations across different guidelines. There are tools that will assist us with each of these processes. There are also a variety of freely accessible resources that help with the process itself. For example, the Registered Nurses Association of Ontario provides a guide that can be downloaded free of charge and used to facilitate the phases of guideline implementation. The guide addresses selecting CPGs, identifying and engaging stakeholders, assessing your environmental readiness, choosing implementation strategies, evaluating the impacts, and dealing with resource issues (www.rnao.org/Storage/12/668_BPG_Toolkit.pdf). The Web site and tool kit also come with supporting tools that assist with identifying indicators, resources, and stakeholders. The Canadian Medical Association also produces a guide that deals with implementation issues (www.cma.ca//multimedia/CMA/Content_Images/ClinicalResources/PDF/English/CPGHandbook.pdf).

In general, CPGs are best performed in situations in which the team recognizes that care could be improved, that the guideline offers an opportunity to improve care, and that the frontline clinical treatment team is involved in making decisions about what aspects of an evidence-based guideline will be implemented in practice. Organizational support for this process as a quality improvement initiative—not as a means for managing resources—is more likely to generate better collaboration. With proper motivation, the individual clinician or multidisciplinary team can access the resources outlined in this chapter to plan their CPG implementation.

Guideline Implementability Appraisal

After considering quality, guideline users may wish to consider the implementability of a guideline or its recommendations. The Guideline Implementability Appraisal (GLIA) is an appraisal instrument that is intended to provide information about a guideline's implementability. It can be used by developers to ensure that guidelines are created in a manner that facilitates their implementation by users. The developers have created a GLIA Web site from which the tool can be freely downloaded after registering (http://gem.med.yale.edu/glia/login.htm). The Web site also provides eGLIA—a Web-based version of the GLIA instrument—that allows groups to work at a distance to evaluate guideline implementability.

For users, GLIA focuses on the intrinsic factors that individuals or organizations might wish to consider. Although extrinsic factors are important, they are site specific and not addressed by the instrument. GLIA does address the following (Table 11-5):

- Executability—Exactly what to do
- Decidability—Precisely under what conditions action should be taken
- Validity—The degree to which the recommendation reflects the intent of the developer and the strength of evidence
- Flexibility—The degree to which a recommendation permits interpretation and allows for alternatives in its execution
- Effect on process of care—The degree to which the recommendation impacts upon the usual workflow in a typical care setting
- Measurability—The degree to which the guideline identifies markers or end points to track the effects of implementation of this recommendation
- Novelty/innovation—The degree to which the recommendation proposes behaviors considered unconventional by clinicians or patients
- Computability—The ease with which a recommendation can be operationalized (in an electronic information system) is only applicable when an electronic implementation is planned

When using GLIA, there is a global dimension to consider and the tool also directs the user to decisions about individual recommendations. GLIA questions 1 through 9 (global dimension) relate to the guideline document as a whole. The remaining dimensions of GLIA consider recommendations individually. It is to be expected that certain recommendations within a guideline might be implementable, whereas others may not. This process, whether guided by a structured instrument or not, is critical because prioritizing or staging the process of change can reduce the resistance or barriers to change. The instrument purposely divides recommendations into two types. A conditional recommendation is one that defines the action to be taken under a certain set of circumstances or for a certain subset of individuals. An imperative recommendation states one or more actions to be performed for all members of the target population. Guidelines typically can contain both types of recommendations. The dimension of executability (GLIA questions 10 to 11) focuses on the recommended action and can apply to both imperative and conditional recommendations. The dimension of decidability (GLIA questions 12 to 14) only applies to imperative recommendations as the evaluator decides whether there are clear specifications about the conditions under which a specific course of action should be taken. Although an individual may use GLIA when deciding to change his or her own practice, the most common use of this instrument is when a team or organization is planning to implement changes based on existing guidelines. GLIA developers suggest that at least one clinician and one implementation expert be involved in the process of evaluating guidelines for implementation. Again, in our experience, individual clinicians find a multidimensional assessment challenging. Although clinicians may not feel that they can use GLIA in a formal structured process, it is often advisable to perform a less formal evaluation with the tool as a general guide to identifying and resolving issues around implementation. Individual clinicians can use GLIA criteria to identify recommendations that are most implementable in their clinic.

Appraisers answer each question using the following responses:

- The recommendation meets this criterion fully.
- The recommendation does not meet this criterion.

Table 11-5

The Guideline Implementability Appraisal Tool to Evaluate Implementability of Guidelines

GLOBAL ITEMS (CONSIDERED FOR THE GUIDELINE AS A WHOLE)
1. Does the guideline clearly define the target patient population?
2. Does the guideline clearly define its intended audience (i.e., types of providers)?
3. Are the settings in which the guideline is to be used clearly described?
4. Do the organization(s) and author(s) who developed the guideline have credibility with the intended audience of the guideline?
5. Does the guideline suggest strategies for implementation or tools for application (e.g. a summary document, a quick reference guide, educational tools, patients' leaflets, online resources, or computer software)?
6. Is it clear in what sequence the recommendations should be applied?
7. Is the guideline internally consistent; that is, without contradictions between recommendations?
8. Are all recommendations easily identifiable (e.g., summarized in a box, bold text, underlined, etc.)?
9. Are all recommendations (and their discussions) concise?
RECOMMENDATION ITEMS/EXECUTABILITY (EXACTLY WHAT TO DO): CONSIDERED FOR EACH RECOMMENDATION INDIVIDUALLY
10. Is the recommended action (what to do) stated specifically and unambiguously?
11. Is sufficient detail provided or referenced about how execute the recommendation in order to allow the intended audience to perform the recommended action?
DECIDABILITY (PRECISELY UNDER WHAT CONDITIONS TO DO SOMETHING)
12. Would the guideline's intended audience consistently determine whether each condition in the recommendation has been satisfied?
13. Are all reasonable combinations of conditions addressed?
14. If this recommendation contains more than one condition, is the logical relationship (ANDs and ORs) between conditions clear?
VALIDITY (THE DEGREE TO WHICH THE RECOMMENDATION REFLECTS THE INTENT OF THE DEVELOPER AND THE QUALITY OF EVIDENCE)
15. Is the justification for the recommendation stated explicitly?
16. Is the quality of evidence that supports each recommendation stated explicitly?
FLEXIBILITY (THE DEGREE TO WHICH A RECOMMENDATION PERMITS INTERPRETATION AND ALLOWS FOR ALTERNATIVES IN ITS EXECUTION)
17. Is the strength of each recommendation stated explicitly?
18. Does the recommendation specify patient characteristics that require or permit individualization?
19. Does the recommendation specify practice that requires or permits modification?

(continued)

Table 11-5 (continued)
<h1 style="text-align:center">The Guideline Implementability Appraisal Tool to Evaluate Implementability of Guidelines</h1>
EFFECT ON PROCESS OF CARE (THE DEGREE TO WHICH THE RECOMMENDATION IMPACTS THE USUAL WORKFLOW OF A CARE SETTING)
20. Can the recommendation be carried out without substantial disruption in current workflow?
21. Can the recommendation be pilot tested without substantial resource commitment?
MEASURABILITY (THE DEGREE TO WHICH MARKERS OR ENDPOINTS CAN BE IDENTIFIED TO TRACK THE EFFECTS OF IMPLEMENTATION OF THIS RECOMMENDATION)
22. Can adherence to this recommendation be measured?
23. Can outcomes of this recommendation be measured?
NOVELTY/INNOVATION (THE DEGREE TO WHICH THE RECOMMENDATION PROPOSES ACTIONS CONSIDERED UNCONVENTIONAL BY CLINICIANS OR PATIENTS)
24. Can the recommendation be performed by the guideline's intended users without acquisition of new knowledge or skills?
25. Is the recommendation consistent with existing attitudes and beliefs of the guideline's intended audience?
26. Is the recommendation consistent with patient expectations?
COMPUTABILITY (THE EASE WITH WHICH A RECOMMENDATION CAN BE OPERATIONALIZED IN AN ELECTRONIC INFORMATION SYSTEM; ONLY APPLICABLE WHEN AN ELECTRONIC IMPLEMENTATION IS PLANNED FOR A PARTICULAR SETTING)
27. Are all patient data needed for this recommendation available electronically in the system in which it is to be implemented?
28. Is each condition of the recommendation defined at a level of specificity suitable for electronic implementation?
29. Is each recommended action defined at a level of specificity suitable for electronic implementation?
30. Is it clear by what means a recommended action can be executed in an electronic setting (e.g., creating a prescription, medical order, or referral; creating an electronic mail notification; or displaying a dialog box)?

From "The GuideLine Implementability Appraisal: Development of an Instrument to Identify Obstacles to Guideline Implementation," by R. N. Shiffman, J. Dixon, C. Brandt, A. Essaihi, A. Hsiao, G. Michel, & R. O'Connell, 2005, *BMC Medical Informatics and Decision Making, 5,* p. 23. Reprinted with permission.

- Rater is unable to address this question because of insufficient knowledge or experience in this area.
- N/A—Criterion is not applicable to this recommendation.

When the evaluator decides that a given recommendation does not meet a criterion, the reason(s) it fails the criterion should be recorded in the comment section. The tool provides a location to record barriers and suggested solutions so that the raters can improve the implementability of the guideline.

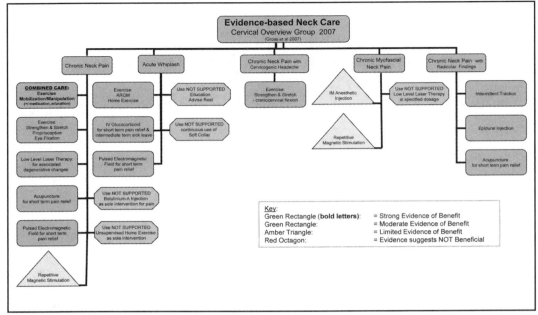

Figure 11-1. An example algorithm developed to summarize evidence on managing neck pain with current best evidence. (From "Conservative Management of Mechanical Neck Disorders: A Systematic Review," A. R. Gross, C. Goldsmith, J. L. Hoving, et al., 2007, *Journal of Rheumatology, 34*(3), pp. 1083-1102. Adapted with permission.)

ALGORITHMS

Algorithms are "written guidelines for stepwise evaluation and management strategies that require observations to be made, decisions to be considered, and actions to be taken" (Hadorn, McCormick, & Diokno, 1992). They can be formulated by taking information from CPGs and arranging it in a decision tree format. For example, the algorithm in Figure 11-1 summarizes a large volume of evidence performed by the Cervical Overview Group (Gross et al., 2007) to indicate which treatment choices are most evidence based by diagnostic subcategory. Some algorithms are designed to synthesize information from diagnostic test results to formulate an overall diagnosis. This can be particularly valuable for clinical diagnostic tests because therapists often perform multiple tests and use them to make an overall diagnosis. Algorithms can be based on evidence alone or a combination of evidence and clinical reasoning/experience. For example, Cools, Cambier, and Witvrouw (2008) used an algorithm to demonstrate a clinical reasoning process for screening athletes with shoulder impingement symptoms into different diagnostic subgroups (Figure 11-2). Subsequently, Ellenbecker and Cools (2010) provided an algorithm for evidence-based treatment that summarized information from a systematic review.

The development of an algorithm can be a straightforward way to implement CPGs and pathways. Furthermore, whereas CPGs can be large unwieldy documents, algorithms can be straightforward diagrams that focus on action. Algorithms help clarify the key decision points requiring action. Algorithms are easiest to devise when courses of action can be defined based on clearly specified criteria. For example, if a cluster of clinical examination criteria can strongly differentiate patients with a specific diagnosis or benefiting from a specific treatment, an algorithm might provide a pictorial method of communicating this that could be readily followed by clinicians. Algorithms can be useful methods for communicating evidence in a way that facilitates implementation.

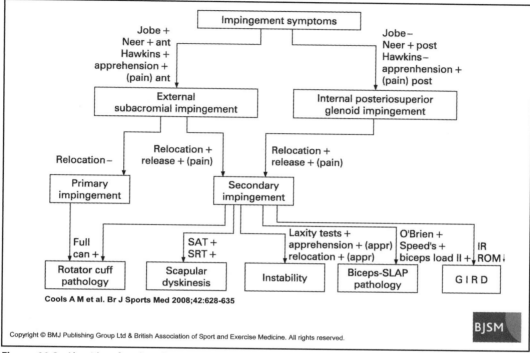

Figure 11-2. Algorithm for clinical reasoning in the examination of impingement-related shoulder pain. (From "Screening the Athlete's Shoulder for Impingement Symptoms: A Clinical Reasoning Algorithm for Early Detection of Shoulder Pain," by A. M. Cools, D. Cambier, & E. E. Witvrouw, 2008, *British Journal of Sports Medicine, 42*(8), pp. 628-635. Reprinted with permission.)

Algorithms can be based on formally developed CPRs. Some algorithms communicate the overall findings of a systematic review that differentiates which type of patients should receive different interventions. Some algorithms are based on decision analysis where the uncertainty of different events is characterized based on data derived from existing literature and a decision tree is identified. The steps in creating a decision tree are (a) the clinical scenario is defined; (b) possible methods of examination, testing, and treatment are listed; (c) probabilities are assigned; and (d) outcomes are listed and matched with probabilities (Greep & Siezenis, 1989). As clinical problems become more complex, it may be difficult to assign probabilities. Under these circumstances, decision trees may or may not include probabilities. Decision trees can be used to represent how the clinician should proceed with diagnosis and management under a set of conditions as dictated by the patient's clinical and diagnostic test findings.

CLINICAL PREDICTION RULES

CPRs, also known as *clinical decision tools*, are evidence-based tools that quantify the contributions of relevant patient characteristics and clinical findings to provide numeric indices that assist clinicians in making decisions about diagnosis or predictions about treatment response or outcome. In a prediction rule study, investigators identify a cohort of patients and measure suspected diagnostic or prognostic indicators and then determine the outcome (diagnosis or treatment response). Statistical analyses are used to determine which of the possible diagnostic or prognostic indicators have clinical utility. CPRs can be communicated in a variety of ways including text summaries indicating what findings must appear together in order to achieve the specified outcome, or as algorithms or decision trees with specified probabilities. CPRs are commonly used to describe the likelihood of the presence or absence of a condition, assist in determining patient prognosis, and help in the classification of patients for treatment. They usually compose of variables—obtained from the history, physical examination, and simple diagnostic tests—that show strong predictive value.

CPRs should be differentiated by their purpose into three distinct groups: (a) diagnostic, (b) prognostic, and (c) prescriptive. CPRs that focus on factors that differentiate patients with a specific diagnosis are known as diagnostic CPRs. Some diagnostic CPRs are used to assist with determination of when additional diagnostic tests such as imaging or biopsy might be warranted. Others focus on determining the specific diagnostic label. CPRs that identify factors that can predict future outcome such as treatment success or return to work are considered prognostic; these CPRs can also predict future adverse events like stroke (Shah, Metz, & Edlow, 2009). CPRs designed to target the most effective interventions based on presenting criteria are prescriptive CPRs. The latter should be derived from RCTs. CPRs of all three types are becoming increasingly prevalent in rehabilitation. One of the most well-known and most commonly implemented (Dowling & Wishart, 2011) diagnostic CPR is the Ottawa Ankle Rules, which is used to differentiate which patients presenting with ankle pain require an x-ray, with fracture being the diagnosis of interest. A CPR has also been developed to help with diagnosis of carpal tunnel syndrome by combining different diagnostic features (Wainner et al., 2005). Prognostic CPRs have been used to determine outcomes in a variety of areas of practice including neurological, musculoskeletal, and pediatric. For example, a CPR consisting of age and four neurological tests has been used to predict ambulation following spinal cord injury (van Middendorp et al., 2011). Prescriptive CPRs have been used to describe patients who would respond to different interventions; for example, for neck and back pain (Childs et al., 2004; Cleland et al., 2010). An indicator of the increasing role of CPRs is the publication of a physical therapy textbook on CPRs (Glynn & Weisbach, 2011).

McGinn et al. (2000) proposed the following stages in development of a CPR: derivation (analyzing a data set to establish a rule with predictive power); narrow validation (evaluating the rule in a similar clinical setting and population); broad validation (evaluating the rule in multiple clinical settings); and impact analysis (determining whether the rule changes clinicians' behaviors, improves patient outcomes, or reduces costs). Derivation is the stage where the CPR is first proposed and tested on at initial data set. One might expect CPRs to work best within data sets where the rules have been devised. Therefore, it is important that a preliminary CPR be validated in other research studies.

The first stage of validation would involve testing the CPR in a similar independent sample and then proceeding to broader (different) patient samples. If the CPR can be demonstrated to be generalizable to other patients, they can be considered to have reached Level 2. The highest level of validation is Level 1 and occurs when CPRs have undergone an impact analysis that demonstrates positive effects on clinician behaviors, outcomes, and cost-effectiveness of care. For example, the Ottawa Ankle Rules have been shown to decrease utilization of radiographs without resulting in missed fractures (Knudsen, Vijdea, & Damborg, 2010) and provide a mechanism for patients to self-assess their need for emergency treatment (Blackham, Claridge, & Benger, 2008) but do not reduce time in the emergency room (Fan & Woolfrey, 2006). CPRs that reach Level 1 validation can be used in a wide array of settings with confidence that their use will be beneficial (McGinn et al., 2000).

Despite the increased acceptance of CPRs into rehabilitation practice, they are not without controversy. Systematic reviews indicate that few have undergone sufficient validation (Beneciuk, Bishop, & George, 2009). Furthermore, there is limited study of their impact within controlled trials (Stanton, Hancock, Maher, & Koes, 2010). A number of developmental studies have been conducted on samples of convenience and the rules have not been adequately validated across different clinical contexts. Furthermore, analytical techniques designed to identify positive predictors may increase the risk of identifying predictors unique to that data set. Thus, it can be uncertain whether a CPR will work in another clinical situation. One should be particularly cautious when considering a prescriptive CPR to choose an intervention because, in addition to the limitations cited previously, these are subject to additional methodological concerns. That is, many of the studies addressing this type of CPR are unable to differentiate between predictors of response to a specific treatment and general predictors of outcome. Patients who are most likely to respond to any of the treatments studied within a prescriptive CPR may be those most likely to recover because of inherent positive predictive factors. Thus, it can be difficult to attribute the positive outcomes to the intervention. At present, few CPRs have reached the Level 1 validation they should have before considered appropriate for widespread implementation. Therapists should consider CPRs carefully, evaluating the quality of their development and the extent that they could be generalized to their patient population (McGinn et al., 2000) before implementing them. However, given the rapid emergence of evidence in this area and its potential benefit to practice, it is important to continue this research and eventually identify the smaller subset of CPRs that will reach a Level 1 validation. When this subset is identified, they can be used with confidence to make more efficient evidence-based decisions.

CLINICAL PATHWAYS

CPs, also termed *critical pathways* or *integrated care pathways*, use accepted benchmark goals to enhance outcomes and contain costs within a constrained clinical intervention.

CPs have defined processes that have been described and developed differently across different contexts (Currie & Harvey, 1998; McKenna et al., 2006). In the United States, the concept of a CP has been commonly used as a framework for balancing costs and quality, whereas in the United Kingdom, CPs are viewed as a way of achieving a continuum of care across care settings (integrated care pathways). Pathways have been utilized in the American health care system since the late 1980s when Dr. Karen Zander of the Center for Case Management developed a patented model named CareMap. The model applied the engineering project management principles used in manufacturing to a nursing and case management initiative in Boston's New England Medical Center. Later, American health care organizations started to define clusters of patients/clients with similar conditions called *case mixed groups* or *diagnostic-related groups*. Then the system moved to capping service by dictating maximum costs based on the projected episode of care in a model known as *managed care*.

In some cases, CPs are evidence based; in others, they are not. Differences in how they are defined are evident from the literature (Kinsman, Rotter, James, Snow, & Willis, 2010). A systematic review identified 84 definitions (De Bleser, De Waele, Vanhaecht, Vlayen, & Sermeus, 2006). The review suggested the following definitions:

- A care pathway can be defined as a complex intervention for the mutual decision making and organization of care processes for a well-defined group of patients during a well-defined period.
- The aim of a care pathway is to enhance the quality of care across the continuum by improving risk-adjusted patient outcomes, promoting patient safety, increasing patient satisfaction, and optimizing the use of resources.

Defining characteristics of care pathways include the following:

- An explicit statement of the goals and key elements of care based on evidence, best practice, and patients' expectations and their characteristics.
- Facilitation of communication among team members and with patients and their families.

- Coordination of the care process by coordinating the roles and sequencing the activities of the multidisciplinary care team, patients, and their relatives.
- Documentation, monitoring, and evaluation of variances and outcomes.
- Identification of the appropriate resources.

The CP is a tool that sets locally agreed-upon clinical standards, based on the best available evidence, for managing specific groups of clients. It can form part or all of the clinical record and enables the care given by members of the multidisciplinary team—together with the progress and outcome—to be documented. Variations from the pathway are recorded and analysis allows a continuous evaluation of the effectiveness of clinical practice. Information obtained is used to revise the pathway to improve the quality of client care (Kitchiner & Bundred, 1996, 1999). Five characteristics have been used to define a CP:

1. The intervention is a structured multidisciplinary plan of care.
2. The intervention is used to translate guidelines or evidence into local structures.
3. The intervention details the steps in a course of treatment or care in a plan, pathway, algorithm, guideline, protocol, or other inventory of actions.
4. The intervention has time frames or criteria-based progression.
5. The intervention aimed to standardize care for a specific clinical problem, procedure, or episode of health care in a specific population.

Systematic reviewers have used attainment of three of these criteria as sufficient evidence to indicate that an intervention constituted a CP (Kinsman et al., 2010).

The pathway process is expected to contribute to the following potentially valuable consequences:
- Define specific expected clinical behaviors to reduce practice variation.
- Provide mechanisms to help clinicians assimilate large amounts of rapidly evolving scientific evidence.
- Provide a vehicle for the public, clinicians, and administrators to participate in joint decision making around clinical processes.
- A respectable process to respond to the demands of third-party funding and quality monitoring agents for standards around appropriate rehabilitation practice.

Clinical pathway models have a matrix listing interventions along one axis and a time frame along another. Interventions typically include the spectrum of relevant diagnostic, treatment, and outcome interventions that should be specified for that caseload (Figure 11-3). CP elements can include consultations and referral, assessments/observations, tests, treatments, measurements/diagnostics, nutrition, medication, activity and mobility, safety, patient/client and family education/teaching, and discharge planning. Within the time line, benchmarks may be identified, as well as typical problems, desired clinical outcomes, intermediate goals or key indicators, and physician orders. Some pathways include variance tracking records to identify the reasons why actions were not taken or benchmarks were not achieved. The pathway may also include admission and discharge indicators/status, as well as key indicator and outcome records (clinical and client/patient). Pathways are typically identified for areas with an appropriate blend of the following characteristics: high volume, high cost, high risk, high practice variability, potential for improvement, potential to cross multiple settings and disciplines in continuum, predictable course, provider interest/initiative, and acceptance of the development/implementation process.

The evidence around CPs is complicated by variations between studies on what constitutes a care pathway (Vanhaecht et al., 2011). Despite variations, there is more evidence suggesting that CPs can improve the process of care in comparison to evidence suggesting that they have the ability to improve outcomes. For example, the prevention pathway methodology was useful to define inefficiencies and quality problems in the occupational health practices around chemical risk assessment and biomonitoring (Godderis, Vanhaecht, Masschelein, Sermeus, & Veulemans, 2004). In a systematic review, 22 studies of CPs developed for total joint arthroplasty and administered to a total sample of 6,316 patients did not demonstrate differences in discharge status or time but did find that there were significantly fewer patients suffering postoperative complications in the CP group compared to the standard care group. Furthermore, pathway patients had a shorter length of stay and lower costs during their hospital stay (Barbieri et al., 2009). A systematic review conducted on 27 studies involving 11,398 participants evaluated the impact of CPs with usual care. These studies indicated a reduction in in-hospital stay and improved documentation with CPs (Rotter et al., 2010). There was no evidence of differences in readmission to the hospital or in-hospital mortality. The primary indicators used to study the impact of a CP are related to process (Rotter et al., 2010). Thus, there is more information on their impact on process. Clinical pathway implementation is common in lower extremity arthroplasty (see Figure 11-3), where it has been shown to result in significant reduction in the length of stay (reducing costs) without compromising outcome (Pennington, Jones, & McIntyre, 2003). The use of CPs in above- or below-knee amputation indicated that more patients were able to return home from acute care and rehabilitation with a CP (Schaldach, 1997). Implementation of a CP was also reported to reduce health care costs without impairing quality of care in the treatment of decubitus ulcer patients (Dzwierzynski, Spitz, Hartz, Guse, & Larson, 1998). CPs have been used commonly in stroke rehabilitation; however, a recent systematic review concluded:

> Care pathways should, intuitively, improve the quality of stroke care; however, surprisingly, evidence does not support this conclusion. It is not clear why this occurs. Care pathways may simply reinforce rather than change practice. This suggests that imposing a blueprint of care, rather than individualizing treatment, does not improve outcomes. Therefore, although organized interdisciplinary stroke rehabilitation units have been shown to improve outcomes, care pathways do not appear to be contributing to this success. (StrokEngine, 2013)

Pathway Development

It is important that the development team selects the specific client group for the pathway to ensure interest and enthusiasm for the task at the front line rather than solely at an administrative level. Many excellent pathways have failed simply because those affected by the tool were not involved with its formulation and implementation. As a result, they were disinterested and did not see the importance of the work. Interested participants who are involved in the actual care delivery must be identified and selected to form working groups. If the literature search identifies relevant CPGs, the CPGs can become the foundation for the pathway. It is important that people who understand the evidence and the frontline operations cooperate on developing the pathway. It is preferable if patients are consulted in the process to ensure that meaningful patient considerations are included in the CP.

Ideally there should be a congruence between CP tools and non-pathway tools such as flowcharts and outcome measures. When they were first developed, CPs were tools used only as a guide, often housed in policy and procedure manuals. With some pathways, staff were asked to sign off at the end of a shift. Others were used in conjunction with flow sheets to facilitate compiling information over an episode of care. With a move toward electronic records, there is an increasing ability to incorporate CPs into documentation. The existence of a CP can facilitate the move to a charting-by-exception model, resulting in efficiencies in the amount of time spent on documentation versus direct patient care.

PATIENT'S NAME: _____   CLINICAL PATHWAY - TOTAL KNEE   November, 1998

Date: _____
Date: _____

	Preadmission	Preop/Same Day Admission Day 1 Pre	Preop/Same Day Admission Day 1 Post	Day 2 Post Op Day 1	Day 3 Post Op Day 2	Day 4 Post Op Day 3	Day 5 Post Op Day 4	Day 6/Day 7 Post Op Day 5/6
Consults/Referrals	Mandatory • Nursing • Physio • Pharmacy • Orthopaedic Resident Optional • OT G • Medical consult (may have been pre-arranged) G • Anaesthesia consult G • Pastoral Care G • Social Work G • Dietician G • CCAC G • Rehabilitation G	• Pastoral Care	• Physio referral	• Chest physio if needed • Pastoral Care if required	Ongoing Physio for ambulation & ROM --------->	---------> • OT Assessment * if needed for ADLs • Assess need for Outpatient, Physio or CCAC Physio or Rehab	• CCAC if required ---------> • Pharmacist (if anticoagulant required upon discharge) ---------> --------->	---------> ---------> --------->
Patient/Family Teaching	• Give Total Knee Booklet G • PCA sheet G • Pharmacy anticoag teaching G • Nursing preop teaching (counselling) G - SDA - DB&C • Physio G • Give Pastoral Care flyer G	• PCA Sheet G • Physio Sheet G • OR Record G • DB/C • Reinforce PCA-teaching	---------> --------->	• Isometric exercises • leg on pillow avoiding knee flexion and heel pressure	• Don't sit for longer than 1 h at a time • Review s/s infection and DVT • WBAT • Sit in chair with feet on floor to encourage knee flexion (may use stool if necessary)	• Physio reviews mobility equipment needs • OT for ADLs * --------->	• If patient requires anticoagulant at home, arrange pharmacist to see patient family if previous or current DVT, PE) • Arrange for GP to monitor INRs • Assess knowledge and understanding of knee exercises/positioning • Make sure patient has necessary equipment for home	• Review S/S infection/DVT • Stress importance of exercises, mobility and appropriate rest ---------> • Review proper positioning - review discharge sheet - have patient sign and take copy
Tests	• CBC • S S ± • U/A • CXR ± • EKG ± • Knee x-ray ±	• CBC, SS (if not done Preadmission) • U/A • CXR ± • EKG ± • Knee x-ray ±	• knee x-ray in OR post OP	• CBC • SS • INR • Oxygen saturation (if on oxygen)	• INR	• CBC, SS, INR	• INR	
Treatments	• Explain Hibitane scrub and give sponge to take home	• Hib scrub if not done at home • DB/C • Start IV	• Oxygen as ordered • Skin care q4h • CSM q1h x4 then q4h • HMV - monitor and empty and record q12h (if no HMV - monitor dressing and reinforce as needed) • Maintain IV at rate ordered • I and O - q shift or more often as needed • VS q 1/2h on return from PACU x2 then q4h x 48hrs • may have femoral block which may effect CSM	• D/C HMV • monitor dressings q shift and PRN • CSM Q4h • VS q4h • I and O q shift • D/C oxygen if sat >92 • IV as ordered • Turn Q4h with skin care • Assess for abdominal and bladder distention q4h • Change to light dressing • Document drainage • Physio to initiate ROM exercises 2 times per day unless patient's pain uncontrolled	• Turn q4h with skin care • D/C IV/PCA if oral intake adequate and good pain control • CSM q4h • VS q4h • Assess for Homan's sign and edema	• Monitor wound/dressing: change PRN and document appearance of wound / drainage • VS q shift • CSM q shift • Turn Q4h with skin care while in bed	• Monitor wound/dressing - change PRN and document appearance of wound / drainage • VS daily • CSM q shift • Turn Q4h with skin care while in bed (teach how to turn independently) • Encourage independent turning while in bed every four hours --------->	• Change dressing to light and assess wound before discharge • Give staple remover with instructions for G.P. to remove 2 weeks post op • VS before discharge >
Medication	• Pharmacist to provide anticoagulant teachings and give Coumadin, for night before OR • List patient's meds • Advise patient which of own meds to take with sips in a.m. of OR according to Dr's orders	• Give pre-op meds as ordered • Antibiotic IV on call if ordered • Coumadin @ HS if ordered • Post op Coumadin (7.5 mgms) at HS	• Antibiotic IV x 24h • PCA - monitor pain relief (If no PCA offer analgesia q4h) • Continue home meds as ordered • Coumadin at HS	---------> ---------> --------->	• Begin oral analgesia once PCA D/C'd (offer 1/2 hour before physio to see) • Continue home meds as ordered • Offer laxative as ordered per bowel routine	---------> ---------> --------->	---------> ---------> --------->	---------> • Scripts for analgesic and/or any new medication started in hospital and to continue at home • D/C Coumadin
Diet	N/A	• NPO at 2400 day before OR	• Diet as tolerated (start with clear fluids)	• DAT - advance as tolerated • Encourage fluids	• DAT • Push fluids	• DAT	• DAT	• DAT
Activity	N/A		• Bed rest • Commode privileges	• Physio to see - up in chair as tolerated x2 • Encourage foot and ankle exercises and quad setting • Wear proper foot wear • Physio to see regarding ambulation WBAT and begin knee ROM • Document progress on physio sheet at bedside 2x day	---------> ---------> ---------> ---------> --------->	• Ambulation/endurance in hall x2 • Teach independent transfers • Knee ROM with physio x2	• Continue to increase length of ambulation with supervision only • Attempt stairs • Continue knee ROM • Assess need for continuing physio at home	• OT D/C if needed • Independent with walking aid and with stairs • Physio/D/C • Referral for Outpatient physio or home care physio if needed • Independent with home exercise program
Discharge Plan	• Community supports available (Booklet for seniors if needed) • Home resources • Make patient aware of expected length of stay • Convalescent care to be explored if required (Social Work) • Patient to get commitment from family members for assistance at discharge for ADLs/IADLs • Prepare and freeze meals ahead of time • Stress Home Care is generally not indicated but is available based on specific needs • Staple remover (check with GP's office if one available)				• Clarify home supports and discharge plans (ensure follow-up)	• Make appropriate referrals to Rehab/Social Work if required • Contact family if necessary regarding home supports • Instruct patient in TKA Home Exercise Program	• Reinforce discharge planning • Plan specific D/C day based on patient's progress to date • Assess need for continuing physio and arrange Outpatient or CCAC physio	• Discharge by 1000 • Follow-up appointment with surgeon for six weeks • Outpatient physio referral if required • Discharge sheet of exercises from physio
Other	• Nursing assessment/data collection (esp. previous mobility status); anaesthetic questionnaire; consent signed • HT/WT							
Expected Outcomes	• Patient and family verbalize understanding of pre-op teaching		• Chest clear • VS stable (within normal limits) • Able to dorsi flex (unless had spinal / block anaesthesia) • Patient verbalizes reasonable pain control	• Patient learns how to transfer bed/chair with assistance • Patient understands importance of turning q4h to maintain skin integrity --------->	• Patient able to transfer bed/chair with one assistant • in chair for all three meals if able • begin to ambulate short distance in room with walker/crutches • Perform isometric exercises and ROM of knee (dorsi flexion and quads setting) with physio 2x day and independently 3x day	• Bed/Chair transfers with minimal assistance • Ambulate to BR in room with one assistant and walking aid • Performs isometric exercises independently and continue to improve knee ROM independently • Identifies need for mobility aids	• Bed/Chair transfers with minimal assistance / independent • Ambulate in hall with supervision and walking aid • Walk to bathroom / supervision • Attempt stairs • Patient verbalizes readiness for discharge • D/C plans in place • Home support in place • Discharge plans made with community if required --------->	• Manages stairs, transfers and ambulation independently • Independent with walking aid and with stairs • Patient and/or family independent with ADL's • Patient has all needed mobility equipment • Home has been modified for safety • Achieves ROM as outlined by physician --------->
Signatures								

Figure 11-3. An example clinical pathway for total knee arthroplasty.

VARIANCE TRACKING SHEET

Date of Admission: **Clinical Pathway Name:**

Date of Discharge:

		VARIANCE		SOURCE			
Date	Actual Care Path Day	SPECIFY VARIANCE	Category (Select A to D)	Reason (Select 1-16)	Specify Reason for Variance	Sig./Status	

CATEGORY

A. Patient/Family

B. Care Giver/Clinician

REASON

01-Patient condition
02-Pt/family decision
03-Pt/family availability
04-Pt/family other

05-Physician order
06-Caregiver(s) decision
07-Caregiver(s) response time
08-Caregiver other

CATEGORY

C. Hospital

D. Community

REASON

09-Bed/appt time availability
10-Information/date availability
11-Supplies/equipment availability
12-Dept. overbooked/closed

13-Hospital other
14-Placement/Home Care availability
15-Transportation availability
16-Community other

Figure 11-3 (continued). An example clinical pathway for total knee arthroplasty.

Inherent in the definition of a CP is the process of tracking variance data. A *variance* is the difference between what is expected and what actually happens. Variances can be the result of client, practitioner, or system issues and can be either positive or negative.

Factors usually resulting in a variance include the following:

- The client's condition can cause an unexpected complication or unanticipated rapid progress.
- The support network of informal or formal supports can facilitate or impose restrictions.
- A provider or agency issue, such as presence of a wait list or availability of test results.
- Provision of equipment and supplies (e.g., delivery, availability).
- Environmental issues (e.g., unsanitary conditions, lack of water, heat, electricity, food, telephone).

If the recording and reporting system is computerized, it may be possible to track variances concurrently (at the same time the variance is identified) and address the variance immediately. Variances that focus on the program include factors such as length of stay, number and frequency of visits, readmission rates, infection rates, and length of time waiting for service. The example in this chapter includes a variance tracking record used for total knee arthroplasty.

Clinical Pathway Appraisal

In deciding to implement a CP developed by others, a process of critically evaluating the CP should be undertaken. A guide for the development and evaluation of integrated care pathways has been published by National Leadership and Innovation Agency for Healthcare (Davis, 2005).

The Integrated Care Pathway Appraisal Tool (Whittle, McDonald, & Dunn, 2004) was developed for pathway appraisal. Example questions include the following:

- Does the CP have an identified start point?
- Are there clear instructions on how to use the documentation?
- Is there a record of the decisions made and discussion concerning the content of the pathway?
- Has an ongoing training program for the staff users been established?
- Is someone nominated to maintain the CP?

A content analysis of seven different appraisal tools identified 17 core characteristics. The resulting Integrated Care Pathway Appraisal Tool can be used to assess CP (Vanhaecht, De Witte, Depreitere, & Sermeus, 2006).

The appraisal tool has subscales that address the following dimensions:

- Dimension 1: Is it an integrated care pathway (ICP)?
- Dimension 2: The ICP documentation
- Dimension 3: The ICP development process
- Dimension 4: The ICP implementation process
- Dimension 5: Maintenance of the ICP
- Dimension 6: The role of the organization

The Care Process Self-Evaluation Tool (CPSET; Vanhaecht et al., 2007) is a 29-item self-evaluation scale to evaluate the organization of the care process from the multidisciplinary point of view. It contains five subscales: patient-focused organization (6 items), coordination of the care process (7 items), communication with patients and family (4 items), collaboration with primary care (3 items), and follow-up of the care process (9 items). The CPSET can be used in the audit and accreditation of care processes by managers and clinicians to better understand how care processes are organized (Vanhaecht et al., 2007). This can be useful to monitor the outcomes of a CP in terms of process. Tracking information on CPs may help define optimal steps in clinical processes, reduce unnecessary variation in these processes, and provide data for continuous quality and process improvement. This instrument has been used to evaluate how health care teams perceive the organization of care processes with respect to CPs. A cross-sectional, multicenter study was performed composed of 309 health care workers, 103 care processes, and 49 hospitals using the CPSET to score care processes according to their organization. Care processes supported by CPs had the highest CPSET scores (Vanhaecht, De Witte, Panella, & Sermeus, 2009).

For more information, researchers can consult the European Clinical Pathway Association (www.e-p-a.org/about-epa/index.html), which is a nonprofit organization that is entirely focused on CPs and provides definitions, a variety of resources, and opportunities around CPs. Membership is free of charge.

PATIENT DECISION AIDS

All of the evidence-based knowledge synthesis tools discussed previously have focused on clinicians or organizations as a decision maker. Evidence can also be synthesized and presented in a way to support decision making by patients. PDAs are evidence-based tools that help people become involved in decision making by providing information about options and outcomes and typically encourage patients to reflect on these through the lens of their own personal values. They are generally most useful in situations where there is sufficient time to reflect on options and there are differential outcomes and risks/side effects. For example, non-urgent interventions or diagnostic tests may benefit from the use of a PDA. Implementation of PDAs/decision support can be motivated by wanting to be more patient centered, recognizing an area where patients are struggling to make decisions, and wanting to improve the quality or satisfaction associated with decision making (for quality or medical–legal reasons).

There are now more than 500 DAs available, and the scientific literature around developing, appraising, and implementing these tools is increasing. There is no consensus on the nature or role of PDAs (Holmes-Rovner et al., 2007), but there is an increased focus on understanding them. Decision aids (DAs) can be generic tools to support the decision process or can be more specific evidence-based tools that incorporate data about the specific risks and benefits of different options for specific decisions. Generic tools can be useful during a patient–clinician interaction if the therapist is willing and able to present evidence-based considerations to the patient and then use the tool to facilitate integration of evidence and values. Specific tools can be beneficial because the clinician does not need to locate the evidence but can provide it in a prepackaged format.

The (Ottawa) decision aids Web site provides a host of resources with respect to DAs, learning materials, and resources for developing and evaluating PDAs (http://decisionaid.ohri.ca/). It includes generic DAs (http://decisionaid.ohri.ca/docs/das/OPDG.pdf), the "Ottawa Personal Decision Guide," and a downloadable file of specific DAs (http://decisionaid.ohri.ca/cochinvent.php).

The International Patient Decision Aid Standards Collaboration is a group of researchers, practitioners, and stakeholders from around the world. Appraisal of a PDA can be conducted using a structured appraisal tool available free of charge (www.ipdasi.org/2006%20IPDAS%20Quality%20Checklist.pdf). This tool was developed using criteria evaluated through international consensus (Elwyn et al., 2006; http://ipdas.ohri.ca/IPDAS_checklist.pdf).

Evidence synthesis tools that focus on patients are bringing to the forefront concepts such as health literacy, theoretical foundations of decision making (Elwyn, Stiel, Durand, & Boivin, 2011), cultural/contextual variation in values and preferences, and issues around communication. Health literacy is an individual's ability to read, understand, and use health care information to make decisions and follow instructions for treatment. PDAs ideally can be a tool to facilitate incorporating evidence and values in the decision-making process and should incorporate best practices in health literacy. Health literacy goes beyond reading and incorporates the ability to understand the evidence that is presented, including understanding the risks and benefits. A variety of ways of presenting information including risk and benefit have been investigated and have led to greater use of graphic images to display risk and benefit in PDAs. Variations in how information is presented to affect recall and understanding of risk–benefit (Martin, Brower, Geralds, Gallagher, & Tellinghuisen, 2011) have become an emerging area of research that links health literacy with communication of evidence. A criticism of DAs has been that they have not been sufficiently culturally sensitive and may contain text that is too difficult according to health literacy standards (Thomson & Hoffman-Goetz, 2007).

A systematic review of 55 RCTs investigating the impact of PDAs determined that the outcomes measured were variable: 69% of studies included at least one effectiveness measure (O'Connor et al., 2007). Measures of decision quality were knowledge scores (27 trials), accurate risk perceptions (12 trials), and value congruence with the chosen option (3 trials). PDAs improved knowledge scores relative to usual by approximately 15%. The findings also were supportive of specific PDAs in that detailed PDAs were about 5% more effective than simple PDAs and were associated with better value congruence. Risk perception was better if data were provided. The review concluded that PDAs improve the perception of being informed and decision quality, although the size of the effect varied across studies (O'Connor et al., 2007). Overall, this suggests that using a generic evidence-based PDA can improve the process of informed consent; however, the inclusion of specific evidence has a small impact on patients. Reviews have noted that the large variability in impact suggests that as we better understand PDAs and how to use them effectively, we may obtain more consistent results.

Computerized Clinical Decision Support Systems

Clinical decision support systems are active knowledge systems that use two or more items of patient data to generate case-specific advice and typically integrate medical knowledge, patient data, and a computer-based inference analysis to generate case-specific advice. Electronic decision support is becoming increasingly prevalent with the advent of electronic medical records and the development of computer technologies. Decision support systems can take advantage of a variety of knowledge management strategies including findings from evidence syntheses and analysis of large data sets including strategies such as network analysis or artificial intelligence to support decision making. They can be used for administrative purposes such as clinical coding and documentation, authorization of procedures, and referrals. They can also be used to manage clinical complexity by including specific information protocols or care pathways. They are sometimes used as cost-control mechanisms to monitor the use of medications or diagnostic tests. With respect to evidence-based practice, they can be used to implement evidence arising from evidence syntheses around assessment, prognosis, or treatment implementation that come from condition-specific CPGs. They have evolved to a greater extent in medicine given the focus on coding, diagnostic procedures, and medications.

Computerized decision support has been investigated in a systematic review in the context of the multidisciplinary management of chronic disease management. Of 55 included trials, 87% measured impact on the process of care and 52% of those demonstrated statistically significant improvements. Sixty-five measured the impact on patient outcomes and, of these, 31% demonstrated benefits (Roshanov et al., 2011). Similar findings were reported for acute care management (Sahota et al., 2011), drug prescribing (Hemens et al., 2011), and prevention (Souza et al., 2011). At the time of this book's publication, there has been limited study of the use of clinical decision support systems in rehabilitation.

Implementation of Evidence Synthesis Tools

Although evidence synthesis tools are designed to facilitate implementation of evidence into practice, we know that development of the tool itself is not sufficient to change practice. Implementation or knowledge translation is addressed in a separate chapter. We will merely summarize what is known about knowledge translation with respect to evidence synthesis tools. The first important step in identification of an appropriate tool is determining that it is strongly grounded in evidence before investigating implementability. Table 11-6 has a summary of the tools and products. We know that active engagement of the users throughout the process of identifying and evaluating the evidence synthesis process can facilitate buy-in. We know that there are a variety of tools that can assist with evaluation of the quality of different evidence synthesis tools. Our personal experience tells us that clinicians often find these difficult to navigate and may require initial support from experts on how to use the tools. Appraisal tool developers recommend that both clinicians and methodological experts be involved in the appraisal and selection of evidence synthesis tools or specific recommendations from them. We know that simple dissemination of these recommendations has minimal impact on practice. Rather, more active and multipronged efforts are needed. These are more clearly articulated in the chapter on knowledge translation.

TAKE-HOME MESSAGES

✓ Evidence can be incorporated into tools that facilitate implementation of evidence-based clinical decisions.

✓ A large number of resources have been directed to development of evidence-based CPGs in a variety of professions including multidisciplinary and rehabilitation-specific CPGs.

✓ CPGs can lead to other evidence-based tools such as algorithms, CPs, and DAs.

✓ There are standardized processes for development and appraisal of CPGs, CPs, and DAs.

✓ Implementation can be facilitated by the use of these tools but requires an active ongoing process to facilitate better patient outcomes being achieved.

✓ CPG development and evaluation is facilitated by the use of AGREE.

✓ Algorithms can be useful to communicate or implement decision making.

✓ CPs can result in improvements in process, but improvements in outcome are less consistently demonstrated.

✓ DA can improve patients' involvement in evidence-based decision making and reduce decision regret, but effects are inconsistent.

LEARNING ACTIVITIES

1. Explore the following Web sites to find examples of different evidence synthesis products described in this chapter.

2. Explore Google and professional Web sites to find evidence-based tools and discuss with other clinicians whether they could be implemented into your practice.

3. Perform a critical appraisal of a CPG using AGREE II; compare with a colleague.

4. Choose five recommendations from a CPG guideline and evaluate their implementability using the GLIA tool. Discuss with others whether this facilitated defining an implementation plan and whether key issues were missed.

5. Practice using a PDA with a colleague and discuss what types of decisions in your practice might benefit from this tool.

Table 11-6

An Overview of Evidence Synthesis Products

CLINICAL PRACTICE GUIDELINES	
Question	*Answer*
What is it?	Clinical practice guidelines are "systematically developed statements to assist practitioners and patient decisions about appropriate health care for specific clinical circumstances" (Field & Lohr, 1992). In evidence-based practice, it is implied that guidelines are systematically developed using a synthesis of the best quality evidence and a structured process for making recommendations that may include the input of a panel of clinical experts and methodologists.
Why are they needed?	In all areas of health care practice, a consistent finding is that there is tremendous practice variation. Practice patterns indicate that evidence-based treatments are underutilized and ineffective ones continue to be used. This indicates that consistent use of best practice is not achieved in most areas of health care practice. It is assumed that if one can synthesize the evidence to make evidence-based recommendations about best practices, these could be communicated to clinicians to reduce the variations and practice patterns, providing both more effective and more efficient management of health conditions.
What is the evidence?	There is moderate evidence that guidelines can reduce practice variation or process of care and limited evidence and that they improve patient outcomes within specific contexts (Bahtsevani et al., 2004; Lugtenberg, Burgers, & Westert, 2009). A systematic review of trials evaluating guideline impact identified 20 studies (Lugtenberg et al., 2009). In 17 of 19 studies that measured the effects on the process or structure of care, significant improvements were reported; 6 of 9 studies that measured patient health outcomes showed significant but small improvements as a result of the use of clinical guidelines.
When to use?	Can be helpful in defining an approach when encountering a new health problem to get a broad overview of best practice or can be useful to define variations between best practices and current practice for an existing caseload.
What are the challenges?	The quality of guideline recommendations is dependent on the quality of existing research. There is evidence that clinicians who develop CPGs without adequate balance from expert methodologists are more likely to depart from the evidence (Savoie et al., 2000; van der Sanden et al., 2004). However, involvement of clinicians is also critical to relevance and acceptance. There is evidence that written guidelines without accompanying dissemination activities have little clinical impact. Changes in practice are more easily achieved with simple decisions/interventions such as prescribing practices compared to more complex management issues such as rehabilitation, which is a complex intervention. The quality of CPGs is variable but increasing. CPG are often not updated every 3 years as suggested.
How to optimize?	Engagement of multiple stakeholders including a variety of disciplines, as well as experts in guideline development, patients, researchers, practicing clinicians, and professional associations in the development and implementation process. Use of recognized methods for collection and synthesis of evidence, as well as for achieving consensus (Woolf, DiGuiseppi, Atkins, & Kamerow, 1996). Clear recommendations (GRADE); specific and actionable recommendations. Provide supporting tools for implementation. Use AGREE II to select between competing guidelines, APAPTE to adapt existing guidelines, and GLIA to assess implementability.
Where to Find	National Guideline Clearinghouse

(continued)

Table 11-6 (continued)

An Overview of Evidence Synthesis Products

CLINICAL/CRITICAL PATHWAYS	
Question	*Answer*
What is it?	Clinical pathways (care pathways/critical pathway/integrated care pathways/care maps) are structured multidisciplinary tools used to manage the specific tasks and time lines required to implement evidence-based recommendations for a specific group of patients in a specific context who are expected to follow a predictable clinical course over a specific time interval. The pathway defines the different tasks (interventions) performed by the care team and typically provides targets for modification of the care plan in achieving target outcomes.
Why are they needed?	To reduce practice variations; coordinate multidisciplinary care and clarify roles; define benchmarks and monitor variations in achieving the expected processes and outcomes of care.
What is the evidence?	There is limited evidence that CPs improve outcomes, but a substantial amount of evidence suggests that they improve the process of care (fewer complications, more timely or cost-effective care).
When to use?	CPs can be useful when a sufficient number of patients who have a relatively consistent health problem or intervention are being managed by a multidisciplinary team and there is a sufficient body of evidence that allows one to define the optimal things to do. Ideally, a CPG is used to develop a CP.
What are the challenges?	There can be considerable staff time to develop a CP because these must be context specific. CPs are not necessarily transferable across contexts. Commercially promoted pathways are common and it is unknown whether they offer the same advantages of a locally driven pathway. Without motivation of the frontline staff, implementation is problematic.
How to optimize?	Engagement of a multidisciplinary team, including frontline staff, to develop or adapt the CP is critical to its implementation. Specific tasks, time lines, and roles must be clearly defined. Patients should be included to identify patient-based barriers. Process and outcome indicators should be clearly identified. Monitoring of variances to improve the quality and process of care should be transparent and done with a spirit of quality improvement.
Where to find?	CPs are context specific. Information about CPs can be found at www.e-p-a.org/000000979b08f9803/index.html

PATIENT DECISION AIDS	
Question	*Answer*
What is it?	Tools developed to assist patients in making specific decisions using available evidence where it is important to weigh potential benefits and risks or different options and their potential outcomes. Tools should incorporate patient values and preferences in the decision tool.

(continued)

Table 11-6 (continued)

An Overview of Evidence Synthesis Products

Why are they needed?	Patients are often unable to filter/understand evidence about risks and benefits of different interventions, particularly where these vary across different choices and involve short-term and longer-term differential risks/benefits. Health care providers are not always effective at communicating with patients about decisions or the existing evidence. Patients and providers are often unclear about how to incorporate values and preferences into decision making.
What is the evidence?	Overall, patient DAs have been shown to have a small to moderate impact on improving knowledge, decision quality, and the perception of being informed or understanding values; however, there is considerable variation across studies (O'Connor et al., 2009). Despite positive attitudes about PDAs (Adam, Khaw, Thomson, Gregg, & Llewellyn-Thomas, 2008), intention to use is low (Graham & Tetroe, 2007).
When to use?	When there are one or more reasonable investigational or treatment options with varying types of effects or risks/complications.
What are the challenges?	There are limited number of PDAs relevant to rehabilitation practice. Cultural, readability, and other aspects of health literacy may not be adequately addressed.
How to optimize?	Use a guide to assist with development of a PDA or search for DAs that are already developed. Consider use of the generic Ottawa Patient DA if there is none available. Follow quality criteria (Elwyn et al., 2006) for DAs.
Where to find	The Cochrane Library provides a decision aid library (https://decisionaid.ohri.ca/DALI/); Ottawa decision aid resource (http://decisionaid.ohri.ca/)

CLINICAL DECISION/PREDICTION RULES	
Question	*Answer*
What is it?	A specific kind of DA for clinicians containing variables from the history, physical examination, or simple diagnostic tests that are used in combination to make a decision. There are three types: diagnostic, predictive, and prescriptive.
Why are they needed?	It can be difficult to incorporate multiple pieces of evidence-based information into an overall decision. It can be difficult to recognize how clusters of information combine without the use of special analyses to identify it. These rules have potential to optimize identification of patterns or clusters of characteristics that indicate specific diagnoses, outcomes, or response potential.
What is the evidence?	Studies suggest that the use of well-developed clinical decision rules results in better medical decision making (Perry & Stiell, 2006). Their use in rehabilitation is starting to emerge but is currently inconclusive. Overall, the quality of many of the existing CPRs is insufficient for implementation in practice.
When to use?	When there is a Level 1 CPR (shown to have positive effects on provider behavior and/or patient outcomes across a broad spectrum of patients and clinical contexts) that has been validated for patients similar to those in your practice.

(continued)

Table 11-6 (continued)

An Overview of Evidence Synthesis Products

Where to find?	Particularly useful for combining clinical tests, imaging, or other diagnostic tests into an overall diagnosis. Also useful for making decisions about ordering additional tests particularly imaging. The classic example is the Ottawa Ankle Rules (Keogh, Shafi, & Wijetunge, 1998; Leddy, Smolinski, Lawrence, Snyder, & Priore, 1998; Mann, Grant, Guly, & Hughes, 1998). In physical therapy, has been used to classify patients most likely to respond to interventions.
How to optimize?	Use of rigorous methodology to develop (McGinn et al., 2000; Shapiro, 2005, 2006; Stiell & Wells, 1999); involvement of stakeholder in setting the priority for an implementation of the clinical decision rules.
Where to find?	

COMPUTER DECISION SUPPORT FOR CLINICIANS	
Question	*Answer*
What is it?	Technology-enabled decision support utilizes information from evidence, patient specifics, and technology-enabled algorithms/monitoring to assist practitioners in decision making.
What is the evidence?	There is insufficient supporting current evidence to be confident about effects; the variability of what computer-based decision support is composed of must be considered as a limitation in the evidence. A variety of systematic reviews have been conducted and indicated no benefit or a small benefit.
When to use?	Computer decision support for clinicians is best used when evidence is clear, the indicators and appropriate responses are clear, and they can easily be incorporated into standard practice such as an electronic medical record.
How to optimize?	Careful implementation and accuracy reaching verification. Monitoring of process and outcomes.

KEY WEB LINKS

Clinical Practice Guidelines Web Sites

* www.guideline.gov

  National Guidelines Clearinghouse provides a look-up and sign-up service that has extensive coverage and evaluation of CPGs. A standardized format presents information on development and access to guidelines. The user may request regular updates. The majority of guidelines are medically oriented; some include recommendations around rehabilitation and few specifically focus on rehabilitation.

* www.openclinical.org/guidelines.html

  OpenClinical is a nonprofit organization that provides resources on advanced knowledge management methods, technologies, and applications for health care. The link summarizes information about CPGs.

- www.health.uottawa.ca/rehabguidelines/en/login.php

  School of Rehabilitation Sciences' Evidence-Based Practice Web Site contains a developing database of CPGs for rehabilitation.

- www.asha.org/members/guidelines.aspx

  The American Speech Language Hearing Association has compiled a list of relevant CPGs that have been evaluated by their staff using the AGREE framework.

- www.orthopt.org/ICF.php

  CPGs developed by the American Physical Therapy Association–Orthopedic Division.

- www.caot.ca/default.asp?pageid=2130

  Position statement by the Canadian Occupational Therapy Association on CPGs.

- www.g-i-n.net/

  This is the Web site of the Guidelines International Network (G-I-N), founded in 2002. G-I-N is an organization dedicated to the development and implementation of guidelines. It has grown to compose of 90 organizations and 92 individual members and contains a variety of resources that can be useful for development or implementation of CPGs.

- www.g-i-n.net/document-store/adapte-resource-toolkit-guideline-adaptation-version-2

  ADAPTE describes a process and provides supporting tools for adaptation of guidelines.

- http://gem.med.yale.edu/glia/login.htm

  The GLIA Web site; the tool can be downloaded free of charge.

Clinical Pathways

- www.e-p-a.org/index2.html

  European CP association contains a variety of resources for pathway development and appraisal.

- www.wales.nhs.uk/sitesplus/documents/829/integratedcarepathways.pdf

  A free online guide for the development and evaluation of integrated care pathways.

Patient Decision Aids

- http://decisionaid.ohri.ca/

  The (Ottawa) decision aids Web site provides a host of resources with respect to DAs, learning materials, and resources for developing and evaluating PDA.

- www.ipdasi.org/2006%20IPDAS%20Quality%20Checklist.pdf

  The International Patient Decision Aid Standards Collaboration appraisal of a PDA tool.

- www.openclinical.org/dss.html

  Decision support tools for clinicians.

REFERENCES

Adam, J. A., Khaw, F. M., Thomson, R. G., Gregg, P. J., & Llewellyn-Thomas, H. A. (2008). Patient decision aids in joint replacement surgery: A literature review and an opinion survey of consultant orthopaedic surgeons. *Annals of the Royal College of Surgeons, 90*, 198–207.

The AGREE Collaboration. (2001). Appraisal of guidelines for research and evaluation (AGREE) instrument. Retrieved from www.agreecollaboration.org

The AGREE Collaboration. (2003). Development and validation of an international appraisal instrument for assessing the quality of clinical practice guidelines: The AGREE project. *Quality and Safety in Health Care, 12*, 18–23.

Atkins, D., Eccles, M., Flottorp, S., Guyatt, G. H., Henry, D., Hill, S., et al. (2004). Systems for grading the quality of evidence and the strength of recommendations I: Critical appraisal of existing approaches The GRADE Working Group. *BMC Health Services Research, 4*, 38.

Bahtsevani, C., Uden, G., & Willman, A. (2004). Outcomes of evidence-based clinical practice guidelines: A systematic review. *International Journal of Technological Assessmennt in Health Care, 20*, 427–433.

Barbieri, A., Vanhaecht, K., Van, H. P., Sermeus, W., Faggiano, F., Marchisio, S., et al. (2009). Effects of clinical pathways in the joint replacement: A meta-analysis. *BMC Medicine, 7*, 32.

Beneciuk, J. M., Bishop, M. D., & George, S. Z. (2009). Clinical prediction rules for physical therapy interventions: A systematic review. *Physical Therapy, 89*, 114–124.

Berrigan, L., Marshall, S., McCullagh, S., Velikonja, D., & Bayley, M. (2011). Quality of clinical practice guidelines for persons who have sustained mild traumatic brain injury. *Brain Injury, 25*, 742–751.

Bitzer, E.M., Klosterhuis, H., Dorning, H., and Rose, S. (2003). Developing an evidence based clinical guideline on cardiac rehabilitation--Phase 2: comparative analysis of the present level of service provision in cardiac rehabilitation based on the KTL statistics. *Rehabilitation* (Stuttg), 42, 83-93.

Blackham, J. E., Claridge, T., & Benger, J. R. (2008). Can patients apply the Ottawa Ankle Rules to themselves? *Emergency Medicine Journal, 25*, 750–751.

Brooks, D., Solway, S., MacDermid, J.C., Switzer-McIntyre, S., Brosseau, L., Graham, I. (2005) The quality of clinical practice guidelines in physical therapy. *Physiotherapy Canada, 57*, 123-134,

Brosseau, L., Graham, I.D., MacLeay, L., Cleaver, S., Dumont, A.M., Gravel, M., March, A., and McGowan, J. (2004). What is the quality of clinical practice guidelines accessible on the World Wide Web for the treatment of musculoskeletal conditions in physiotherapy? *Physiotherapy Theory and Practice, 5*, 18.

Brouwers, M. C., Kho, M. E., Browman, G. P., Burgers, J. S., Cluzeau, F., Feder, G., et al. (2010a). AGREE II: Advancing guideline development, reporting and evaluation in health care. *Canadian Medical Association Journal, 182*, E839–E842.

Brouwers, M. C., Kho, M. E., Browman, G. P., Burgers, J. S., Cluzeau, F., Feder, G., et al. (2010b). Development of the AGREE II, part 1: Performance, usefulness and areas for improvement. *Canadian Medical Association Journal, 182*, 1045–1052.

Brouwers, M. C., Kho, M. E., Browman, G. P., Burgers, J. S., Cluzeau, F., Feder, G., et al. (2010c). Development of the AGREE II, part 2: Assessment of validity of items and tools to support application. *Canadian Medical Association Journal, 182*, E472–E478.

Browman, G.P. (2000). Improving clinical practice guidelines for the 21st century. Attitudinal barriers and not technology are the main challenges. *International Journal of Technology Assessment in Health Care, 16*, 959-968.

Brozek, J. L., Akl, E. A., Alonso-Coello, P., Lang, D., Jaeschke, R., Williams, J. W., et al. (2009). Grading quality of evidence and strength of recommendations in clinical practice guidelines. Part 1 of 3. An overview of the GRADE approach and grading quality of evidence about interventions. *Allergy, 64*, 669–677.

Brozek, J. L., Akl, E. A., Compalati, E., Kreis, J., Terracciano, L., Fiocchi, A., et al. (2011). Grading quality of evidence and strength of recommendations in clinical practice guidelines part 3 of 3. The GRADE approach to developing recommendations. *Allergy, 66*, 588–595.

Cabana, M. D., Rand, C. S., Powe, N. R., Wu, A. W., Wilson, M. H., Abboud, P. A., et al. (1999). Why don't physicians follow clinical practice guidelines? A framework for improvement. *Journal of the American Medical Association, 282*, 1458–1465.

Canadian Medical Association (1994). *Guidelines for Canadian clinical practice guidelines*. Ottawa, Canada.

Childs, J. D., Fritz, J. M., Flynn, T. W., Irrgang, J. J., Johnson, K. K., Majkowski, G. R., et al. (2004). A clinical prediction rule to identify patients with low back pain most likely to benefit from spinal manipulation: A validation study. *Annals of Internal Medicine, 141*, 920–928.

Cleland, J. A., Mintken, P. E., Carpenter, K., Fritz, J. M., Glynn, P., Whitman, J., et al. (2010). Examination of a clinical prediction rule to identify patients with neck pain likely to benefit from thoracic spine thrust manipulation and a general cervical range of motion exercise: Multi-center randomized clinical trial. *Physical Therapy, 90*, 1239–1250.

Cools, A. M., Cambier, D., & Witvrouw, E. E. (2008). Screening the athlete's shoulder for impingement symptoms: A clinical reasoning algorithm for early detection of shoulder pathology. *British Journal of Sports Medicine, 42*, 628–635.

Cuello Garcia, C. A., Pacheco Alvarado, K. P., & Perez, G. G. (2011). Grading recommendations in clinical practice guidelines: Randomised experimental evaluation of four different systems. *Archives of Disease in Childhood, 96*, 723–728.

Currie, V. L., Harvey, G. (1998) Care pathways development and implementation. *Nursing Standard, 12*:3, 35-38.

Davis N., ed. (2005). Integrated Care Pathways: A Guide to Good Practice, Wales. National Leadership and Innovation Agency for Healthcare. Available at: http://www.wales.nhs.uk/sitesplus/documents/829/integrated-carepathways.pdf. Accessed September 18, 2013.

Davis, D. (2006). Continuing education, guideline implementation, and the emerging transdisciplinary field of knowledge translation. *Journal of Continuing Education in the Health Professions, 26*, 5–12.

De Bleser, L.D.R., De Waele, K., Vanhaecht, K., Vlayen, J., Sermeus, W. (2006) Defining pathways. *Journal of Nursing Management, 14*:553-563.

Dowling, S. K., & Wishart, I. (2011). Use of the Ottawa Ankle Rules in children: A survey of physicians' practice patterns. *Canadian Journal of Emergency Medical Care, 13*, 333–338.

Dzwierzynski, W.W., Spitz, K., Hartz, A., Guse, C., and Larson, D.L. (1998). Improvement in resource utilization after development of a clinical pathway for patients with pressure ulcers. *Plastic and Reconstructive Surgery, 102*, 2006-2011.

Eccles, M. P., & Grimshaw, J. M. (2004). Selecting, presenting and delivering clinical guidelines: Are there any "magic bullets"? *Medical Journal of Australia, 180*, S52–S54.

Ellenbecker, T. S., & Cools, A. (2010). Rehabilitation of shoulder impingement syndrome and rotator cuff injuries: An evidence-based review. *British Journal of Sports Medicine, 44*, 319–327.

Elwyn, G., O'Connor, A., Stacey, D., Volk, R., Edwards, A., Coulter, A., et al. (2006). Developing a quality criteria framework for patient decision aids: Online international Delphi consensus process. *BMJ, 333*, 417.

Elwyn, G., Stiel, M., Durand, M. A., & Boivin, J. (2011). The design of patient decision support interventions: Addressing the theory–practice gap. *Journal of Evaluation in Clinical Practice, 17*, 565–574.

Fan, J., & Woolfrey, K. (2006). The effect of triage-applied Ottawa Ankle Rules on the length of stay in a Canadian urgent care department: A randomized controlled trial. *Academic Emergency Medicine, 13*, 153–157.

Farquhar, C.M., Kofa, E.W., and Slutsky, J.R. (2002). Clinicians' attitudes to clinical practice guidelines: a systematic review. *Medical Journal of Australia, 177*, 502-506

Field, M., & Lohr, K. E. (1992). *Guidelines for clinical practice: From development to use*. Washington, DC, National Academy Press.

Fortney, J., Rost, K., Zhang, M., & Pyne, J. (2001). The relationship between quality and outcomes in routine depression care. *Psychiatric Services, 52*, 56–62.

Fritz, J. M., MacDermid, J. C., & Snyder-Mackler, L. (2011). Counting what counts. *Journal of Orthopaedic & Sports in Physical Therapy, 41*, 907–908.

Garfield, F.B. and Garfield, J.M. (2000). Clinical judgment and clinical practice guidelines. *International Journal of Technology Assessment in Health Care, 16*, 1050-1060.

Glynn, P. E., & Weisbach, P. C. (2011). *Clinical prediction rules: A physical therapy reference manual*. Sudbury, MA: Jones and Barlett Publishers.

Godderis, L., Vanhaecht, K., Masschelein, R., Sermeus, W., & Veulemans, H. (2004). Prevention pathways: Application of the critical path methodology in occupational health services. *Journal of Occupational and Environmental Medicine, 46*, 39–47.

Goldsmith, C. H., Gross, A. R., MacDermid, J., Santaguida, P. L., & Miller, J. (2011). What does the evidence tell us about design of future treatment trials for whiplash-associated disorders? *Spine (Philadelphia), 36*, S292–S302.

Graham, I. D., Calder, L. A., Hebert, P. C., Carter, A. O., & Tetroe, J. M. (2000). A comparison of clinical practice guideline appraisal instruments. *International Journal of Technological Assessment in Health Care, 16*, 1024–1038.

Graham, I. D., & Tetroe, J. (2007). Some theoretical underpinnings of knowledge translation. *Academic Emergency Medicine, 14*, 936–941.

Greep, J. M., & Siezenis, L. M. (1989). Methods of decision analysis: Protocols, decision trees, and algorithms in medicine. *World Journal of Surgery, 13*, 240–244.

Grimshaw, J., Eccles, M., & Tetroe, J. (2004). Implementing clinical guidelines: Current evidence and future implications. *Journal of Continuing Education in the Health Professions, 24*(Suppl. 1), S31–S37.

Grimshaw, J.M. & Hutchinson, A. (1995). Clinical practice guidelines--do they enhance value for money in health care? *British Medical Bulletin, 51*, 927-940.

Gross, A. R., Goldsmith, C., Hoving, J. L., Haines, T., Peloso, P., Aker, P., et al. (2007). Conservative management of mechanical neck disorders: A systematic review. *Journal of Rheumatology, 34*, 1083–1102.

Gross, A. R., Kay, T. M., Kennedy, C., Gasner, D., Hurley, L., Yardley, K., et al. (2002). Clinical practice guideline on the use of manipulation or mobilization in the treatment of adults with mechanical neck disorders. *Manual Therapy, 7*, 193–205.

Gulich, M., Engel, E.M., Rose, S., Klosterhuis, H., and Jackel, W.H. (2003). Development of a guideline for rehabilitation of patients with low back pain-- phase 2: analysis of data of the classification of therapeutic procedures. *Rehabilitation* (Stuttg), 42, 109-117.

Guyatt, G. H., Oxman, A. D., Vist, G. E., Kunz, R., Falck-Ytter, Y., Alonso-Coello, P., et al. (2008). GRADE: An emerging consensus on rating quality of evidence and strength of recommendations. *BMJ, 336*, 924–926.

Hadorn, D. C., McCormick, K., & Diokno, A. (1992). An annotated algorithm approach to clinical guideline development. *Journal of the American Medical Association, 267*, 3311–3314.

Harris, S.R., Hugi, M.R., Olivotto, I.A., and Levine, M. (2001). Clinical practice guidelines for the care and treatment of breast cancer: 11. Lymphedema. *Canadian Medical Association Journal*, 164, 191-199.

Hemens, B. J., Holbrook, A., Tonkin, M., Mackay, J. A., Weise-Kelly, L., Navarro, T., et al. (2011). Computerized clinical decision support systems for drug prescribing and management: A decision-maker–researcher partnership systematic review. *Implementation Science, 6*, 89.

Hillier, S., Grimmer-Somers, K., Merlin, T., Middleton, P., Salisbury, J., Tooher, R., et al. (2011). FORM: An Australian method for formulating and grading recommendations in evidence-based clinical guidelines. *BMC Medical Research Methodology, 11*, 23.

Holmes-Rovner, M., Nelson, W. L., Pignone, M., Elwyn, G., Rovner, D. R., O'Connor, A. M., et al. (2007). Are patient decision aids the best way to improve clinical decision making? Report of the IPDAS Symposium. *Medical Decision Making, 27*, 599–608.

Hurdowar, A., Graham, I. D., Bayley, M., Harrison, M., Wood-Dauphinee, S., & Bhogal, S. (2007). Quality of stroke rehabilitation clinical practice guidelines. *Journal of Evaluation in Clinical Practice, 13*, 657–664.

Hurkmans, E. J., Jones, A., Li, L. C., & Vliet Vlieland, T. P. (2011). Quality appraisal of clinical practice guidelines on the use of physiotherapy in rheumatoid arthritis: A systematic review. *Rheumatology, 50*, 1879–1888.

Johnston, M. V., Wood, K., Stason, W. B., & Beatty, P. (2000). Rehabilitative placement of poststroke patients: Reliability of the Clinical Practice Guideline of the Agency for Health Care Policy and Research. *Archives of Physical Medicine and Rehabilitation, 81*, 539–548.

Keogh, S. P., Shafi, A., & Wijetunge, D. B. (1998). Comparison of Ottawa Ankle Rules and current local guidelines for use of radiography in acute ankle injuries. *Journal of the Royal College of Surgeons, 43*, 341–343.

Kinsman, L., Rotter, T., James, E., Snow, P., & Willis, J. (2010). What is a clinical pathway? Development of a definition to inform the debate. *BMC Medicine, 8*, 31.

Kitchiner, D.J. and Bundred, P.E. (1996). Integrated care pathways. *Archives of Disease in Childhood, 75*, 16-168.

Kitchiner, D.J. and Bundred, P.E. (1999). Clinical pathways. *Medical Journal of Australia, 170*, 54-55.

Knudsen, R., Vijdea, R., & Damborg, F. (2010). Validation of the Ottawa Ankle Rules in a Danish emergency department. *Danish Medical Bulletin, 57*, A4142.

Leddy, J. J., Smolinski, R. J., Lawrence, J., Snyder, J. L., & Priore, R. L. (1998). Prospective evaluation of the Ottawa Ankle Rules in a university sports medicine center. With a modification to increase specificity for identifying malleolar fractures. *American Journal of Sports Medicine, 26*, 158–165.

Lugtenberg, M., Burgers, J. S., & Westert, G. P. (2009). Effects of evidence-based clinical practice guidelines on quality of care: A systematic review. *Quality and Safety in Health Care, 18*, 385–392.

MacDermid, J. C. (2004). The quality of clinical practice guidelines in hand therapy. *Journal of Hand Therapy, 17*, 200–209.

MacDermid, J. C., Brooks, D., Solway, S., Switzer-McIntyre, S., Brosseau, L., & Graham, I. D. (2005). Reliability and validity of the AGREE instrument used by physical therapists in assessment of clinical practice guidelines. *BMC Health Services Research, 5*, 18.

Mann, C. J., Grant, I., Guly, H., & Hughes, P. (1998). Use of the Ottawa Ankle Rules by nurse practitioners. *Accident and Emergency Medicine, 15*, 315–316.

Martin, R. W., Brower, M. E., Geralds, A., Gallagher, P. J., & Tellinghuisen, D. J. (2011). An experimental evaluation of patient decision aid design to communicate the effects of medications on the rate of progression of structural joint damage in rheumatoid arthritis. *Patient Education and Counseling.*

McGinn, T. G., Guyatt, G. H., Wyer, P. C., Naylor, C. D., Stiell, I. G., & Richardson, W. S. (2000). Users' guides to the medical literature: XXII: Gow to use articles about clinical decision rules. Evidence-Based Medicine Working Group. *Journal of the American Medical Association, 284*, 79–84.

McKenna, H.P., Keeney, S., Currie, L., Harvey, G., West, E., Richey, R.H. (2006). Quality of care: a comparison of perceptions of health professionals in clinical areas in the United Kingdom and the United States. *Journal of Nursing Care Quality, 21*(4):344-351.

McPoil, T. G., Martin, R. L., Cornwall, M. W., Wukich, D. K., Irrgang, J. J., & Godges, J. J. (2008). Heel pain—Plantar fasciitis: Clinical practice guildelines linked to the international classification of function, disability, and health from the orthopaedic section of the American Physical Therapy Association. *Journal of Orthopaedic and Sports Physical Therapy, 38*, A1–A18.

Moulding, N. T., Silagy, C. A., & Weller, D. P. (1999). A framework for effective management of change in clinical practice: Dissemination and implementation of clinical practice guidelines. *Quality in Health Care, 8*, 177–183.

O'Connor, A. M., Bennett, C., Stacey, D., Barry, M. J., Col, N. F., Eden, K. B., et al. (2007). Do patient decision aids meet effectiveness criteria of the international patient decision aid standards collaboration? A systematic review and meta-analysis. *Medical Decision Making, 27*, 554–574.

O'Connor, A. M., Bennett, C. L., Stacey, D., Barry, M., Col, N. F., Eden, K. B., et al. (2009). Decision aids for people facing health treatment or screening decisions. *Cochrane Database of Systematic Reviews,* CD001431.

Pagliari, C. and Grimshaw, J. (2002). Impact of group structure and process on multidisciplinary evidence-based guideline development: an observational study. *Journal of Evaluation in Clinical Practice, 8*, 145-153.

Pennington, J.M., Jones, D.P., and McIntyre, S. (2003). Clinical pathways in total knee arthroplasty: a New Zealand experience. *Journal of Orthopaedic Surgery and Research* (Hong Kong), 11, 166-173.

Perry, J. J., & Stiell, I. G. (2006). Impact of clinical decision rules on clinical care of traumatic injuries to the foot and ankle, knee, cervical spine, and head. *Injury, 37*, 1157–1165.

Prior M., Guerin, M., Grimmer-Somers, K. (2008) The effectiveness of clinical guideline implementation strategies--a synthesis of systematic review findings. *Journal of Evaluation in Clinical Practice, 14*(5):888-97.

Rodin, M., Saliba, D., & Brummel-Smith, K. (2006). Guidelines abstracted from the Department of Veterans Affairs/Department of Defense clinical practice guideline for the management of stroke rehabilitation. *Journal of the American Geriatrics Society, 54*, 158–162.

Roshanov, P. S., Misra, S., Gerstein, H. C., Garg, A. X., Sebaldt, R. J., Mackay, J. A., et al. (2011). Computerized clinical decision support systems for chronic disease management: A decision-maker–researcher partnership systematic review. *Implementation Science, 6*, 92.

Rotter, T., Kinsman, L., James, E., Machotta, A., Gothe, H., Willis, J., et al. (2010). Clinical pathways: Effects on professional practice, patient outcomes, length of stay and hospital costs. *Cochrane Database of Systematic Reviews,* CD006632.

Rutten, G. M., Degen, S., Hendriks, E. J., Braspenning, J. C., Harting, J., & Oostendorp, R. A. (2010). Adherence to clinical practice guidelines for low back pain in physical therapy: Do patients benefit? *Physical Therapy, 90,* 1111–1122.

Rutten, G. M, Kremers, S., Rutten, S., & Harting, J. (2009). A theory-based cross-sectional survey demonstrated the important role of awareness in guideline implementation. *Journal of Clinical Epidemiology, 62,* 167–176.

Sahota, N., Lloyd, R., Ramakrishna, A., Mackay, J. A., Prorok, J. C., Weise-Kelly, L., et al. (2011). Computerized clinical decision support systems for acute care management: A decision-maker–researcher partnership systematic review of effects on process of care and patient outcomes. *Implementation Science, 6,* 91.

Savoie, I., Kazanjian, A., & Bassett, K. (2000). Do clinical practice guidelines reflect research evidence? *Journal of Health Services Research and Policy, 5,* 76–82.

Schaldach, D.E. (1997). Measuring quality and cost of care: evaluation of an amputation clinical pathway. *Journal of Vascular Nursing,* 15, 13-20.

Scholten-Peeters, G. G., Bekkering, G. E., Verhagen, A. P., Der Windt, D. A., Lanser, K., Hendriks, E. J., et al. (2002). Clinical practice guideline for the physiotherapy of patients with whiplash-associated disorders. *Spine, 27,* 412–422.

Shah, K. H., Metz, H. A., & Edlow, J. A. (2009). Clinical prediction rules to stratify short-term risk of stroke among patients diagnosed in the emergency department with a transient ischemic attack. *Annals of Emergency Medicine, 53,* 662–673.

Shapiro, S. E. (2005). Evaluating clinical decision rules. *Western Journal of Nursing Research, 27,* 655–664.

Shapiro, S. E. (2006). Guidelines for developing and testing clinical decision rules. *Western Journal of Nursing Research, 28,* 244–253.

Souza, N. M., Sebaldt, R. J., Mackay, J. A., Prorok, J. C., Weise-Kelly, L., Navarro, T., et al. (2011). Computerized clinical decision support systems for primary preventive care: A decision-maker–researcher partnership systematic review of effects on process of care and patient outcomes. *Implementation Science, 6,* 87.

Stanton, T. R., Hancock, M. J., Maher, C. G., & Koes, B. W. (2010). Critical appraisal of clinical prediction rules that aim to optimize treatment selection for musculoskeletal conditions. *Physical Therapy, 90,* 843–854.

Stergiou-Kita, M. (2010). Implementing clinical practice guidelines in occupational therapy practice: recommendations from the research evidence. *Australian Occupational Therapy Journal,* 57(2):76-87.

Stiell, I. G., & Wells, G. A. (1999). Methodologic standards for the development of clinical decision rules in emergency medicine. *Annals of Emergency Medicine, 33,* 437–447.Thomson, M. D., & Hoffman-Goetz, L. (2007). Readability and cultural sensitivity of web-based patient decision aids for cancer screening and treatment: A systematic review. *Medical Informatics & the Internet in Medicine, 32,* 263–286.

StrokEngine (2013). Retrieved October 9, 2013. Available at: http://strokengine.ca/intervention/index.php?page=topic&id=53

Thomson MD, Hoffman-Goetz L. (2007) Readability and cultural sensitivity of web-based patient decision aids for cancer screening and treatment: a systematic review. *Medical Informatics and the Internet in Medicine,* 32(4):263-286.

van der Sanden, W. J., Mettes, D. G., Plasschaert, A. J., Grol, R. P., & Verdonschot, E. H. (2004). Development of clinical practice guidelines: Evaluation of 2 methods. *Journal of the Canadian Dental Association, 70,* 301.

van Middendorp, J. J., Hosman, A. J., Donders, A. R., Pouw, M. H., Ditunno, J. F., Jr., Curt, A., et al. (2011). A clinical prediction rule for ambulation outcomes after traumatic spinal cord injury: A longitudinal cohort study. *Lancet, 377,* 1004–1010.

Vanhaecht, K., De Witte, K., Depreitere, R., & Sermeus, W. (2006). Clinical pathway audit tools: A systematic review. *Journal of Nursing Management, 14,* 529–537.

Vanhaecht, K., De Witte, K., Panella, M., & Sermeus, W. (2009). Do pathways lead to better organized care processes? *Journal of Evaluation in Clinical Practice, 15,* 782–788.

Vanhaecht, K., De Witte, K., Depreitere, R., van Zelm, R., De Bleser, L., Proost, K., et al. (2007). Development and validation of a care process self-evaluation tool. *Health Services Management Research, 20,* 189–202.

Vanhaecht, K., Ovretveit, J., Elliott, M. J., Sermeus, W., Ellershaw, J. E., & Panella, M. (2011). Have we drawn the wrong conclusions about the value of care pathways? Is a Cochrane review appropriate? *Evaluation & the Health Professions*.

Wainner, R. S., Fritz, J. M., Irrgang, J. J., Delitto, A., Allison, S., & Boninger, M. L. (2005). Development of a clinical prediction rule for the diagnosis of carpal tunnel syndrome. *Archives of Physical Medicine and Rehabilitation, 86*, 609–618.

Whittle, C.L., MacDonald, P., Dunn, L., & de Luc, K. (2004). Developing the integrated care pathway appraisal tool (ICPAT): a pilot study. *Journal of Integrated Care Pathways*, 8:77-81.

Woolf, S. H., DiGuiseppi, C. G., Atkins, D., & Kamerow, D. B. (1996). Developing evidence-based clinical practice guidelines: Lessons learned by the US Preventive Services Task Force. *Annual Review of Public Health, 17*, 511–538.

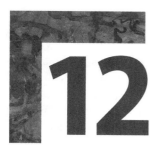

COMMUNICATING EVIDENCE TO
CLIENTS, MANAGERS, AND FUNDERS

Linda Tickle-Degnen, PhD, OTR/L, FAOTA

LEARNING OBJECTIVES

After reading this chapter, the student/practitioner will be able to:

- Recognize the role that effective communication about evidence plays in being an evidence-based practitioner.
- Understand the various clinical roles of potential decision makers.
- Critically evaluate the body of evidence on a clinical situation, including distinguishing between different types of evidence.
- Use appropriate communication techniques to discuss the evidence and make treatment decisions based on the persons involved.

Imagine that next Monday you have your first appointment with Mr. Davis, a man with Parkinson's disease. As an evidence-based practitioner, you would seek recent research evidence on the daily lives of persons with this disease to supplement the knowledge you have accrued through your clinical experience and training. One important clinical outcome of gathering this evidence is that you would become a more knowledgeable practitioner. The evidence would hopefully inform your own practice actions. For example, during the appointed meeting time, you might have a list of issues to discuss with Mr. Davis and his family that is expanded beyond what you normally would have addressed. More important, beyond informing your own practice actions, you would possibly be able to expand Mr. Davis's knowledge in a manner that would enable him to become a collaborative partner in the clinical process. Just as important is your ability to expand the relevant knowledge of informal (i.e., family and friends) and formal (i.e., health care providers and policy makers) care partners. The more Mr. Davis and his social and health care partners know about how others with similar circumstances manage their lives and health, the more they can make reasoned choices that are effectively supportive.

Law M., & MacDermid, J. C.
*Evidence-Based Rehabilitation: A Guide
to Practice, Third Edition* (pp 275–304).
© 2014 SLACK Incorporated.

The point of the aforementioned scenario is to demonstrate that the purpose of evidence gathering does not stop with the personal edification of the practitioner. The evidence is put to use to achieve many purposes, some of which require direct communication with others about the content of the evidence. A collaborative relationship requires this direct communication so that the client and important people in the lives of the client become informed clinical partners. They are active rather than passive (i.e., they act with as much autonomy as possible and the least amount of dependency); clients and those acting on their behalf must be informed rather than uninformed or misinformed.

As an expert consultant, the therapist must directly communicate about evidence with other decision makers besides clients and their family and friends. The therapist talks about evidence with managers and funders of services so that management and funding decisions are informed. The focus of this chapter is on communicating research evidence so that decision makers can make informed decisions that relate to clients' lives and the provision of rehabilitation services.

EFFECTIVELY COMMUNICATING EVIDENCE

Talking about evidence alone will not guarantee that decision makers will become more informed. The therapist must take steps to effectively communicate about the evidence while understanding that communication is bidirectional among stakeholders and creates new knowledge for decision making (Brouwers, Stacey, & O'Connor, 2010). An effective communication regarding practice evidence is one in which messages are exchanged, understood, and acted upon, a process called *knowledge utilization* (Canadian Institutes of Health Research, 2011; Sudswad, 2007). A therapist may talk about evidence, but if the message is irrelevant, not framed in a manner that enables decision making and action, or incomprehensible, it will not be listened to, comprehended, and acted upon. Messages that are relevant, framed to enable decision making and action, and comprehensible are most effective for making a communication bridge between sender and receiver. Effective communication during a rehabilitation encounter involves the therapist and client fluidly exchanging the roles of sender and receiver through verbal and nonverbal behavior. For example, clients who play an active role in communication, such as initiating and asking questions, are more likely to have their perspectives, beliefs, and values understood by the practitioner (Street & Haidet, 2011). With an underlying premise that it is a therapist's role to facilitate a bidirectional exchange of information for knowledge creation and decision making, this chapter describes the following four steps on the path to effective evidence-based communication:

1. Identify the clinical role of the decision maker with respect to the therapist.

2. Identify the decisions that the decision maker will be involved in making with the therapist.

3. Gather and interpret research evidence that is guided by the information needs of the decision maker and the clinical population of interest.

4. Translate the evidence into a comprehensible communication to facilitate an informed discussion with the decision maker.

Step 1: Identify the Clinical Role of the Decision Maker With Respect to the Therapist

This chapter addresses three types of decision makers with whom therapists are likely to communicate—client or family and friend care partners, manager, and funder. Effective communication begins with identifying the distinctions between the communication recipients' clinical roles and the contexts surrounding the performance of those roles. Different clinical roles generate different perspectives and needs. People are more likely to understand and respond to communication messages that are consistent with their own experiences and perspectives and based on their own needs, objectives, and preferences (Coulter & Ellins, 2007).

The clinical role of clients and family members is to receive therapy services to improve their lives. Communication with clients and family members often occurs face-to-face in periodic and repeated appointments. The clinical role of managers is to develop therapy programs; allocate resources such as space, budget, materials, and staff support; and guide the therapist's provision of services. Managers must work within a set of multiple and complex organizational objectives (e.g., provide effective and efficient services to a particular population); initiatives (e.g., increase client satisfaction while increasing therapists' caseload); and constraints (e.g., limited building space). Communication with managers may occur frequently and informally or infrequently and formally and is often face-to-face. The clinical role of funders is to decide whether to fund the development of future clinical programs and the provision of current services from an array of possible services and programs. Communication with funders is often formal and in written form.

Step 2: *Identify the Decisions That the Decision Maker Will Be Involved in Making With the Therapist*

The therapist has a clinical role that intersects with the decision maker's clinical role, and together these roles determine what types of decisions will be important to communicate about. In rehabilitation, the therapist and client are concerned with helping the client to participate more competently and with more satisfaction in daily living and valued activities that occur in the home, community, and society at large. Throughout the chapter, the term *participation* is used to mean this activity and societal participation. The therapist and decision maker engage in the following three decision-making tasks with respect to client participation outcomes:

1. Description task: Determine and describe participation issues that are relevant to a particular client population.

2. Assessment task: Select assessment procedures to measure client attributes related to participation.

3. Intervention task: Plan and implement intervention to maintain or improve client participation.

There are other tasks as well; however, these central ones are useful as a basis for demonstrating what types of information, or evidence, therapists will be most likely to communicate with decision makers. Decision making is required around all of these tasks, whether the decision making occurs in the context of direct service provision to clients, in the context of program development or resource allocation discussions with managers, or in the context of written communication with funders around program funding and service compensation.

- Clients and their care partners need *descriptive* information from the therapist about the importance of participation in their lives. With this information they can begin to understand and give voice to their life experiences and begin to plan an adaptive course of action in response to their own rehabilitation needs. They need *assessment* and *intervention* information to make informed decisions related to choosing assessment and intervention procedures.

- Managers need *descriptive* information about participation from the therapist in order to develop and support clinical programs that are likely to be responsive to client rehabilitation needs. They need *assessment* and *intervention* information to decide which assessment and intervention procedures should be supported and provided by the organization.

- Funders need *descriptive* information about participation from the therapist in order to determine, if in the planning phase, whether or not a clinical program addresses or will address important client rehabilitation needs. They need to determine whether there is a reasonable

Table 12-1		
Organizing the Search for Descriptive Evidence to Discuss With Different Decision Makers		
DECISION MAKER	**DECISION MAKER'S USE OF EVIDENCE**	**QUESTION THAT GUIDES SEARCH FOR EVIDENCE**
Client and family members	To understand and give voice to one's own life experience and to begin to plan an adaptive course of action.	What factors are associated with high quality of life and life satisfaction among 75-year-old men with Parkinson's disease?
Manager	To develop and support clinical programs that are likely to be responsive to client rehabilitation needs.	What factors are associated with high quality of life and life satisfaction among persons with Parkinson's disease?
Funder	To determine whether a clinical program will address important client rehabilitation needs.	What factors are associated with high quality of life and life satisfaction among persons with Parkinson's disease?

rationale for funding. They need *assessment* information to determine whether or not assessment procedures currently or will effectively document important attributes of clients and their responses to rehabilitation intervention. Finally, they need *intervention* information to decide whether or not the current or predicted level of effectiveness and feasibility of a clinical intervention program is worth funding.

Step 3: Gather and Interpret Research Evidence That Is Guided by the Needs of the Decision Maker and the Clinical Population of Interest

Steps 1 and 2 provide a general conceptual territory for the kind of evidence that the therapist will have to gather to meet the needs of decision makers. At Step 3, the therapist begins to narrow this territory to address the specific and unique needs of decision makers and the client population that is involved in the decisions. The therapist creates a clinical question to guide the retrieval of information (Straus, Richardson, Glasziou, & Haynes, 2005). As the therapist gathers and interprets information, the therapist formulates possible answers to the question. The therapist then presents these possible answers to the decision maker for discussion.

Tables 12-1 through 12-3 show sample questions for organizing the gathering and interpretation of descriptive, assessment, and intervention evidence separately for different types of decision makers. Each question is composed of at least three elements: the type of evidence that is being sought, an attribute related to participation, and a description of a clinical population. Keeping in mind this chapter's opening clinical scenario involving Mr. Davis, all of the questions in the tables are about the clinical population with Parkinson's disease. The questions that guide the search for evidence for communicating with clients and their family members are written with the specific attributes of the client in mind (e.g., age and gender are specified). The questions that guide the search for evidence for communicating with managers and funders are written with a more general clinical population in mind. Based on the particular context and timing of decision-making activities, the therapist can develop the wording of the questions independently or in collaboration with the decision maker. The questions can be written with as much specificity or generality as is needed for decision making, as long as two conditions are met: The questions cannot be written so specifically that the evidence will be extremely restricted and hard to find (e.g., a question about quality

Table 12-2

Organizing the Search for Assessment Evidence to Discuss With Different Decision Makers

DECISION MAKER	DECISION MAKER'S USE OF EVIDENCE	QUESTION THAT GUIDES SEARCH FOR EVIDENCE
Client and family members	To make informed decisions about participating in assessment procedures.	Is the Activity Card Sort a more reliable and valid method for assessing social participation, compared to the Parkinson's Disease Questionnaire-39, among 75-year-old men with Parkinson's disease?
Manager	To decide which assessment procedures should be supported and provided by the organization.	What are the most reliable and valid methods for assessing social participation among persons with Parkinson's disease?
Funder	To determine whether or not assessment procedures will effectively document important attributes of clients and their responses to rehabilitation intervention.	What are the most reliable and valid methods for assessing social participation among persons with Parkinson's disease?

Table 12-3

Organizing the Search for Intervention Evidence to Discuss With Different Decision Makers

DECISION MAKER	DECISION MAKER'S USE OF EVIDENCE	QUESTION THAT GUIDES SEARCH FOR EVIDENCE
Client and family members	To make informed decisions about participating in intervention procedures.	What are the most effective and feasible rehabilitation interventions for increasing social participation among 75-year-old men with Parkinson's disease?
Manager	To decide which intervention procedures should be supported and provided by the organization.	What are the most effective and feasible rehabilitation interventions for increasing social participation among persons with Parkinson's disease?
Funder	To decide whether or not the predicted level of effectiveness and feasibility of a clinical intervention program is worth funding.	What are the most effective and feasible rehabilitation interventions for increasing social participation among persons with Parkinson's disease?

of life [QOL] for 75-year-old men with Parkinson's disease who live in Minnesota and are retired bankers). Nor can they be written so generally that they would require lengthy evidence searching and synthesizing and be of no particular consequence to the decision makers (e.g., a question about concerns of clients living in the community).

The questions vary across the three tables in terms of the type of evidence and the attribute of interests that are involved. The descriptive questions in Table 12-1 involve evidence about associations and attributes related to QOL and life satisfaction. The assessment questions in Table 12-2 involve evidence about reliability, validity, and attributes related to health-related QOL and participation. The intervention questions in Table 12-3 involve evidence about effectiveness and feasibility and attributes related to participation. The attributes in all of these questions are the measured or outcome variables of interest in the research studies that the therapist retrieves in the literature search.

The emphasis in this chapter is on communicating about information from published research articles. This source of information is particularly important when the therapist does not have readily available data that have been systematically collected in his or her own setting. It should be noted, however, that in actuality therapists will most likely draw upon a variety of information sources for meeting the decision-making needs of clients, managers, and funders. They can gather information by talking to clinical experts and clients, recalling their own practice experience and training, and systematically collecting data in their practice setting (Straus et al., 2005).

Using keywords or related words and synonyms in the questions to search the literature, the therapist retrieves research articles. Table 12-4 shows some possible terms that could be used to search for evidence relevant to the sample questions in Tables 12-1 through 12-3. The most effective and efficient use of the therapist's time is to first search for research syntheses and meta-analyses (with "synthesis" or "meta-analysis" as keywords). These types of research articles describe a whole body of research that might be relevant to answering a clinical question. Their strength is that they amass evidence in one location; however, this strength is the limitation of the research synthesis in that it may provide evidence that is highly summarized and general. Therefore, it is often useful to supplement synthesis and meta-analytic articles with research articles that report the findings from single studies to find detailed evidence about situations and issues related to the clinical population of interest. Once retrieved, the therapist must interpret the findings before communicating about them. A later section in this chapter, "Examples of Interpreting and Communicating Evidence," provides details about how to interpret findings from sample research articles found in response to the questions in Tables 12-1 through 12-3. Chapter 7 also provides more information about systematic reviews and evidence.

Step 4: Translate the Evidence Into a Comprehensible Communication to Facilitate an Informed Discussion With the Decision Maker

Once the therapist has gathered and interpreted the evidence, it is time to have the direct face-to-face or written communication. By following Steps 1 through 3, the therapist has assured that the evidence collected is important and relevant to the decision maker. Now the therapist must help make the evidence comprehensible. Individuals understand and retain information better when the content and presentation of the communication has the following attributes:

- Nontechnical, simple, and concrete language with simple grammatical structure and words with few syllables, presented orally if possible.

- Terms that cross cultures and perspectives. The words and images have the same meaning for the sender and receiver of the communication. The communication is tailored to the decision maker's own words, messages, context, and preference for information format (e.g., words, pictures, or numbers).

- Brevity, with just enough detail for decision making. Limit the number of ideas expressed in the communication to three or less.

- Checks for confusion or lack of comprehension, perhaps by having the decision maker repeat back the information in his or her own words.

- Suggestions for concrete actions or choice options related to the information.

Table 12-4

Search Terms for the Sample Questions in Tables 12-1, 12-2, and 12-3

	TYPE OF EVIDENCE		PARTICIPATION ATTRIBUTE		CLIENT POPULATION	
Table	*Keywords*	*Related Words*	*Keywords*	*Related Words*	*Keyword*	*Related Words*
12-1	association	correlation regression descriptive qualitative cross-sectional longitudinal	quality of life life satisfaction	well-being coping happiness time use daily activities depression	Parkinson's disease	neurological older adult gerontology geriatric rehabilitation
12-2	reliability validity	consistency trustworthiness assessment outcome measure instrument development	Activity Card Sort Parkinson's Disease Questionnaire-39 social participation	self-report social activity quality of life leisure	Parkinson's disease	neurological older adult gerontology geriatric rehabilitation
12-3	effectiveness feasibility rehabilitation intervention	efficacy outcome rehabilitation treatment experiment randomized trial quasi-experiment	social participation	self-report social activity quality of life leisure	Parkinson's disease	neurological older adult gerontology geriatric rehabilitation

These attributes and tools for implementing them are discussed in the patient education and health literacy literature and Web sites (Agency for Healthcare Research & Quality, 2011; O'Connor, Stacey, & Jacobsen, 2011; Redman, 2007; Rudd, 2011; Rudd, Anderson, Oppenheimer, & Nath, 2007). They apply to persons regardless of their level of education or comprehension. Although it is always best to use common, everyday language and simple phrasing, the therapist should be prepared to give more details should the listener ask for this information.

For clients who have comprehension disabilities, limited education, or a primary language other than the therapist's, the therapist should adjust the language, use of probability, and other forms of numeracy appropriately (Golbeck, Paschal, Jones, & Hsiao, 2011; Griffin, McKenna, & Tooth, 2006). In these cases, pictures, visual images, videotapes, and interactive computer characters are helpful (Bickmore, Pfeifer, & Jack, 2009; Houts, Doak, Doak, & Loscalzo, 2006; Rudd et al., 2007). It is important to keep distractions at a minimum and create a comfortable communication environment. Despite the listener's level of comprehension and scientific background, the therapist should allow enough time for the listener to absorb and discuss the communicated information before engaging in any decision making.

The most important attribute of the communication to keep in mind is that the therapist is providing possible answers, not the one correct answer, to a clinical question. Research with human beings is based on a model of tendencies and variations in living organisms and complex events, not on determined facts. As a result, the therapist offers information to discuss, not to dictate. Examples for how to communicate about a body of evidence are given in the following sections.

EXAMPLES OF INTERPRETING AND COMMUNICATING EVIDENCE

Using a case of a person with Parkinson's disease is useful for communicating about evidence because participation evidence relevant to this disease is only recently emerging. Such is the case with many of the populations with whom therapists work. Despite this challenge, there is hope for the evidence-based therapist who works with populations about whom there is seemingly little research evidence. There is a growing body of research on QOL and life satisfaction descriptions, assessments, and interventions for persons with chronic illness and disability. The terms *quality of life* and *life satisfaction* tap into aspects of persons' lives related to their everyday participation in activities and satisfaction with their activities. Knowledge that these terms are highly relevant to therapists is one of the first steps in bridging the communication gaps that face the evidence-based therapist. In the next few sections, the case of Mr. Davis as an individual client and Parkinson's disease as a clinical population is used to demonstrate how the research literature is interpreted and communicated to clients and their family members, managers, and funders. Three types of evidence are discussed: descriptive, assessment, and intervention. There are two illustrations for each of these areas of evidence: one from an article that is a synthesis of more than one study and one from an article on a single study.

To begin to interpret the evidence given in each article, the therapist—let us call him or her Therapist Foster—must first determine whether the research participants are relevant to Mr. Davis or the general population of clients with Parkinson's disease with whom he or she works at the clinic. For the findings to be highly relevant for discussion with Mr. Davis and his family, some of the research participants should be similar to him with respect to important attributes that could affect the answers to the clinical questions. These attributes of interest may be disease severity, gender, age, cultural background, marital status, and socioeconomic status. For the findings to be relevant for discussions with managers and funders, the participants should be similar to the Parkinson's disease population seen in Therapist Foster's own clinic. Table 12-5 summarizes the fictional characteristics of the case of Mr. Davis, as well as the therapist's Parkinson's disease caseload

Table 12-5

Characteristics of the Therapist's Clinical Population and the Reviewed Studies' Research Participants

CHARACTERISTIC	MR. DAVIS	THERAPIST FOSTER'S PARKINSON'S CASELOAD	PINQUART AND SÖRENSEN (2000)	BUCHMAN ET AL. (2010)	DEN OUDSTEN ET AL. (2007)	DUNCAN AND EARHART (2010)	GOODWIN ET AL. (2008)	TICKLE-DEGNEN ET AL. (2010) AND WHITE ET AL. (2008)
Health condition	Parkinson's	Parkinson's	Well and ill	Older adults including 13 with Parkinson's	Parkinson's	Parkinson's	Parkinson's	Parkinson's
Degree of disability	Moderate, community living	Mild to severe, inpatient and outpatient rehabilitation	None to severe	Diverse ability, retirement facilities, and subsidized housing	NR	Mild to severe	Mild to severe (primarily moderate)	Mild to moderate, community dwelling
Age (in years)	75	> 50	> 55	Average of 80	NR	Average of 70	NR	Average of 66
Gender	Man	70% men 30% women	Men and women	245 men 740 women	Men and women	35 men 27 women	282 men 141 women 72 NR	82 men 35 women
Race and ethnicity	Black, United States	Primarily White, United States	Race NR, North America, Europe	Race NR, United States	Race NR, several countries	NR	Race NR, several countries	97% White United States
Social network	Lives with disabled wife (post-stroke), with adult children near	Diverse	Diverse	Average social networks size of 7	NR	NR	NR	81% had spouse or partner; 83% living with family or friend
Work status	Retired banker	Retired	Diverse	NR	NR	NR	NR	NR
Socioeconomic status	16 years education	Diverse	Diverse	14 years education	NR	NR	NR	85% college educated

NR = not reported or unable to infer from the article.

Table 12-6

Study Results That Provide Probable Answers to Different Types of Questions

TYPE OF QUESTION	DATA ANALYTIC RESULTS
Descriptive	• General and unique qualitative themes, categories • Means, medians, modes • Frequency distributions, ranges, variances • Sign and magnitude of measures of association (e.g., r) and difference (e.g., d)
Assessment[a]	• Reliability coefficients • Validation coefficients and measures of difference (e.g., d, t, F)
Intervention	• Mean and variation of change scores • Magnitude of difference between intervention change and control change (e.g., r or d)[b] • Confidence intervals • Tests of significance (e.g., t, F)

[a]See Tables 12-7, 12-8, and 12-9 for more information.
[b]See Table 12-10 for more information.

and the actual characteristics of research participants in research articles that are reviewed in the following sections. Second, the therapist should determine what possible answers each research paper gives to the clinical questions that guided the search for the evidence. Therapist Foster will be concerned with answering those questions listed in Tables 12-1 through 12-3. Table 12-6 shows the types of data analytic findings that would most likely provide answers to the questions. Third, and finally, the therapist should determine the strength of the evidence in answering the questions by evaluating the quality of the study design, procedures, and measures.

EVIDENCE THAT DESCRIBES THE LIVES AND NEEDS OF CLIENTS WITH PARKINSON'S DISEASE

Interpretation of a Synthesis of Descriptive Studies

Using the clinical questions in Table 12-1 to organize a literature search, Therapist Foster found an article by Pinquart and Sörensen (2000) that reported the findings of a meta-analysis on subjective well-being in later life. As of 2011, this paper continued to be one of the most highly cited meta-analytic studies in this area. Subjective well-being is a construct that encompasses QOL and life satisfaction concepts. The meta-analysis combined the findings of 286 research studies that examined well-being in relation to socioeconomic status; quantitative and qualitative aspects of older persons' social networks; and competence, defined as skills to manage basic, instrumental, and leisure daily life activities.

Therapist Foster begins the interpretation of this meta-analytic study by determining how relevant it is to Mr. Davis's case and to Therapist Foster's larger Parkinson's disease caseload. Table 12-5 shows that the meta-analysis included studies that had research participants similar to Mr. Davis in many respects. Although the meta-analysis included studies with participants who were chronically ill, it did not report information about specific diseases. However, some findings were reported separately for men and women and separately for participants of different age groups. Therefore, Therapist Foster could pay attention to the findings for men and the oldest adults for communicating with Mr. Davis.

Therapist Foster, having determined that the meta-analytic report is relevant, turns to locating the findings that will help to answer the clinical questions. Table 12-6 shows the types of findings that are often important to descriptive evidence. In the case of Pinquart and Sörensen's report (2000), correlations are the primary findings of interest. It was found that the higher the participants' socioeconomic status, the higher their life satisfaction ($r = 0.17$), but this association was smaller for adults who were 75 years and older ($r = 0.10$). The quality of social contacts had a higher association with life satisfaction ($r = 0.22$) than quantity of contacts ($r = 0.12$). The quality of contacts association was highest for participants over the ages of 70 ($r = 0.29$). Finally, the higher the participants' competence in basic and instrumental daily living skills, the higher their life satisfaction ($r = 0.23$) regardless of age. In general, the differences between genders in the associations appeared to be less relevant to Mr. Davis's case than the differences between different ages, so gender differences are not discussed here.

Two important pieces of evidence to note from the correlations described previously are their signs and magnitude (i.e., how big they are). The signs are positive, indicating that on average participants tended to have higher life satisfaction when they had higher socioeconomic status, stronger social networks, and more competence in performing daily living activities. As far as magnitude is concerned, Cohen (1988) suggested that descriptive correlations with absolute values of about .10 are of a small magnitude, of about .30 are of a medium magnitude, and of about .50 or higher are of a large magnitude. Using these criteria, the magnitude of the correlations in the meta-analytic report of Pinquart and Sörensen (2000) were of a small to medium magnitude. Another important piece of evidence is the statistical significance of the findings. The correlations and comparisons between correlations reported in the previous paragraph were reported to be statistically significant below the traditional level of .05. This statistical significance indicates that the findings were strong enough, given the sample size, to feel confident in ruling out chance as the factor responsible for the strength. Studies that have large sample sizes, such as meta-analyses (this one having thousands of research participants represented), often have significant findings, thus effectively ruling out chance as an explanation for the magnitude of the findings.

Therapist Foster can take away from this examination of the Pinquart and Sörensen (2000) meta-analysis the following possible answer to the questions in Table 12-1: high quality of social contacts, continued competence in daily living activities, and socioeconomic status may be important aspects of life satisfaction for clients with Parkinson's disease. For Mr. Davis, in particular, socioeconomic status may not be an important factor unless he has financial concerns at this time. This possibility is based on the meta-analytic findings that socioeconomic status was not an important QOL factor for participants who were at least 75 years old, the age of Mr. Davis. Mr. Davis's age may make his well-being particularly vulnerable to poor quality social contacts or, in other words, particularly protected by higher quality social contacts.

Descriptive evidence, unless it is derived from experimental (including randomized controlled trials) or, sometimes, from longitudinal studies, does not usually give strong indication of causality. The associations found in the Pinquart and Sörensen (2000) meta-analysis are not causal patterns despite the authors' questionable use of the word *influence* in the title and throughout the text, a word that implies causality. The quality of social contacts could affect a person's life satisfaction, but the reverse could be true as well. A person who feels satisfied may engender high-quality social interactions. There may be a different, unmeasured factor that may explain why both life satisfaction and quality of contacts are high together or low together—perhaps good physical and mental health. Descriptive evidence helps the therapist to understand possible patterns that exist in human behavior and experience, but it does not provide definitive prescriptions for intervention. Intervention decisions require evidence of a causal nature, as when individuals are randomly assigned to intervention and control conditions or when interventions are systematically provided and withdrawn. Descriptive evidence, on the other hand, helps a therapist recognize potentially important client issues and to have a language for discussing and exploring these issues with clients, managers, and funders.

Interpretation of a Single Descriptive Study

From Pinquart and Sörensen's (2000) review, Therapist Foster learned about several factors related to subjective well-being in aging, and among these was the importance of the quality social contacts. Recently studies have found that social participation and loneliness are fundamental to older adults' emotional and physical health (Buchman et al., 2009, 2010; Holt-Lunstad, Smith, & Layton, 2010). For example, Buchman et al. (2010) followed the rate of motor decline in older adults for up to 12 years. They found that feelings of loneliness and social activity at baseline predicted the rate of motor decline as measured through a single composite score from a motor battery that included testing of upper extremity strength, speed of gait, lower extremity endurance, balance, and fine motor speed and coordination. With each additional point of loneliness on a 5-point scale, motor decline was 40% more rapid and there was a 50% increased risk of death. Social activity showed similar findings, with social activity and loneliness both contributing independently and statistically significantly to the prediction of the rate of motor decline. The statistical significance suggests that the magnitude of the findings were not attributable to chance. Social network size did not contribute to the prediction. Table 12-5 shows that the participants in this study were similar to Mr. Davis in age and amount of education. Yet participants were primarily women, and only a small percentage of participants had Parkinson's disease. However, the findings were similar for men and women, and the removal of participants with Parkinson's from the analysis did not change the findings, suggesting that the results are applicable to older adults in general and probably to people like Mr. Davis. The study appears also to be relevant for Therapist Foster's broader Parkinson's disease caseload.

The study methods involved mixed-effect models with control of covariates. Many quantitative descriptive studies of QOL and health use complex and multivariate analyses because QOL and health are complex constructs that involve many facets. The therapist, however, need not be an expert in multivariate analysis to glean evidence from the article.

Buchman et al. (2010) present clear descriptions of the statistical analyses and provide clear graphs and basic descriptive statistics and correlations to illustrate the findings. The authors provide some basic means and standard deviations that might be informative to the therapist. For example, they show that the research participants had a baseline average body mass index of weight in kilograms divided by height in meters squared of 27.35 with a standard deviation of 5.25. One property of a normal distribution of scores, described in any statistics textbook (e.g., Portney & Watkins, 2009), is that 68% of the sample's scores fall within one standard deviation, in either direction, of the average score. Another property is that 95% of the sample scores fall within two standard deviations. Assuming that the scores are distributed normally, then 95% of older adult scores fall within the range of 16.85 [27.35 − (2 × 5.25)] to 37.85 [27.35 + (2 × 5.25)]. This range indicates that the sample represents a population that varies across all categories of body mass, from underweight through obese (adult standards found at http://www.cdc.gov/healthyweight/assessing/bmi/adult_bmi/index.html).

Pinquart and Sörensen (2000) suggested misleadingly that the factors they described "influence" subjective well-being. However, Buchman et al. (2010) did not incorrectly draw causal implications from their predictive association study. Instead, they explored several explanations for the findings including prospective causality (e.g., social activity may be protective against neurotoxic damage) or reverse causality (e.g., motor decline causes reduction in social activity). That the research design was a prospective longitudinal study with control for various covariates strengthens the argument for prospective causality but does not eliminate the reverse causality explanation. This latter causality explanation could be challenged more directly with an experiment in which participants are randomly allocated to different levels of social activity and their motor decline is measured prospectively. This experimental design may not be easy to implement in an ethical manner. Therapist Foster can take away from this examination of Buchman et al.'s (2010) findings the following possible answer to the questions in Table 12-1: older adult clients' feelings of loneliness and their social participation may be important components of QOL that are associated with physical health.

Communication Examples for Descriptive Evidence

Therapist Foster would probably want to peruse other research articles about QOL and Parkinson's disease, but the two reviewed in this section provide enough evidence to compose initial communications to Mr. Davis, managers, and funders. The following example might be a way to begin a discussion with Mr. Davis:

> I would like to get to know you better. Recent research suggests that older adults and people with Parkinson's enjoy being with friends and family members, have loving and good times with them, and give one another useful support and help. People who are not lonely and do their social activities are likely to protect their strength and ability to move their hands and legs. What do you think about your family life and social activities? [Discuss.] Communication can be a problem of Parkinson's disease. Is this a concern for you? [Discuss, and raise other remaining issues in a similar fashion.] Are there any changes in your day-to-day life that would make your life more satisfying to you, your wife, and others who are important to you?

The wording in this communication example may be too complex or too simple for Mr. Davis. One way to assess the complexity of this example, as described by health literacy experts (Rudd et al., 2007), is to type out the communication and score its readability using Microsoft Word's readability calculations under the spelling and grammar check tool. Using this tool, the previous example contains 116 words outside of the brackets, has 16.5 words per sentence on the average, and requires a comprehension level at the eighth-grade level in the United States. In comparison, reading levels of ninth and tenth grade were found in a study of written occupational therapy education material for older clients (Griffin et al., 2006). Therefore, the communication example discussed is simpler than what is generally found in occupational therapy. However, some health literacy advocates advise that oral and written patient education material be presented at no more than the fifth-grade level, even for individuals who have higher comprehension ability (Wilson, 2003). The following example is a modified and less complex version of the previous example. It contains 93 words, 10 words per sentence on average, and requires a fifth-grade comprehension level:

> I would like to know you better. Let's start by talking about some studies of older people. These studies find that people feel good about life when they have loving relationships with family and friends. [Discuss.] One study found that doing social activities may help your ability to move. What activities do you do with other people? [Discuss.] Communication can be a problem of Parkinson's. Is this a concern for you? [Discuss, and raise other remaining issues in a similar fashion.] We've talked about what makes you feel good. Are there any changes in your life that would make you and your family feel better?

A communication with a manager or funder could be stated more formally. It could be used to start a discussion about the development of an evidence-based rehabilitation program for a Parkinson's disease population. If the communication is in written form, it is appropriate to include research literature citations and to have more complex wording. The following example contains 116 words, has an average of 29 words per sentence, and requires very high comprehension ability (grade 17.8):

> A research synthesis found that older people, including those with chronic illnesses, reported higher well-being when they had active and high-quality relationships with friends and family members, were able to perform their daily living and leisure activities competently, and were of a higher socioeconomic status. Another study followed older adults and a small subset of people with Parkinson's disease for up to 12 years. The higher the participant's reported loneliness and the lower the social activity at baseline, the higher the participant's rate of motor decline. Together these studies suggest that rehabilitation programs for Parkinson's disease must address social factors related to daily living in order to support quality of life and physical health outcomes.

EVIDENCE THAT GUIDES THE CHOICE AND USE OF ASSESSMENT TOOLS FOR CLIENTS WITH PARKINSON'S DISEASE

Every score or conclusion drawn from an assessment procedure is a measure of several simultaneous elements; the client's performance is only one of those elements. Other elements are called *error* and include the context of the assessment, the attributes of the therapist, and the testing tool itself. For example, a measure of a client's dressing performance could also be a measure of the client's familiarity with the room in which the dressing is performed and with the clothing used; a measure of the therapist's emotions, expectations, and behavior with the client; and a measure of the scale used in scoring. Imagine a client putting on an unfamiliar blouse, in an unfamiliar environment, with a harried therapist who was using a 2-point rating scale (0 = *dependent*, 1 = *independent*) to judge the performance. Now imagine this client putting on a familiar blouse, in a familiar environment, with a relaxed therapist who was using a 5-point scale (graduated from 0, requires another to perform every step to 4, able to perform every step with no assistance) to judge the performance. This client may receive two very different recommendations based on these two testing situations, perhaps a recommendation for further rehabilitation in the first situation and for immediate discharge home in the second. Standardized assessment procedures that are reliable and valid are, by definition, less likely to result in inconsistent and incorrect conclusions compared to unstandardized, low reliability, or low validity procedures. Obviously, therapists, clients, funders, and managers do not want to waste the client's or therapist's time and resources in assessments that will result in incorrect conclusions. More importantly, they want assessments to generate correct clinical recommendations that have the potential for improving client outcomes.

The challenge of the evidence-based practitioner is to use assessment procedures that have demonstrated reliability and validity, are feasible in the therapist's clinical context, and are the right fit for the client. The research literature on the measurement properties of assessment procedures uses a dizzying array of terminology to discuss and report reliability and validity findings. What is most crucial to the selection of an assessment tool is whether or not that tool has been tested for the particular forms of reliability and validity most pertinent to the purpose of the assessment. See Tables 12-7, 12-8, and 12-9 for common forms, methods, and standards derived from a quantitative paradigm that are used with many assessments relevant to rehabilitation.

Table 12-7

A Reliability Primer

FORM OF RELIABILITY	TESTED WHEN THE SCORE OR ASSESSMENT CONCLUSION IS EXPECTED TO BE CONSISTENT ACROSS DIFFERENT ...	EXAMPLES OF ASSESSMENTS THAT SHOULD DEMONSTRATE AN ADEQUATE DEGREE OF THIS FORM OF RELIABILITY	THE DEGREE OF RELIABILITY IS COMMONLY SUMMARIZED WITH A COEFFICIENT THAT REPRESENTS THE CONSISTENCY BETWEEN DIFFERENT RATERS, TIMES, OR ITEMS, SUCH AS ...	WHAT IS AN "ADEQUATE" DEGREE OF RELIABILITY?
Interrater	Therapists or raters	Therapist's judgment of ADL independence from observing client's performance. Therapist's summary of a client's feelings or experiences.	Correlation (e.g., intraclass) Cohen's kappa percentage agreement	> .70 > .40 > 80%
Test–retest	Testing times, as long as the client has not changed	Client's ADL performance before receiving intervention. An interest checklist.	Correlation (e.g., intraclass) Difference in standard deviation units (e.g., d)	> .70 < .20
Internal consistency	Items of measure	A 20-item short-term memory test. A 10-item self-esteem questionnaire.	Cronbach's alpha correlation	> .40 > .70

Reliability testing methods and standards vary across different research areas. See a research methods textbook (e.g., Portney & Watkins, 2009) for general and common methods and interpretation standards.

Table 12-8

Validity Primer I

GENERAL FORM OF VALIDITY	TESTED WHEN THE SCORE OR ASSESSMENT CONCLUSION IS EXPECTED TO BE A VALID (TRUE) MEASURE OF ...	WHY TESTED?	SPECIFIC FORMS OF VALIDITY TESTING (SEE TABLE 12-9)
Descriptive	Current client attributes at one point in time, such as current ADL performance or feelings about self.	To see whether the measure differentiates between clients who have different attributes.	Content Criterion-related Construct
Predictive	Client attributes in the future, such as ability to successfully perform work activities or to adjust to disability.	To see whether the current measurement predicts future attributes.	Content Criterion-related Construct
Evaluative	Change over time in client attributes, such as change in ADL performance or change in feelings of self-efficacy.	To see whether the measure is responsive to a change in the client.	Content Criterion-related Construct

Validity testing terminology, methods, and standards vary across different research areas (see Portney & Watkins, 2009).

Table 12-9

Validity Primer II

SPECIFIC FORM OF VALIDITY	ADDRESSES THE QUESTION ...	EXAMPLE	HOW THIS FORM OF VALIDITY IS ASSESSED	WHAT IS AN "ADEQUATE" DEGREE OF VALIDITY?
Content	Does the content of the measure cover all aspects or elements of the attribute being measured?	Does a basic ADL instrument measure all important self-care activities?	• Documented expert opinion • Comparison with relevant theory	Relative congruence between content and expert opinion There is a logical direct relationship between the measure and theory
Criterion-related	Does the score or conclusion drawn from the measure relate to a score or conclusion drawn from a valid criterion?	Does the score from a new ADL instrument (the one that is yet to be validated) lead to the same conclusions as a score from an established ADL instrument? Do clients with brain damage have a different score on a cognitive test than clients without brain damage? Do clients who are known to have improved their ability to drive show this improvement in a new driving test?	• Administration of both new and established measure to clients and calculation of correlation between the two measures • Administration of the test to different populations of clients and comparison of the scores • Administration of a test before and after an intervention and comparison of the two scores	A level of association that should theoretically exist between the two (e.g., $r > .60$). A difference that should theoretically exist between the two (e.g., $d > .30$). A difference that should theoretically exist between the two (e.g., $d > .80$)
Construct (convergent and discriminant)	Does the score or conclusion drawn from the measure relate more to validated measures of the same attribute than to validated measures of a different attribute?	Does a dementia test relate more to another dementia test than it does to a test of depression?	• Administration of measures designed to measure similar and different attributes and comparisons of the relationships between the various measures	Larger correlations between similar measures compared to smaller correlations between different measures

Validity is not normally determined by comparison to one absolute standard. It is established through a variety of means that make scientific and theoretical sense and is best determined by comparison with standards in a specific field of research.

Interpretation of a Synthesis of Assessment Studies

Using the clinical questions in Table 12-2 to organize a literature search, Therapist Foster found a systematic review of QOL and related measures used with Parkinson's disease (Den Oudsten, Van Heck, & De Vries, 2007). The researchers summarized findings from 36 studies that evaluated the measurement properties of 16 questionnaires, including the Parkinson's Disease-39 (PDQ-39), one of the most highly used and studied health-related QOL measures in Parkinson's disease. The review is relevant to Therapist Foster's caseload and Mr. Davis in that participants with Parkinson's disease were highly represented in the reviewed studies (see Table 12-5). However, the researchers gave little information about the participants in the reviewed studies. A perusal of the reference list shows that diverse cultures and ethnicities are represented.

The PDQ-39 (Peto, Jenkinson, & Fitzpatrick, 1998) items generate a summary index score that is the average of eight domain scores: *mobility, activities of daily living* (ADL), *emotional well-being, stigma, social support, cognitions, communication,* and *bodily discomfort.* A higher index or domain score indicates more self-perceived frequency of health problems and participation restrictions in the past month that are due to the disease, with 0 indicating *never a problem* and 100 *always a problem.* Den Oudsten et al. (2007) categorized the PDQ-39 as a measure of perceived health status and activity functioning. They distinguished it from other measures in their review that more centrally assess life and activity satisfaction. Using the reliability and validity categories in Tables 12-7 through 12-9, the review findings are summarized as follows:

- Interrater reliability: Not evaluated because it is not relevant for self-report questionnaires about subjective experiences related to QOL.
- Test–retest reliability: Adequate for all scores except *social support.*
- Internal consistency: Adequate alpha levels for all scores. However, confirmatory factory analysis suggests lower internal consistency for *social support* and *emotional well-being.*
- Descriptive validity
  - ○ Content—Floor effects particularly for *social support,* suggesting that respondents either have few concerns as measured in this domain or that it is not sensitive to differences in social support concerns among the respondents. In addition, many times respondents do not fully complete the social support items as missing, suggesting problems with the content.
  - ○ Criterion-related—Demonstrates adequate correlation with other health-related QOL measures.
  - ○ Construct—Convergent validity is shown but discriminant validity is not reported. The researchers note that the PDQ-39 is the only reviewed instrument that has social support items and one of two that has cognitive functioning items. Yet it lacks items on sexual activity and financial consequences of the disease, and almost half of the PDQ-39 items concentrate on physical concerns.
- Predictive validity: Not reported.
- Evaluative validity
  - ○ Content—Not reported.
  - ○ Criterion-related—Change over time in the PDQ-39 score is correlated with change in another health-related QOL measure.
  - ○ Construct—*Mobility, ADL, stigma,* and *social support* are sensitive to deterioration in health status. The researchers noted that the PDQ-39 is one of the few instruments that has documented evaluative validity.

Den Oudsten et al. (2007) suggested that users of QOL types of measures choose first whether or not to assess client perceived health status and function (as in the PDQ-39) or client satisfaction with life domains. Next, users must choose whether or not to use a generic instrument that can be used with many health conditions or a disease-specific instrument that is used with one disease or health condition (as in the PDQ-39). Finally, users must make a decision as to whether or not the quality of the instrument's psychometric properties warrants its use. Because the PDQ-39 is used frequently as an outcome measure for health interventions including rehabilitation outcomes (e.g., Tickle-Degnen, Ellis, Saint-Hilaire, Thomas, & Wagenaar, 2010), and it compares favorably to the other reviewed instruments with respect to psychometric properties, it is a reasonable choice for use in Therapist Foster's practice.

With respect to answering the clinical questions in Table 12-2, the PDQ-39 measures elements relevant to social participation (e.g., community mobility, instrumental activities of daily living, stigma, social support, and communication) with reliability and validity. Although it compares favorably to similar instruments, it is weighted toward assessing participation with physical functioning items and not satisfaction with one's participation. The review did not compare the PDQ-39 to the Activity Card Sort and, as a result, the evidence did not answer the portion of the question related to this comparison.

Interpretation of a Single Assessment Study

Therapist Foster has heard of the Activity Card Sort (ACS; Baum & Edwards, 2008) and knows that although it has not yet been used in as many studies as the PDQ-39, it has a much broader range of older adult activities that it assesses compared to the PDQ-39 and has the content and format to potentially identify a variety of components of social participation in a flexible manner that suits client rehabilitation needs. It can be used as a generic or disease-specific instrument, which can be desirable in practices that serve a variety of older adult clinical populations. However, Therapist Foster knows little about its reliability and validity.

A search for relevant evidence retrieved a paper by Duncan and Earhart (2010) that specifically studied the validity of the ACS as a measure of participation in the Parkinson's population. The study was relevant to Therapist Foster's caseload and Mr. Davis as shown in Table 12-5. The ACS contains photographs of individuals performing activities in four activity domains: 20 photographs of instrumental activities, 35 of low-physical-demand leisure activities, 17 of high-physical-demand leisure activities, and 17 of social activities. For Duncan and Earhart's (2010) study the individuals sorted cards to identify which activities were retained since the onset of their illness. Scores were total percentage of retained activity in each activity domain and overall. What Therapist Foster learns about the reliability and validity from the study and the literature review is the following:

- Interrater reliability: Not evaluated because not relevant for self-report questionnaires about subjective experiences related to QOL.
- Test–retest reliability: Not tested in this study, but the researchers noted that the ACT developers had established this form of reliability in a small sample.
- Internal consistency: Not tested in this study or reported.
- Descriptive validity
  - Content—The researchers reported that the ACS includes items from all domains of the *International Classification of Functioning, Disability and Health* (ICF), a cross-culturally derived framework that guides assessment in rehabilitation and other health fields (World Health Organization, 2001).
  - Criterion-related—Although this Parkinson's sample had less retained activities relative to the published healthy older patient sample, the Parkinson's sample had more retained

activities compared to published multiple sclerosis and stroke samples. The Parkinson's sample performed closer to the healthy sample and not as closely to the neurological samples as would be predicted if the ACS were sensitive to changes in participation due to neurological illness. Note that the researchers referred to this analysis as "discriminant validity." Table 12-9 refers to this form of validity as criterion-related. Either is correct in this case.

    ◦ Construct—This study found that the total percentage of retained activities measured in the ACT held statistically significant and medium to large associations with constructs relevant to participation including QOL concerns as measured by the PDQ-39; disability and disease severity as measured by the Movement Disorders Society Unified Parkinson's Disease Rating Scale (MDS-UPDRS); physical mobility as measured by a number of performance measures related to balance and walking speed and capacity; and a self-reported gait freezing measure. The largest associations, all statistically significant, were with self-report measures related to community mobility/leisure, instrumental and basic activities of daily living, and communication (e.g., PDQ-39, mobility, $r = -0.75$; MDS-UPDRS II, *ADL*, $r = -0.72$; PDQ-39, ADL, $r = -0.57$; and PDQ-39, communication, $r = -0.56$). Thus, the largest convergent validity was demonstrated with self-report measures about participation concerns. The more retained activities as measured on the ACS, the less self-reported concerns with participation in daily life. The next largest set of convergent associations, all statistically significant, were with the mobility performance measures (ranging from $r = 0.27$ to $r = 0.49$). The more retained activities as assessed with the ACS, the better the participants' balance, the less their freezing, and the better their walking capacity. Direction of causality cannot be determined in this study (i.e., whether retaining activities leads to better mobility performance or vice versa). The researchers assumed that mobility performance influenced activity participation; however, this study's correlational design was not designed to test causality.

- Predictive validity: Not reported.
- Evaluative validity: Not reported.

This study builds the repertoire of possible answers to the questions in Table 12-2; the ACS compares favorably to the PDQ-39 as an assessment of participation. The evidence from this study does not suggest that the ACS is a better or worse measure of participation in terms of reliability and validity. The therapist can use other factors that distinguish the two measures to judge the merits of the use of one or the other. For example, the PDQ-39 addresses concerns with attempting activities but does not evaluate which specific activities are retained or not kept up, whereas the ACS can be used to identify specific activities in these categories.

Communication Examples of Assessment Evidence

Mr. Davis and his wife have come to the rehabilitation appointment today. In their past discussion about QOL and social activities, the couple had expressed a concern with not getting out of the house enough and visiting with friends and family. In other words, they are concerned about staying socially and physically active. They do not know how to get more involved given Mr. Davis's weakness due to Parkinson's and Mrs. Davis's weakness due to a stroke. Therapist Foster might begin a discussion of the assessment evidence with them in order to facilitate their engagement in the decision making around assessment procedures that would be most meaningful to them. The following communication example includes 80 words, has 8.8 words per sentence on average, and requires a fifth-grade comprehension level. The terms *validly* and *reliably* have not been included in this example because they require a high level of technical understanding and are not needed to convey the information necessary for decision making. Rather, the word *good* is used to convey the quality of the assessment procedure:

> Rehabilitation helps you do activities that you would like to do. First, we need to learn about your current activities. One good method is to fill out a questionnaire about living with Parkinson's. [Discuss and show the PDQ-39.] This questionnaire tells us only about Mr. Davis's activities. Another good method can involve both of you. You look at pictures of activities. You divide them up. Then we talk about which ones you would like to do. [Discuss and show the ACL.] Which of these methods would you like to try?

A communication with a manager or funder could be spoken more formally, as in the following example, to start a discussion about the development of assessment tools in rehabilitation with a Parkinson's disease population. Citations could be included in a written form of this communication. The example contains 194 words, has 24.2 words per sentence on average, and a 15.5-grade comprehension level:

> The Parkinson's disease literature has demonstrated that the Parkinson's Disease Questionnaire (the PDQ-39) is one reliable and valid procedure for assessing clients' concerns about daily activities and participation due to the disease. The questionnaire assesses concerns in eight domains: mobility, activities of daily living, emotional well-being, stigma, social support, cognitions, communication, and bodily discomfort. One of its strengths is that it can be filled out with or without a therapist. One limitation of the PDQ-39 is that it does not address specific activities that the client has lost or retained due to the disease. The Activity Card Sort (ACS), on the other hand, uses concrete pictures of older adults performing 89 different activities including instrumental, leisure, and social activities. The client sorts the cards into different categories that yield scores for percentage of activities retained following the onset of disease. A strength of the ACS is that the pictures may help people with lower health literacy be able to talk about their activity and participation needs. The ACS correlates with the PDQ-39, suggesting that both are measuring participation and quality of life issues, and both create scores that are useful for rehabilitation planning.

EVIDENCE THAT GUIDES THE CHOICE OF INTERVENTIONS USED WITH CLIENTS WITH PARKINSON'S DISEASE

Suppose that Mr. Davis decides to fill out the PDQ-39 and, with his wife, the ACL. Through the assessment procedure and a discussion with him and his wife, Therapist Foster finds that Mrs. Davis gets out more than Mr. Davis and is involved in volunteer activities in the local elementary school. She is concerned that he does not get out enough and that he is losing his strength and endurance. Mr. Davis has not found social activities that meet his needs. He played tennis regularly until the age of 68 and enjoyed social activities that involved physical activity. Over the years, as his Parkinson's disease progressed, he found that he becomes easily fatigued and has difficulty communicating clearly with others. Mr. Davis tells the therapist that he would like to get out of his home on a regular basis and become more involved in activities with other people. Next, based on the clinical question in Table 12-3, the therapist searches for the latest evidence on interventions suitable for improving community mobility and social participation among individuals like Mr. Davis.

Interpretation of a Synthesis of Intervention Studies

To start to develop possible answers to these questions, Therapist Foster retrieves a recent meta-analysis and qualitative research synthesis published in the rehabilitation literature that examined the effectiveness of exercise interventions for persons with Parkinson's disease (Goodwin, Richards, Taylor, Taylor, & Campbell, 2008). This study quantitatively summarized the findings of randomized controlled trials (RCTs), which are designed to test the causal effects of interventions. RCTs provide stronger evidence for causality than do descriptive studies, and a meta-analysis of RCTs provides the strongest evidence for the average effectiveness of interventions in a clinical population.

Table 12-5 demonstrates that the participants in the studies included in the meta-analysis are similar to the therapist's Parkinson's disease population in many respects. After determining that the meta-analysis is relevant to this population, the therapist looks for the major meta-analytic results, which are the average effect size estimates for each relevant outcome. Meta-analysts convert every relevant statistical finding to an effect size that can be averaged across all studies. Tests of significance (such as t or F and their p values) cannot be compared across studies because their magnitudes are a function of both the size of the effect and the sample size (Rosenthal & Rosnow, 2007). Common estimates of effect size used in the rehabilitation and psychological literature are the effect size r and the effect size d. Table 12-10 shows interpretations and calculations for these effect sizes. The magnitude of the effect size (i.e., how big it is) is an estimate of the degree to which two conditions (such as intervention versus control) differ in terms of their therapeutic effectiveness. Alternatively, the magnitude is the degree to which involvement in intervention had a more successful or beneficial outcome for research participants than involvement in a control condition. Better average outcomes for the intervention versus control conditions are indicated by a positive effect size, equal average outcomes by a 0 effect size, and worse average outcomes by a negative effect size, regardless of whether the effect size is measured as an r or a d.

Goodwin et al. (2008) found the average effect size of 9 RCTs was $d = .47$ for the effect of exercise on physical functioning in Parkinson's disease (scored client performance in the physical domain), with a 95% confidence interval (CI) ranging from the effect size of .12 to .82. The average effect size of the results can be compared to the d column in Table 12-10. In that column, there is a d of .50, which is very close to .47. Such a magnitude of d is considered to be of "medium" size for intervention effects (Cohen, 1988). The CI indicates that it is reasonable to be confident that the true average effect size of exercise studies including those that are not in this meta-analysis would be likely to fall within the range of a "small" effect (.12) to a "large" effect (.82). Given that the CI does not include $d = 0$ (no effect), chance is not likely to be an explanation for the effect found by Goodwin et al. (2008).

The effect size d is the difference between the means of the outcomes for two conditions in standard deviation units. A d of .47 indicates that the average intervention outcome was nearly one-half of a standard deviation (0.50) more beneficial than the average control outcome. Table 12-10 shows that a d of .50 is equivalent to an effect size r of 0.24. The effect size r is a point-biserial correlation or partial correlation coefficient that indicates the degree to which the independent variable (intervention versus control) is associated with the outcome scores. It can be computed directly to or from d (see Tickle-Degnen [2001] for details). Rosenthal and Rubin (1982) have shown that the magnitude of the r, when multiplied by 100%, can most easily be understood as an estimate of the change in success rates across two conditions. They created a practical tool, called the Binomial Effect Size Display, for translating the effect size r into intervention success rates. Success is defined here as receiving a score that is higher than the combined average of both conditions and failure as receiving a lower-than-average score. Table 12-10 shows that for a medium size r of 0.24 (approximately $d = .50$), 62% of the participants who received exercise intervention had a successful outcome relative to 38% of the participants in the control condition who had a

Table 12-10

Effect Sizes and Success Rates

Magnitude of Effect[a]	d	*d* SUCCESS RATES			r	*r* SUCCESS RATES		
		Control (%)	Intervention (%)	Change (%)		Control (%)	Intervention (%)	Change (%)
Zero	0	50	50	0	0	50	50	0
Small	.20	46	54	8	0.10	45	55	10
Medium	.50	40	60	20	0.24	38	62	24
Large	.80	34	66	32	0.37	32	69	37
Very large	2.00	16	84	68	0.71	15	86	71

[a]Based on Cohen (1988) and Rosenthal and Rosnow (2007). See Tickle-Degnen (2001) for calculation details.

successful outcome. Because 62% minus 38% is equal to 24%, the success rate increases by 24% from the control to the intervention conditions. These success rates, which are generally equivalent to those for the $d = .47$ meta-analytic results, indicate that exercise intervention was successful for more people with Parkinson's disease than the control condition was, and the failure rate was lower for the intervention than control condition.

It is important to note that there were still a number of clients, approximately 38% to 40% on average, for whom rehabilitation intervention was not successful, and a number of clients, also approximately 38 to 40%, for whom the control condition was successful. Research evidence provides probabilistic answers to clinical questions. Although it is probable that exercise intervention will be effective with the Parkinson's population, it is not guaranteed that it will be effective for every single member of that population.

Goodwin et al. (2008) also studied meta-analytically the effect of exercise intervention on health-related QOL outcomes (client self-reported functioning in multiple domains of concern) and found the average effect size of four RCTs was $d = .27$ with a 95% CI ranging from the effect size of .04 to .51. A d of .27 indicates that the average intervention outcome was slightly over one-quarter of a standard deviation (0.25) higher than the average control outcome, and the range in the population of exercise intervention studies in Parkinson's disease could be very small (0.04) to medium in magnitude (0.51). Other findings indicated that there was insufficient evidence from RCTs that exercise intervention had significant effects on fall reduction or depression in Parkinson's disease. Further studies were needed in all areas.

The findings of the meta-analysis offer possible answers to the questions in Table 12-3: It is likely that it would be beneficial for Mr. Davis, specifically, and Therapist Foster's population of Parkinson's clients in general, to take part in an exercise intervention. The exercise intervention may have more effect on physical function than on broader areas of social participation. However, as with many forms of intervention, there is no guarantee that rehabilitation will provide a greater benefit to all clients than no treatment or other forms of treatment.

Interpretation of a Single Intervention Study

Therapist Foster may continue to search the literature for evidence specifically related to Mr. Davis's desire to improve social participation and find the results of an RCT on the effect of interdisciplinary self-management rehabilitation on health-related QOL and walking function (Tickle-Degnen et al., 2010; White, Wagenaar, Ellis, & Tickle-Degnen, 2009). Table 12-5 shows that participants were similar to Mr. Davis and representative of Therapist Foster's caseload. Participants on optimal neurological care and medication were randomly assigned to one of three conditions for 6 weeks of intervention: 0 hours of rehabilitation; 18 hours of clinic group rehabilitation, plus 9 hours of attention control social sessions (lower "dose" of rehabilitation) and 27 hours of rehabilitation, with 18 in clinic group rehabilitation and 9 hours of rehabilitation in the home and community (higher dose of rehabilitation). The rehabilitation was provided by physical, occupational, and speech therapists with client-centered skill training in self-managing performance and satisfaction in three functional activity domains: mobility, ADL, and communication. For example, participants engaged in training for how to initiate movement using auditory and visual cues; to do exercises designed specifically for improving strength, endurance, and participation; to adapt self-care and instrumental activities of daily living according to their own preferences and needs; to coordinate their respiration and speech during participation; and to problem-solve "like a therapist" to achieve their own participation goals using a person–task–environment model of performance.

The researchers tested the dose effect of rehabilitation (0 versus 18 versus 27 hours) of rehabilitation at 6 weeks' (post) and at 2 months' and 6 months' follow-up. At 6 weeks there was a beneficial effect of increased rehabilitation hours on health-related QOL measured with the PDQ-39 summary index (eta = 0.23, 95% CI = 0.05–0.40, P = .01; Tickle-Degnen et al., 2010). In this case, the eta is an effect size measure equivalent to the effect size r and is commonly reported when there are more than two conditions being compared. Comparing this eta to the r column in Table 12-10 shows the effect of self-management rehabilitation on participation as measured by the PDQ-39 to be generally of "medium" magnitude. The difference between 18 and 27 hours was not significant. There was marginal evidence suggesting that one reason for no significant difference between the 18- and 27-hour conditions of rehabilitation was that the 9 hours of social control group added to the 18-hour rehabilitation condition was effective in improving participant's QOL in psychosocial domains (decreased feelings of stigma, improved emotional well-being). Rehabilitation benefits in health-related QOL that were found at 6 weeks persisted at 6 months after the completion of the rehabilitation.

Tickle-Degnen et al. (2010) presented PDQ-39 means and standard deviations and several forms of effect sizes for helping clinicians to use the results in decision making. Combining the two rehabilitation conditions, the researchers reported that clinically relevant improvement occurred at a greater rate for 18 and 27 hours (54% improved) than for 0 hours (18% improved), a significant 36% difference in improvement rates between rehabilitation versus no rehabilitation. Effects were largest in communication and mobility domains. Participants with more problematic mobility or ADL at baseline benefitted from rehabilitation in their mobility and ADL, respectively, to a statistically significantly greater degree than participants who had low problems in these domains. Similarly, walking endurance (as reported in White et al., 2009) was improved by rehabilitation primarily for individuals who had low walking endurance at baseline. Effects were nonsignificant for those who already had high walking endurance. Alternatively, rehabilitation was more effective in increasing the time spent in walking activity for participants who spent more time in walking at baseline than participants who spent little time in walking. These findings suggest that interventions should be tailored to client needs and not applied in a one-method-fits-all approach.

Goodwin et al.'s (2008) meta-analysis found that exercise interventions produced medium effects on physical functioning outcomes and small effects on QOL. Alternatively, the self-management rehabilitation trial produced small effects on physical walking parameters when not taking into account individual client needs and medium effects on QOL outcomes (Tickle-Degnen et al., 2010; White et al., 2009). Interventions, such as exercise, that target physical functioning specifically may have larger effects on walking function than QOL interventions, perhaps because of more intense targeting of a focused domain, whereas QOL interventions that provide training on problem solving in multiple domains may have more generalized effects on reducing participation concerns. From this evidence, Therapist Foster can derive a possible answer to the questions in Table 12-3: Mr. Davis and others in the therapist's caseload are likely to be able to improve social participation by participating in rehabilitation that addresses domains that are particularly problematic from the participant's perspective. Because Mr. Davis has concerns about physical functioning, an exercise intervention may be a good intervention option and a group exercise intervention may be of particular value to him for meeting his social needs. However, an intervention that provides him with tools for managing participation in several domains of living may be more beneficial for him.

COMMUNICATION EXAMPLES OF INTERVENTION EVIDENCE

The therapist might begin the communication with Mr. Davis about the intervention evidence in the following manner. This communication involves 55 words, has an average of 11 words in a sentence, and requires almost an eighth-grade comprehension level.

> Studies show that exercise helps people who have physical concerns like you. Group exercise may meet your physical and social needs. [Discuss.] Or you could do rehabilitation that teaches you a variety of skills. It might include exercise, how to communicate clearly with others, or how to do daily activities more easily. What do you think?

Health literacy experts suggest that clients receive both an oral presentation and supplementary handouts presented in user-friendly format and plain language (Rudd, 2011). One written planning tool that Therapist Foster might find helpful for using with Mr. Davis is the Ottawa Personal Decision Guide (O'Connor et al., 2011). It is a one-page questionnaire that helps the client to clarify the decision, explore the benefits and risks of various options, determine the social support needed for the options, assess whether the client's needs for decision making are met, and provides a checklist for planning the next steps.

In all of the client communication examples in this chapter, no numbers have been used. Clients vary in their level of understanding of percentages, proportions, and graphical representations of data (Golbeck et al., 2011; Rudd et al., 2007). Some clients may prefer to know the numbers and the therapist should be comfortable with providing statistical information or gathering it for the client if the client desires it.

Dependent on the needs of the caseload and the resources of the clinic, Therapist Foster can advocate to managers and funders for infrastructure and funding to provide either interventions targeted at improving specific functional domains or interventions that target multiple domains of participation. In the following example, there are 205 words (not including citations), with an average of 29 words per sentence, and the required educational level for comprehension of the message is grade 21. It is likely that such a technically difficult communication would be more appropriate for an audience that has a high degree of fluency in rehabilitation constructs and terminology (e.g., *physical functioning, participation, self-management*):

> Recent rigorous studies have shown that exercise programs benefit physical functioning specifically, whereas interdisciplinary rehabilitation programs that train several sets of skills for managing daily life benefit overall participation and quality of life. A recent meta-analytic study of randomized controlled trials of exercise interventions with Parkinson's disease found exercise to have statistically significantly larger positive outcomes relative to control interventions (Goodwin et al., 2008). The average improvement in physical functioning was approximately one-half standard deviation greater for

exercise participants than control participants. Improvement in quality of life outcomes received smaller beneficial effects of exercise (a difference of one-fourth standard deviation). In an interdisciplinary rehabilitation randomized controlled trial (Tickle-Degnen et al., 2010; White et al., 2009), participants who received mobility, self-care, and communication rehabilitation skill training to self-manage Parkinson's disease during daily participation in the home and community had significantly greater improvements in overall quality of life outcomes than control participants (about one-half standard deviation greater). Physical functioning (walking) effects of self-management rehabilitation were of small magnitude in general but larger for some subgroups of participants. The research evidence suggests that rehabilitation is most effective for people with Parkinson's disease when it is designed to target individual clients' specific functioning and quality of life needs.

EVIDENCE-BASED COMMUNICATION IN THE FACE OF UNCERTAINTY

When the search for evidence has turned up a recent and high-quality published literature review or meta-analysis, the integration that is needed has already been completed by the published author. The therapist need only translate the technical language and presentation of these reviews into language understandable to decision makers. However, if no such review has been found, the therapist must make an accurate integration him- or herself. Such integration takes skill, which develops with the study of research methods and the practice of having to communicate clearly about a body of evidence. Among the guidelines to follow when making an integrated interpretation of a body of evidence are the following:

- Give heavier emphasis to studies that provide more accurate (stronger) evidence than to those studies with potentially less accurate (weaker) evidence. The therapist should refer to the sections of standard research methods textbooks (Portney & Watkins, 2009) that address how to evaluate the internal and external validity, or accuracy, of studies.

- When examining statistics, do not rely solely on significance tests and their P values for determining what the study found unless the study involved a large sample size, roughly about 60 or more participants. Studies that have large sample sizes have more power to detect a statistically significant effect than studies with small sample sizes (Rosenthal & Rosnow, 2007).

It is possible that the findings of two studies may appear to be different. For example, one claims to support the effectiveness of an intervention and the other claims to not support it. The study that claims to fail to support the effectiveness, typically represented as $p > .05$, may have had a small sample size, possibly making it a low power study. The study that claimed to support the effectiveness, with a $P < .05$, may have had a large sample size, enhancing its power to detect a statistically significant effect. Despite the difference in the P values of the two studies, the actual mean scores of the participants may show that participants in both studies derived benefit more from the intervention than the nonintervention condition. Therefore, the P value findings may have led to different conclusions about effectiveness, simply because of power issues, not because of underlying differences in true effectiveness. The integrated interpretation of these two studies would be that they appear to support the effectiveness of the intervention.

When the findings from two high-quality, large-sample studies are in opposite directions, the therapist will find the task of integration more challenging. In this case, the therapist must report to the decision makers that the body of evidence gives conflicting answers to the clinical question. This conflicting evidence will be one factor that therapist and decision makers consider as they discuss the evidence. Conflicts in evidence call upon the therapist to use the highest level of clinical reasoning skills. There is much uncertainty in therapy because every human being is unique and responds to therapy in an individual manner. Nevertheless, there is a great deal of predictable and systematic behavior in human beings as well. The therapist uses reasoning that brings uniqueness and predictability together to make decisions in the face of uncertainty.

Conflicts in evidence call upon therapists to not only tap into their clinical reasoning skills but also to start to develop research questions for an on-site research study. This chapter has addressed how the therapist collects and talks about evidence from published research studies undertaken by researchers other than the therapist. The next logical step in evidence-based practice is to design an on-site study for collecting evidence about one's own clinical population and to use that evidence to help resolve the conflicting findings found in the body of published evidence.

EVIDENCE-BASED COMMUNICATION OPPORTUNITIES IN EVERYDAY PRACTICE

Evidence-based practice requires therapists to keep current in the research findings that are relevant to their clinical populations. To keep current, the therapist must incorporate time for literature searching and reading into clinical practice. The communication about evidence with others will not be an additional time burden if the therapist learns to turn everyday communication opportunities into evidence-based ones.

Communication opportunities with clients arise at the first meeting, at assessment and intervention planning sessions, during the provision of treatment, and at discharge planning sessions. Whenever the therapist is giving recommendations or involving the client in decision making, there is an opportunity for incorporating evidence into the message. Even if the client is not interested in hearing evidence-based information, the therapist can communicate about it in an indirect manner to support the client's development of knowledge and active involvement in decision making. For example, using evidence from research on the effectiveness of microwave ovens in enhancing participation in meal preparation activities, the therapist might say, "Some people find it helpful to do exercise with groups of people. Do you want me to help you find a group in your community that helps people with health conditions like Parkinson's disease?"

With managers and colleagues, group meetings are an ideal forum for disseminating research evidence because the message is discussed among several people at one time in one location. Appropriate types of meetings are team conferences about clients, staff education sessions, and departmental meetings directed at program planning, budget review, and quality assurance. Journal clubs, in which members take turns in reviewing and presenting a summary of a body of research literature, can reduce the individual burden of searching and reading literature. Discussions at journal clubs are relatively unfettered by day-to-day clinical demands. This type of context supports brainstorming and creative thinking that can stimulate the evidence-based modification or development of assessment and intervention procedures.

Any communication with a funder can be an opportunity for the discussion of research evidence, whether face-to-face, via telephone, or by written documentation. One of the more formal communications might be a funding proposal, which requires tight organization and scholarly citations. The more comfortable therapists become with the published research evidence in their area of clinical expertise, the more skillfully they will be able to communicate about that evidence in a brief and understandable format. There is no need to tell the client, the manager, or the funder everything that is known about the evidence unless asked to do so. The therapist communicates enough evidence for informed decision making yet is prepared to communicate about evidence in a more detailed manner.

TAKE-HOME MESSAGES

Communicating Evidence Effectively

✓ Message must be relevant, framed to enable decision making and action, and comprehensible.

✓ Four steps to evidence-based communication:

1. Identify clinical role of decision maker: Client/family and friends, manager, and funder are all potential decision makers.

2. Determine the decisions to be made: Describe relevant client participation issues, select assessment procedures, and choose and plan intervention. The types of information are descriptive, assessment, and intervention.

3. Gather/interpret evidence: Formulate clinical question and research possible answers. Type of evidence being sought; attribute of interest; description of clinical population. Most efficient to search for research synthesis and meta-analysis.

4. Communicate the evidence: For communication with clients use plain language, terms that cross cultures and perspectives, brevity with appropriate amount of detail, repetition and checks for confusion, suggestions for concrete action related to the information.

Interpretation

✓ Assessment tool should have been tested for the particular form of reliability and validity that is needed.

✓ Studies that provide access to both quantitative and qualitative details help in examining similarities and differences in responses.

Uncertainty

✓ If no meta-analysis or systematic review is available, the therapist can perform this function, but it takes a great deal of skill.

✓ Give heavier emphasis to studies that provide more accurate evidence than those with potentially less accurate evidence (internal and external validity).

✓ Do not rely solely on statistical significance tests and their p-values unless there are more than 60 participants in the study; studies with a larger size have more power to detect a statistically significant effect.

✓ When findings are in contradictory directions, report upon conflict and use reasoning skills; opportunity to develop research questions for on-site study.

Everyday Practice

✓ Incorporate time for literature searching and reading.

✓ Take advantage of opportunities for communicating evidence to clients and for utilizing group meetings as a forum for disseminating research evidence.

✓ Therapists maintain balance of communicating just enough evidence for informed decision making while being prepared to communicate about evidence in a more detailed manner.

LEARNING AND EXPLORATION ACTIVITIES

The purpose of this chapter is to demonstrate the important role that effective communication plays in incorporating evidence into practice. The following exercise builds upon the process developed in the chapter to assist the student interpreting research studies and relating them to the individual.

1. Research and Communication

   a. To complete the following exercises, create a case scenario or think of an actual client in your area of clinical interest. Write down a description of the client. Be sure to specify the diagnosis or presenting reasons for coming to the therapist and other attributes of interest about the client, such as those in Table 12-5.

   b. Create a descriptive, an assessment, and an intervention clinical question for guiding the search for evidence and the development of possible answers to discuss with the client or the client's family members.

   c. Create a table like Table 12-5 and, using the following template, include columns for describing the client and research participants from each of the three types of studies: a descriptive, assessment, and intervention study. Complete a preliminary literature search based upon the three clinical questions and locate three studies that appear relevant from their titles. Retrieve and read the articles. Fill in the table by summarizing the research participants' attributes.

   d. Interpret the results from the study that you judge to be most relevant for generating possible answers to one of the clinical questions. Based upon the results, what is the possible answer to the clinical question? Is the study of a quality that makes you feel confident that the possible answer is justifiable? Explain.

Template for Research and Communication Exercise

CLIENT IDENTITY	HEALTH CONDITION	DEGREE OF DIS-ABILITY	AGE	GENDER	RACE AND ETH-NICITY	SOCIAL NET-WORK	WORK STATUS	SOCIO-ECONOMIC STATUS
Case description								
Study #1 (descriptive)								
Study #2 (assessment)								
Study #3 (interven-tion)								

REFERENCES

Agency for Healthcare Research & Quality. (2011). *Questions are the answer. Better communication. Better care.* Retrieved from http://www.ahrq.gov/questions/

Baum, C. M., & Edwards, D. (2008). *Activity Card Sort* (2nd ed.). Bethesda, MD: AOTA Press.

Bickmore, T., Pfeifer, L., & Jack, B. W. (2009). *Taking the time to care: Empowering low health literacy hospital patients with virtual nurse agents.* Paper presented at the ACM SIGCHI Conference on Human Factors in Computing Systems (CHI) 2009, Boston, MA.

Brouwers, M., Stacey, D., & O'Connor, A. (2010). Knowledge creation: Synthesis, tools and products. *Canadian Medical Association Journal, 182*(2), E68–E72. doi:10.1503/cmaj.081230

Buchman, A. S., Boyle, P. A., Wilson, R. S., Fleischman, D. A., Leurgans, S. E., & Bennett, D. A. (2009). Association between late-life social activity and motor decline in older adults. *Archives of Internal Medicine, 169*(12), 1139–1146. doi:10.1001/archinternmed.2009.135

Buchman, A. S., Boyle, P. A., Wilson, R. S., James, B. D., Leurgans, S. E., Arnold, S. E., & Bennett, D. A. (2010). Loneliness and the rate of motor decline in old age: The Rush memory and aging project, a community-based cohort study. *BMC Geriatrics, 10.* doi:10.1186/1471-2318-10-77.

Canadian Institutes of Health Research. (2011). *More about knowledge translation at CIHR. Knowledge translation—Definition.* Retrieved from http://www.cihr-irsc.gc.ca/e/39033.html

Cohen, J. (1988). *Statistical power analysis for the behavioral sciences* (2nd ed.). Hillsdale, NJ: Lawrence Erlbaum.

Coulter, A., & Ellins, J. (2007). Effectiveness of strategies for informing, educating, and involving patients. *BMJ, 335*(7609), 24–27. doi:10.1136/bmj.39246.581169.80

Den Oudsten, B. L., Van Heck, G. L., & De Vries, J. (2007). The suitability of patient-based measures in the field of Parkinson's disease: A systematic review. *Movement Disorders, 22*(10), 1390–1401.

Duncan, R. P., & Earhart, G. M. (2010). Measuring participation in individuals with Parkinson disease: Relationships with disease severity, quality of life, and mobility. *Disability and Rehabilitation, 1*–7. doi:10.3109/09638288.2010.533245

Golbeck, A., Paschal, A., Jones, A., & Hsiao, T. (2011). Correlating reading comprehension and health numeracy among adults with low literacy. *Patient Education and Counseling, 84,* 132–134.

Goodwin, V. A., Richards, S. H., Taylor, R. S., Taylor, A. H., & Campbell, J. L. (2008). The effectiveness of exercise interventions for people with Parkinson's disease: A systematic review and meta-analysis. *Movement Disorders, 23*(5), 631–640.

Griffin, J., McKenna, K., & Tooth, L. (2006). Discrepancy between older clients' ability to read and comprehend and the reading level of written educational materials used by occupational therapists. *American Journal of Occupational Therapy, 60,* 70–80.

Holt-Lunstad, J., Smith, T. B., & Layton, J. B. (2010). Social relationships and mortality risk: A meta-analytic review. *Public Library of Science Medicine, 7*(7), 1–20.

Houts, P. S., Doak, C. C., Doak, L. G., & Loscalzo, M. J. (2006). The role of pictures in improving health communication: A review of research on attention, comprehension, recall, and adherence. *Patient Education and Counseling, 61,* 173–190.

O'Connor, A. M., Stacey, D., & Jacobsen, M. J. (2011). *Ottawa personal decision guide.* Retrieved from http://decisionaid.ohri.ca/index.html

Peto, V., Jenkinson, C., & Fitzpatrick, R. (1998). PDQ-39: A review of the development, validation and application of a Parkinson's disease quality of life questionnaire and its associated measures. *Journal of Neurology, 245*(Suppl. 1), S10–S14.

Pinquart, M., & Sörensen, S. (2000). Influences of socioeconomic status, social network, and competence on subjective well-being in later life. *Psychology and Aging, 15,* 187–224.

Portney, L. G., & Watkins, M. P. (2009). *Foundations of clinical research: Applications to practice* (3rd ed.). Upper Saddle River, NJ: Prentice Hall Health.

Redman, B. K. (2007). *The practice of patient education: A cases study approach* (10th ed.). St. Louis, MO: Mosby.

Rosenthal, R., & Rosnow, R. (2007). *Essentials of behavioral research: Methods and data analysis* (3rd ed.). New York, NY: McGraw-Hill.

Rosenthal, R., & Rubin, D. B. (1982). A simple general purpose display of magnitude of experimental effect. *Journal of Educational Psychology, 74,* 166–169.

Rudd, R. E. (2011). *Health literacy studies: Overview.* Retrieved from http://www.hsph.harvard.edu/healthliteracy/overview/

Rudd, R. E., Anderson, J. E., Oppenheimer, S., & Nath, C. (2007). Health literacy: An update of medical and public health literature. In J. P. Comings, B. Garner, & C. Smith (Eds.), *Annual review of adult learning and literacy: Connecting research, policy and practice* (Vol. 7, pp. 175–203). Mahwah, NJ: Lawrence Erlbaum.

Straus, S. E., Richardson, W. S., Glasziou, P., & Haynes, R. B. (2005). *Evidence-based medicine: How to practice and teach EBM* (3rd ed.). New York, NY: Churchill Livingstone.

Street, R. L., & Haidet, P. (2011). How well do doctors know their patients? Factors affecting physician understanding of patients' health beliefs. *Journal of General Internal Medicine, 26,* 21–27.

Sudsawad, P. (2007). *Knowledge translation: Introduction to models, strategies, and measures.* Austin, TX: Southwest Educational Development Laboratory. Retrieved from http://www.ncddr.org/kt/products/ktintro/

Tickle-Degnen, L. (2001). From the general to the specific: Using meta-analytic reports in clinical decision-making. *Evaluation & the Health Professions, 24,* 308–326.

Tickle-Degnen, L., Ellis, T., Saint-Hilaire, M., Thomas, C. A., & Wagenaar, R. C. (2010). Self-management rehabilitation and health-related quality of life in Parkinson's disease: A randomized controlled trial. *Movement Disorders, 25*(2), 194–204.

White, D. K., Wagenaar, R. C., Ellis, T. D., & Tickle-Degnen, L. (2009). Changes in walking activity and endurance following rehabilitation for people with Parkinson's disease. *Archives of Physical Medicine & Rehabilitation, 90,* 43–50.

Wilson, J. F. (2003). The crucial link between literacy and health. *Annals of Internal Medicine, 139,* 875–878.

World Health Organization. (2001). *International classification of functioning, disability, and health (ICF).* Geneva, Switzerland: Author.

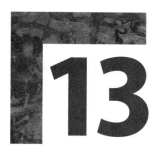

MOVING EVIDENCE INTO PRACTICE
Case Examples of the
Knowledge-to-Action Cycle at Work

*Jocelyn Harris, PhD, OT Reg (Ont); Saurabh Mehta, PT, PhD;
and Joy C. MacDermid, PhD, PT Reg (Ont), FCAHS*

LEARNING OBJECTIVES

After reading this chapter, the student/practitioner will be able to:
- Apply a taxonomy for implementing evidence in practice to rehabilitation evidence-to-practice gaps.
- See exemplars of how evidence can be implemented in rehabilitation practice.

The scientists involved in creating new evidence do not always indulge in disseminating that evidence; or, if they do, their dissemination strategies are not always targeted properly. They may also believe that the knowledge will have spontaneous uptake as soon as it is created. Researchers may not be aware that their work is not having an impact, because they may have no feedback on the downstream impacts of their work. We now know that moving evidence into practice requires concerted effort. In this text we explore knowledge translation, including the knowledge-to-action cycle (Graham & Tetroe, 2007). The knowledge-to-action cycle (see Figure 9-1) consists of an inner circle of knowledge creation that starts with primary research studies. As evidence is synthesized it funnels into evidence-based synthesis such as systematic reviews and meta-analyses (discussed in a separate chapter) and is further synthesized into tools such as the clinical practice guidelines, algorithms, and clinical pathways (discussed in Chapter 11).

In the outer circle of the knowledge-to-action cycle, evidence is customized, barriers to implementation are assessed, implementation occurs, and the outcomes evaluated. The cyclic process should encourage practice-based evidence and experience to feedback into the knowledge creation cycle. The implementation cycle can involve multiple steps and the process by which evidence is contextualized for practice is the focus of these examples. In this chapter we present two cases that highlight this. Two clinician-scientists have been engaged in this cyclic knowledge-to-action process to address areas of practice where we could be doing better. These cases highlight how they used evidence and engaged in knowledge translation to move their findings into practice.

Law M., & MacDermid, J. C.
*Evidence-Based Rehabilitation: A Guide
to Practice, Third Edition* (pp 305–324).
© 2014 SLACK Incorporated.

EXAMPLE #1—USING EVIDENCE TO IMPROVE UPPER LIMB RECOVERY POST-STROKE

What Is the Rehabilitation Problem?

Worldwide, stroke is a leading cause of disability (Lopez, Mathers, Ezzati, Jamison, & Murray, 2006), with approximately 4 million individuals in the United States and Canada living with stroke-related disability (American Heart Association, 2008; Heart and Stroke Foundation of Canada, 2011). Medical advances have significantly lowered the mortality rate but in turn have increased the number of individuals living with stroke-related disability, thus increasing the demand for rehabilitation services.

It is estimated that up to 88% of individuals with stroke experience upper limb paresis during the subacute period of recovery (Duncan, 1994), and of those people it is estimated that 40% will live with residual impairment. The ability to use the upper limb is an important aspect of many daily activities; therefore, residual impairment can negatively impact activities of daily living (ADL), involvement in social and recreational activities, and participation in essential and meaningful life roles (Clarke, Black, Badley, Lawrence, & Williams, 1999; Desrosiers et al., 2003; Nakayama, Jorgensen, Raaschou, & Olson, 1994). In turn, the return of upper limb ability has been identified as an important rehabilitation goal by clients (Barker & Brauer, 2005; Broeks, Lankhorst, Rumping, & Prevo, 1999). Importantly, stroke survivors themselves report that upper limb treatment is often neglected in stroke rehabilitation (Barker & Brauer, 2005).

Despite the importance of upper limb movement for participation in many daily activities, it remains a neglected area of stroke rehabilitation at all stages along the treatment/recovery continuum. In fact, studies have found that upper limb treatment accounted for only 4 to 11 minutes per day of occupational and physical therapy (Bernhardt, Chan, Nicola, & Collier, 2007; Bernhardt, Chitravas, Meslo, Thrif, & Indredavik, 2008). This lack of focus and intensity is also in contrast to both systematic reviews and meta-analysis that indicate that one of the essential components of treatment is intensity (Barreca, Wolf, Fasoli, & Bohannon, 2003; Teasell, Bitensky, Salter, & Bayona, 2005; Urton, Kohia, Davis, & Neill, 2007).

What Do We Know About Upper Limb Recovery Following Stroke?

Upper limb motor deficits (e.g., weakness, poor dexterity, sensory deficits) are some of the most significant predictors of poor performance in activities of daily living in both the subacute and chronic stages of recovery (Desrosiers et al., 2003; Hatakenaka, Miyai, Sakoda, & Yanagihara, 2007; Kwakkel & Kollen, 2007). The most common residual upper limb deficits following stroke are muscle weakness, altered tone, and sensory deficits. It stands to reason that the ability to perform a physical task requires the ability to produce sufficient strength; this ability is compromised in many stroke survivors. Weakness was shown to be the most significant factor for decreased ability to perform ADL (Canning, Ada, Adams, & O'Dwyer, 2004; Harris & Eng, 2007; Mercier & Bourbonnais, 2004). Altered tone can lead to changes in muscle function (e.g., imbalance between agonists and antagonists) and tissue properties (e.g., shortening of tendons), causing difficulty in daily activities. Sensory impairment is common post-stroke, with up to 70% experiencing some form of deficit (Connell, Lincoln, & Radford, 2008; Tyson, Hanley, Chillala, Selley, & Tallis, 2008). These deficits contribute negatively to performance of daily activities, including ability to produce sufficient speed and accuracy (Wagner et al., 2006). Further tasks that require bimanual movement require interaction between the right and left hemisphere and cortical and subcortical structures, thus reflecting the importance of intervention that focuses on coordination, planning, and execution of movement (Hatakenaka et al., 2007; Sainburg & Duff, 2006). However, treatment seldom focuses on the remediation of these elements of movement but rather on compensatory adaptations.

What Do We Know About Upper Limb Treatment Post-Stroke?

One of the most significant interventions formulated for upper limb recovery post-stroke is constraint-induced movement therapy (CIMT; Taub et al., 1993; Wolf, Lecraw, Barton, & Jann, 1989). The key components of this technique are restraint of the unaffected paretic limb and continuous forced use of the paretic limb, in essence increasing the amount of time spent activating the paretic upper in conjunction with several hours of treatment focused on upper limb function. CIMT has proven to be an effective means of promoting the recovery and use of the paretic upper limb post-stroke. The impressive findings from these trials have increased interest in determining the components of upper limb treatment conducive to improved performance and use. There is also an abundance of high-quality evidence that supports the effectiveness of CIMT for improved upper limb performance and use for individuals in the subacute (Boake et al., 2007; Page, Levine, & Leonard, 2005; Wolf et al., 2006) and chronic stages of recovery (Könönen et al., 2011; Rijntjes, Hamzei, Glauche, Saur, & Weiller, 2011; Siebers, Oberg, & Skargren, 2010; Taub et al., 1993).

Systematic reviews of upper limb treatment following stroke concluded that there is sufficient evidence to support repetitive task/exercise-focused techniques (Barreca et al., 2003; Teasell, Foley, et al., 2009; Urton et al., 2007). However, there is still uncertainty regarding whether it is increased time that promotes recovery or type of technique that is the key element; or is it both? For example, Teasell et al. (2009) found that increased time alone regardless of technique used did not produce significant results; however, studies that have looked at both time and technique seem to conclude that it is technique that is the key element (Barecca et al., 2003; Hiraoka, 2001). For example, in a meta-analyses of upper limb treatment, Hiraoka (2001) indicated favorable results for exercise (d = .51) and Harris and Eng (2010) found significant results for strength training on ADL for individuals with moderate impairment (SMD = 0.45, p = .03). Using Sackett's level of evidence, Urton et al. (2007) found level 1 evidence for upper limb exercise and level 2 evidence for electrical stimulation.

In addition, numerous trials have evaluated the effectiveness of electrical stimulation on upper limb recovery, finding positive results for both improved upper limb impairment and performance in ADL (Alon, Levitt, & McCarthy, 2007; Hesse et al., 2005). However, there is conflicting evidence for improved scores on measures of ADL, with studies finding no improved effect (Church et al., 2006; Kowalczewski, Gritsenko, Ashworth, Ellaway, & Prochazka, 2007). Few studies have evaluated bilateral treatment for upper limb recovery; however, contrary to intuition, results have indicated no benefit for performance in ADL (Coupar, Pollock, van Wijck, Morris, & Langhorne, 2010; Desrosiers, Bourbonnais, Corriveau, Gosselin, & Bravo, 2005; Morris et al., 2008). Recently, though, in a randomized controlled trial, Whitall et al. (2011) found improved motor recovery and performance in ADL for the paretic upper limb.

Individuals classified with severe upper limb impairment following stroke have a significantly reduced likelihood of regaining functional use. In addition, interventions have traditionally been designed for generalization and not specific to motor or functional impairment. It appears that those with severe impairment are a distinct population that require specificity for their unique needs. A promising technique for motor recovery in this group of individuals is robotics (Hayward, Barker, & Brauer, 2010; Mehrholz, Platz, Kugler, & Pohl, 2008). However, this technique is not yet feasible for implementation in most rehabilitation settings. However, the specific elements of these interventions can be applied, such as repetitive practice, feedback, and increased time within treatment sessions. A study by Lang et al. (2009) found that in treatment sessions focused on the upper limb, on average 32 repetitions were completed despite severity level; thus, level of intensity is likely not sufficient to promote positive neuroplastic changes in the brain.

Activity Levels of Individuals While on Rehabilitation Units

Patient inactivity during inpatient rehabilitation is a concern. The main goal of a rehabilitation unit is to begin focused and extensive treatment as early as possible, especially when this timing of treatment is linked to positive changes in brain plasticity and outcome (Dobkin, 2004; Nudo, 2003; Teasell et al., 2009). However, studies have shown that individuals spent approximately 10% of the day in contact with therapists (Bernhardt et al., 2007; De Weerdt et al., 2000). This results in individuals being inactive and alone for up to 80% of the day. What remains problematic is that though this trend of inactivity has been shown since 1980 (Keith, 1980), recent studies have found no change in patient activity levels. In inpatient rehabilitation it has been found that upper limb treatment is the focus of intervention for approximately 11 minutes per day. Further, observation of individuals outside of therapy time found that the paretic upper limb was mostly used for bilateral activities (16%) but for 67% of the day it was not used at all (Bernhardt et al., 2007).

In summary, there are several methods used in the rehabilitation of the paretic upper limb post-stroke. A review of the literature seems to favor approaches that are based on principles of motor control and learning as well as neuroplasticity such as CIMT and repetitive practice. Further, it appears that therapy that utilizes repetitive task- and/or goal-oriented methods have significantly greater improvement in motor and functional recovery of the upper limb compared to therapies that use a more passive facilitative approach (e.g., Bobath and Rood). In addition, it appears that approximately 1 hour of upper limb treatment is required to produce significant improvement in impairment, performance, and use of the paretic upper limb. Further, fear that individuals will be overtaxed in rehabilitation if treatment intensity is increased is unfounded. In fact, therapy levels are not even close to reaching proposed therapeutic levels. Many reasons for this disconnect can be related to systemic factors and not usually a reflection of clinician indifference.

What Is Current Practice?

Current guidelines for upper limb rehabilitation post-stroke recommend that interventions focus on repetitive task-/goal-oriented activities that require active movement (Duncan et al., 2005; Teasell et al., 2012). Included in recommendations are statements regarding inclusion of motor learning principles and ecologically valid treatment environments. In addition, many trials evaluating methods to improve upper limb recovery use traditional methods as the control group. This implies that these traditional methods are seen as inferior and not incorporating advancement in theory, techniques, and technology.

For the most part, current practice for upper limb treatment following stroke is based on generalized opinions, expert experience, and anecdotal evidence. However, evidence based on research trials is not always clear and at times can be inconsistent. Survey studies have found that therapists state the importance of evidence-based practice for improved client care yet fail to adopt recommended methods (Gustafsson & Yates, 2009; Walker & Pink, 2009).

Clinicians still use facilitative approaches despite evidence that they are not superior and that active approaches are more meaningful and effective. Bobath techniques are widely accepted as the primary focus of rehabilitation when evidence suggests that treatment focused on motor skills and meaningful activity produced greater functional results. In a large study completed in the United States, the authors found that occupational therapists were not implementing practice guidelines for stroke rehabilitation but rather continued to practice neuromuscular-based approaches (Smallfield & Karges, 2009). Others have found that mean length of treatment sessions fluctuated between 30 and 40 minutes per day (Jette, Warren, & Wirtalla, 2005; Karges & Smallfield, 2009; McNaughton, DeJong, Smout, Melvin, & Brandstater, 2005), with minimal time devoted to the upper limb. Also inherent in current practice is the philosophy that one size fits all, when in fact evidence suggests that interventions need to be and should be tailored to specific impairment levels or patient capacity.

Why Is There an Evidence-to-Practice Gap?

Although there is an apparent gap between evidence and practice, we can account for some of the barriers to implementation. Key components emphasized for improved upper limb performance and use are duration of treatment sessions, overall time spent participating in tasks, and incorporating task-based activities. Some of the most prevalent barriers to implementing these key components is the amount of therapist time allotted per person/session, multitude of treatment focus required by therapists (e.g., walking, ADL, cognition), and lack of time given for treatment planning. In turn, institutional culture can negatively impact evidence-based practice and the time required to implement new guidelines within current clinical decision making. These barriers are evident from acute care through rehabilitation and into the community.

Another area of concern is the heterogeneity of many clinical trials and thus the difficulty in making informed decisions regarding a specific client. In addition, individuality and client-centered practice is not investigated in clinical trials and yet is described as a major proponent of rehabilitation practice. This disconnect is one of the reasons why researchers are designing studies with more homogeneous samples (e.g., groups with the same motor severity level or time since stroke); it is hoped that this will foster more efficient frontline decision making.

Knowledge Translation to Reduce the Evidence-to-Practice Gap

In order to implement evidence into practice and address the gap, interventions must consider the realities of current practice within a systems and clinical perspective. In addition, the inclusion of end-user stakeholders is instrumental in planning such interventions in order to facilitate collaborative partnerships and inform the design of research protocol. The knowledge translation taxonomy will be used to facilitate the design, validation, and uptake of an intervention for improving inpatient upper limb recovery following stroke: GRASP, a Graded Repetitive Arm Supplementary Program.

Increase Awareness of the Problem, Acquisition of New Knowledge, and Provision of Knowledge Synthesis

It was through review of current literature, appraisal of this literature, and clinical experience that we became aware of the poor prognosis of upper limb recovery post-stroke, the limited focus of upper limb treatment within most rehabilitation settings, as well as new evidence that supported a change in practice. Once a comprehensive and systematic review of the literature was completed, synthesis illustrated the key components of intervention required for improved upper limb performance and techniques that were providing promising outcomes. Informal mechanisms were used to explore the awareness of this new information and the most popular techniques used by clinicians. This included presentation at conferences, attendance at journal clubs, and attendance at occupational and physical therapy meetings. In addition, several studies were conducted in order to further define and test the relevance of key components of upper limb intervention (Harris et al., 2007, 2010; Pang, Harris, & Eng, 2006). Information led to the concept of a homework-based exercise program for improving upper limb performance and use following stroke.

When we decided to approach the problem of increasing an individual's time spent doing upper limb exercise while on an inpatient rehabilitation unit, we knew we needed to meet with frontline clinicians and administrators in order to inform us of the current practice culture and potential barriers and/or facilitators. Quickly we found that not all settings were familiar with the newest evidence, suggesting the need for increased time, focus of active and purposeful movement, and the amount of inactivity many patients endure. Subsequently, four in-services were planned and implemented at the major rehabilitation centers across British Columbia, Canada. These in-services were tailored to all clinicians and administrators, not just occupational and physical therapists. At the completion, we were able to collect valuable information for the design of the intervention as well as support for its validation. In turn, we were able to network with appropriate stakeholders and opinion leaders within other health regions in order to expedite the communication of current evidence in this area of stroke rehabilitation. The most informative piece of information was the provision of Web sites where evidence for upper limb treatment post-stroke was synthesized with key points for clinicians, clients and family members (e.g., StrokEngine, Evidence-Based Review of Stroke Rehabilitation). These resources also describe the process used to critically appraise the studies within the synthesis in order for valid recommendations to be made.

SUMMARY OF KEY ISSUES

- Upper limb deficits are prevalent at each stage along the continuum of recovery.
- Upper limb intervention programs need to include a variety of skills and need to be tailored as much as possible to severity of motor impairment.
- Upper limb intervention programs need to increase the number of repetitions during treatment sessions, the number of minutes spent practicing skills daily, and total time spent focused on upper limb activities in rehabilitation settings.
- During inpatient rehabilitation, patients spend most of their time inactive, and when in therapy, levels of intensity are not sufficient to support recovery.
- Often the institutional environment does not support the time for therapists to deliver the required intensity of upper limb programming. In addition, the complexity of stroke rehabilitation requires therapists to focus on multiple skills in order to facilitate recovery and discharge home in a timely manner.

Making a Decision and Adapting Evidence to an Inpatient Treatment Setting

The next step was to integrate the information and evidence collected into a consolidated format. Because this was to be a homework-based program we knew that the format had to be user-friendly not only for therapists but for patients and their family members. Taking the information from clinician experience, well-designed randomized controlled trials, systematic reviews, and meta-analysis we devised an exercise program to promote upper limb recovery. The program consisted of strengthening, range of motion, fine and gross motor skills, and activities based on daily activities. In addition, speed and accuracy were encouraged during target board tasks. From the literature reviews, it appeared that interventions should be tailored to motor severity level; therefore, three programs were designed, for severe, moderate, and mild impairment. Activities in each level were graded within the level by difficulty, number of repetitions and/or repetitions, and incorporation of speed and/or accuracy.

The program was designed to be implemented by a therapist but carried out by the patient and, when possible, with family, outside of regular therapy time. It was unclear whether this type of program would be feasible on an inpatient unit; therefore, a pilot study was completed. Feedback from participants, family members, and clinical staff was collected and changes were made accordingly. To validate the effectiveness of this program, a multisite randomized controlled trial, called GRASP, was completed with positive results (Harris, Eng, Miller, & Dawson, 2009, 2010).

Tools to Facilitate Implementation and Continued Use of GRASP

During and after the study, meetings were held with key stakeholders (e.g., therapists, administrators, and participants who completed the program) to determine continued feasibility and barriers and facilitators to the program and to form a core group of leaders who would champion the program upon completion of the research project. Included in this process was a satisfaction survey completed by the 103 participants involved in the GRASP study; results are summarized in Harris et al. (2009). In turn, we presented the design and results of this study at several conferences throughout British Columbia and Ontario, Canada, through invitation of the Canadian Stroke Network. We received numerous comments, suggestions, and questions that stimulated positive revisions to the program. All feedback was incorporated into the teaching materials (written and Web casts) used to inform clinicians, survivors, and family members on how to use GRASP (http:// neurorehab.med.ubc.ca/grasp/). To further support the use of GRASP, this program was added as part of the 2010 Canada Stroke Guidelines for Upper Limb Treatment (http://www.strokebest-practices.ca). We continue to receive feedback from international users, which has helped us explore ecological validity for other cultures.

Once the feasibility and effectiveness was demonstrated, it was important for GRASP to be easily accessible not only to therapists and other rehabilitation clinicians but also survivors of stroke and their family/caregivers. Presently, the exercise programs are available on the previously mentioned Web site as well as in training manuals and Web videos. In addition, several rehabilitation units across Canada are using the manuals and making them and the exercise equipment available to individuals when they are discharged. Because GRASP was developed for an inpatient setting, several clinicians who work in outpatient centers, community, and long-term care facilities have inquired regarding its efficacy within these environments. Importantly, clinicians have offered valuable information/suggestions on unique issues concerning feasibility within these settings.

Outcome Evaluation and Monitoring

In Canada, the Heart and Stroke Foundation has formulated best practice guidelines (Web site listed previously). In addition, each province has a stroke network that supports these guidelines. It is the responsibility of regional rehabilitation coordinators/educators to teach and support implementation of best practice guidelines. GRASP has been recommended with the best practice guidelines for upper limb rehabilitation. We have been asked by several coordinators to do in-services and to provide ideas on how best to implement the program. To monitor the implementation and continued use of the program, we are in contact with local champions to assist in any way necessary. This has been an invaluable means of monitoring uptake and need for revisions. Because this is a new program, we are in the process of designing more formal means of evaluation through Web site tracking, surveys, and focus groups. Further, there is a large multisite randomized controlled trial within Canada that has evaluated the uptake of the Heart Stroke Foundation of Canada, Best Practice Guidelines, of which GRASP is a part. We will be able to determine how many rehabilitation units have implemented the program. This will also allow us to target units using the program for feedback as well as determine why it is not being used in other units.

REFERENCES

Alon, G., Levitt, A. F., & McCarthy, P. A. (2007). Functional electrical stimulation enhancement of upper extremity functional recovery during stroke rehabilitation: A pilot study. *Neurorehabilitation and Neural Repair, 2,* 207–215.

American Heart Association. (2008). Heart disease and stroke statistics—2008 update. Dallas, TX: Author.

Barker, R. N., & Brauer, S. G. (2005). Upper limb recovery after stroke: The stroke survivors' perspective. *Disability and Rehabilitation, 27,* 1213–1223.

Barreca, S., Wolf, S. L., Fasoli, S., & Bohannon, R. (2003). Treatment interventions for the paretic upper limb of stroke survivors: A critical review. *Neurorehabilitation and Neural Repair, 17,* 220–226.

Bernhardt, J., Chan. J., Nicola, I., & Collier, J. (2007). Little therapy, little physical activity: Rehabilitation within the first 14 days of organized stroke unit care. *Journal of Rehabilitation Medicine, 39,* 43–48.

Bernhardt, J., Chitravas, N., Meslo, I., Thrift, A., & Indredavik, B. (2008). Not all stroke units are the same: A comparison of physical activity patterns in Melbourne, Australia, and Trondheim, Norway. *Stroke, 39,* 2059–2065.

Boake, C., Noser, E. A., Ro, T., Baraniuk, S., Gaber, M., Johnson, R., et al. (2007). Constraint-induced movement therapy during early stroke rehabilitation. *Neurorehabilitation and Neural Repair, 21,* 124–124.

Broeks, J. G., Lankhorst, G. J., Rumping, K., & Prevo, A. J. (1999). The long-term outcome of arm function after stroke: Results of a follow-up study. *Disability & Rehabilitation, 21,* 357–364.

Canning, C. G., Ada, L., Adams, R., & O'Dwyer, N. J. (2004). Loss of strength contributes more to physical disability after stroke than loss of dexterity. *Clinical Rehabilitation, 18,* 300–308.

Church, C., Price, C., Pandyan, A. D., Huntley, S., Curless, R., & Rodgers, H. (2006). Randomized controlled trial to evaluate the effect of surface neuromuscular electrical stimulation to the shoulder after acute stroke. *Stroke, 37,* 2995–3001.

Clarke, P. J., Black, S. E., Badley, E. M., Lawrence, J. M., & Williams, J. I. (1999). Handicap in stroke survivors. *Disability & Rehabilitation, 21,* 116–123.

Connell, L. A., Lincoln, N. B., & Radford, K. A. (2008). Somatosensory impairment after stroke: Frequency of different deficits and their recovery. *Clinical Rehabilitation, 22,* 758–767.

Coupar, F., Pollock, A., van Wijck, F., Morris, J., & Langhorne, P. (2010). Simultaneous bilateral training for improving arm function after stroke. *Cochrane Database of Systematic Reviews, 4,* CD006432.

De Weerdt, W., Selz, B., Nuyens, G., Staes, F., Swinnen, D., van de Winckel, A., et al. (2000). Time use of stroke patients in an intensive rehabilitation unit: A comparison between a Belgian and a Swiss setting. *Disability & Rehabilitation, 10,* 181.

Desrosiers, J., Bourbonnais, D., Corriveau, H., Gosselin, S., & Bravo, G. (2005). Effectiveness of unilateral and symmetrical bilateral task training for arm during the subacute phase after stroke: A randomized controlled trial. *Clinical Rehabilitation, 19,* 581–593.

Desrosiers, J., Malouin, F., Bourbonnais, D., Richards, C. L., Rochette, A., & Bravo, G. (2003). Arm and leg impairments and disabilities after stroke rehabilitation: Relation to handicap. *Clinical Rehabilitation, 17,* 666–673.

Dobkin, B. H. (2004). Neurobiology of rehabilitation. *Annals of the New York Academy of Sciences, 1038,* 148–170.

Duncan, P. W. (1994). Stroke disability. *Physical Therapy, 74,* 399–407.

Duncan, P. W., Zorowitz, R., Bates, B., Choi, J. Y., Glasberg, J. J., Graham, G. D., et al. (2005). Management of adult stroke rehabilitation care: A clinical practice guideline. *Stroke, 36,* e100–e143.

Graham, I. D., & Tetroe, J. (2007). Some theoretical underpinnings of knowledge translation. *Academic Emergency Medicine, 14,* 936–941.

Gustafsson, L., & Yates, K. (2009). Are we applying interventions with research evidence when targeting secondary complications of the stroke-affected upper limb. *Australian Occupational Therapy Journal, 56,* 428–435.

Harris, J. E., & Eng, J. J. (2007). Paretic upper limb strength best explains arm activity in people with stroke. *Physical Therapy, 87,* 88–97.

Harris, J. E., & Eng, J. J. (2010). Strength training improves upper-limb function in individuals with stroke: A meta-analysis. *Stroke, 41,* 136–140.

Harris, J. E., Eng, J. J., Miller, W. C., & Dawson, A. S. (2009). A self-administered graded repetitive arm supplementary program (GRASP) improves arm function during inpatient stroke rehabilitation: A multisite randomized controlled trial. *Stroke, 40,* 2123–2128.

Harris, J. E., Eng, J. J., Miller, W. C., & Dawson, A. S. (2010). The role of care-giver involvement in upper limb treatment in individuals with sub-acute stroke. *Physical Therapy, 90,* 1302–1310.

Hatakenaka, M., Miyai, I., Sakoda, S., & Yanagihara, T. (2007). Proximal paresis of the upper extremity in patients with stroke. *Neurology, 69,* 348–355.

Hayward, K., Barker, R., & Brauer, S. (2010). Interventions to promote upper limb recovery in stroke survivors with severe paresis: A systematic review. *Disability & Rehabilitation, 32*, 1973–1986.

Heart and Stroke Foundation of Canada (2011). 2011 Heart and Stroke Foundation Report on Canadians' Health. Ottawa, Canada.

Hesse, S., Werner, C., Pohl, M., Rueckriem, S., Mehrholz, J., & Lingnau, M. L. (2005). Computerized arm training improves the motor control of the severely affected arm after stroke: A single-blinded randomized trial in two centers. *Stroke, 36*, 1960–1966.

Hiraoka, K. (2001). Rehabilitation effort to improve upper extremity function in post-stroke patients: A meta-analysis. *Journal of Physical Therapy Science, 13*, 5–9.

Jette, D. U., Warren, R. L., & Wirtalla, C. (2005). The relation between therapy intensity and outcomes of rehabilitation in skilled nursing facilities. *Archives of Physical Medicine and Rehabilitation, 86*, 273–279.

Karges, J., & Smallfied, S. (2009). A description of the outcomes, frequency, duration, and intensity of occupational, physical, and speech therapy in inpatient stroke rehabilitation. *Journal of Allied Health, 38*, E1–E10.

Keith, R. A. (1980). Activity patterns of a stroke rehabilitation unit. *Social Science & Medicine - Part A: Medical Psychology & Medical Sociology, 14*, 575–580.

Könönen, M., Tarkka, I. M., Niskanen, E., Pihlajamäki, M., Mervaala, E., Pitkänen, K., et al. (2011). Functional MRI and motor behavioral changes obtained with constraint-induced movement therapy in chronic stroke. *European Journal of Neurology*.

Kowalczewski, J., Gritsenko, V., Ashworth, N., Ellaway, P., & Prochazka, A. (2007). Upper-extremity functional electric stimulation-assisted exercises on a workstation in the subacute phase of stroke recovery. *Archives of Physical Medicine and Rehabilitation, 88*, 833–839.

Kwakkel, G., & Kollen, B. (2007). Predicting improvement in the upper paretic limb after stroke: A longitudinal prospective study. *Restorative Neurology and Neuroscience, 25*, 453–460.

Lang, C. E., Macdonald, J. R., Reisman, D. S., Boyd, L., Jacobson, K. T., Schindler-Ivens, S. M., et al. (2009). Observation of amounts of movement practice provided during stroke rehabilitation. *Archives of Physical Medicine and Rehabilitation, 90*, 1692–1698.

Lopez, A. D., Mathers, C. D., Ezzati, M., Jamison, D. T., & Murray, C. J. (2006). Global and regional burden of disease and risk factors, 2001: Systematic analysis of population health data. *Lancet, 27*, 1747–1757.

McNaughton, H., DeJong, G., Smout, R. J., Melvin, J. L., & Brandstater, M. (2005). A comparison of stroke rehabilitation practice and outcomes between New Zealand and United States facilities. *Archives of Physical Medicine and Rehabilitation, 86*(Suppl. 2), S115–S120.

Mehrholz, J., Platz, T., Kugler, J., & Pohl, M. (2008). Electromechanical and robot-assisted arm training for improving arm function and activities of daily living after stroke. *Cochrane Database of Systematic Reviews, 8*, CD006876.

Mercier, C., & Bourbonnais, D. (2004). Relative shoulder flexor and handgrip and handgrip strength is related to upper limb function after stroke. *Clinical Rehabilitation, 18*, 215–221.

Morris, J. H., van Wijck, F., Joice, S., Ogston, S. A., Cole, I., & MacWalter, R. S. (2008). A comparison of bilateral and unilateral upper limb task training in early post stroke rehabilitation: A randomized controlled trial. *Archives of Physical Medicine and Rehabilitation, 89*, 1237–1245.

Nakayama, H., Jorgensen, H. S., Raaschou, H. O., & Olson, T. S. (1994). Recovery of upper limb function in stroke patients: The Copenhagen stroke study. *Archives of Physical Medicine and Rehabilitation, 75*, 394–398.

Nudo, R. J. (2003). Adaptive plasticity in motor cortex: Implications for rehabilitation after brain injury. *Journal of Rehabilitation Medicine, 41*(Suppl.), 7–10.

Page, S. J., Levine, P., & Leonard, A. C. (2005). Modified constraint-induced therapy in acute stroke: A randomized controlled pilot study. *Neurorehabilitation and Neural Repair, 19*, 27–32.

Pang, M. Y., Harris, J. E., & Eng, J. J. (2006). Community-based upper-extremity group exercise program improves motor function and performance of functional activities in chronic stroke: A randomized controlled trial. *Archives of Physical Medicine and Rehabilitation, 87*, 1–9.

Rijntjes, M., Hamzei, F., Glauche, V., Saur, D., & Weiller, C. (2011). Activation changes in sensorimotor cortex during improvement due to CIMT in chronic stroke. *Restorative Neurology and Neuroscience, 29*, 299–310.

Sainburg, R. L., & Duff, S. V. (2006). Does motor lateralization have implications for stroke rehabilitation? *Journal of Rehabilitation Research and Development, 43*, 311–322.

Siebers, A., Oberg, U., & Skargren, E. (2010). The effect of modified constraint-induced movement therapy on spasticity and motor function of the affected arm in patients with chronic stroke. *Physiotherapie Canada, 62*, 388–396.

Smallfield, S., & Karges, J. (2009). Classification of occupational therapy intervention for inpatient stroke rehabilitation. *American Journal of Occupational Therapy, 63*, 408–413.

Taub, E., Miller, N. E., Novack, T. A., Cook, E. W., Fleming, W. C., Nepomuceno, C. S., et al. (1993). Technique to improve chronic motor deficit after stroke. *Archives of Physical Medicine and Rehabilitation, 74*, 347–354.

Teasell, R., Bitensky, J., Salter, K., & Bayona, N. A. (2005). The role of timing and intensity of rehabilitation therapies. *Topics in Stroke Rehabilitation, 12*, 46–57.

Teasell, R., Foley, N., Salter, K., Bhogal, M., Jutai, J., & Speechley. (2012) Evidence-based review of stroke rehabilitation: executive summary (15th edition). Retrieved from http://www.ebrsr.com

Teasell, R., Meyer, M. J., McClure, A., Pan, C., Murie-Fernandez, M., Foley, N., et al. (2009). Stroke rehabilitation: An international perspective. *Topics in Stroke Rehabilitation, 16*, 44–56.

Tyson, S. F., Hanley, M., Chillala, J., Selley, A. B., & Tallis, R. C. (2008). Sensory loss in hospital-admitted people with stroke: Characteristics, associated factors, and relationship with function. *Neurorehabilitation and Neural Repair, 22*, 166–172.

Urton, M. L., Kohia, M., Davis, J., & Neill, M. R. (2007). Systematic literature review of treatment interventions for upper extremity hemiparesis following stroke. *Occupational Therapy International, 14*, 11–27.

Walker, J., & Pink, M. J. (2009). Occupational therapists and the use of constraint-induced movement therapy in neurological practice. *American Journal of Occupational Therapy, 63*, 408–413.

Wagner, J. M., Lang, C. E., Sahrmann, S. A., Hu, Q., Bastian, A. J., Edwards, D. F., et al. (2006). Relationships between sensorimotor impairments and reaching deficits in acute hemiparesis. *Neurorehabilitation and Neural Repair, 20*, 406–416.

Whitall, J., Waller, S. M., Sorkin, J. D., Forrester, L. W., Macko, R. F., Hanley, D. F., et al. (2011). Bilateral and unilateral arm training improve motor function through differing neuroplastic mechanisms: A single-blinded randomized controlled trial. *Neurorehabilitation and Neural Repair, 25*, 118–129.

Wolf, S. L., Lecraw, D. E., Barton, L. A., & Jann, B. B. (1989). Forced use of hemiplegic upper extremities to reverse the effect of learned nonuse among chronic stroke and head-injured patients. *Experimental Neurology, 104*, 125–132.

Wolf, S. L., Winstein, C. J., Miller, J. P., Taub, E., Uswatte, G., Morris, D., et al. (2006). Effect of constraint-induced movement therapy on upper extremity function 3–9 months after stroke. *JAMA, 296*, 2095–2104.

SUGGESTED READINGS

Ada, L., Dorsch, S., & Canning, C. G. (2006). Strengthening interventions increase strength and improve activity after stroke: A systematic review. *Australian Journal of Physiotherapy, 52*, 241–248.

Eng, J. J. (2004). Strength training in individuals with stroke. *Physiotherapie Canada, 56*, 189–201.

EXAMPLE #2—IMPLEMENTING SCREENING PATIENTS FOR RISK OF ADVERSE OUTCOMES FOLLOWING DISTAL RADIUS FRACTURE

Define the Problem in Rehabilitation

Fall-related injuries have significant personal and economic burden (Roudsari, Ebel, Corso, Molinari, & Koepsell, 2005; Stevens, Corso, Finkelstein, & Miller, 2006; Watson, Clapperton, & Mitchell, 2011). Individuals with fall-related lower extremity injuries including hip fractures receive greater screening for future falls and fractures. Most individuals who sustain hip fractures are admitted to hospital, undergo surgical interventions, and receive extensive rehabilitation for optimizing strength, balance, and mobility. Rehabilitative and preventative programs have been designed specifically to prevent future falls and resultant hip fractures in older adults (Becker et al., 2011; Berggren, Stenvall, Olofsson, & Gustafson, 2008). In this case, the evidence is clear and practice guidelines readily acknowledge the important role of fracture prevention.

There is evidence to suggest, however, that there is knowledge-to-practice gap when it comes to fracture prevention for individuals with upper extremity injuries. The context is different than individuals with lower extremity fall injuries in that the upper extremity fall injuries are mostly managed in outpatient trauma clinics or require a brief hospitalization (Mitchell, Curtis, Watson, & Nau, 2010). Practice guidelines for surgical or rehabilitative management of distal radius fractures (DRFs), the most common upper extremity fall injury, do not recommend preventative screening or treatment for fall prevention. Rather, rehabilitation following a DRF tends to focus on pain and functional status (American Academy of Orthopaedic Surgeons, 2009) and restoring upper extremity strength, motion, and function (Michlovitz, LaStayo, Alzner, & Watson, 2001). Most individuals are not screened or receive treatment for preventing future falls and fall-related injuries following a DRF. Because a fall was the primary reason for their injuries, some of these individuals may have problems with balance impairments that create risk for future falls.

The potential to improve practice is considerable given that the DRFs are the most common upper extremity fall injuries (Mitchell et al., 2010). The incidence of DRF is estimated to be between 200 and 400/100,000 persons per year, which is the highest among fractures (Court-Brown & Caesar, 2006; Hodsman, Leslie, Tsang, & Gamble, 2008; van Staa, Dennison, Leufkens, & Cooper, 2001). Previous studies have indicated that a subset of individuals with DRF have a risk for falls and future fractures. These studies suggest that all patients over 40 to 50 years of age with DRF should be screened for these risks (Endres et al., 2006; Nordell, Kristinsdottir, Jarnlo, Magnusson, & Thorngren, 2005). Though not all falls result in DRFs, those with osteoporosis can have significantly higher risk of sustaining a DRF.

Despite being the focus of interventions, chronic pain and functional impairments are reported in as many as 11% of individuals even 1 year following a DRF (MacDermid, Roth, & Richards, 2003; Moore & Leonardi-Bee, 2008). This is a significant number given the high incidence rates for DRFs. A number of patient-reported measures of pain and functional have been validated for use in patients with DRFs (Hudak, Amadio, & Bombardier, 1996; Kotsis, Lau, & Chung, 2007; MacDermid, Turgeon, Richards, Beadle, & Roth, 1998). However, these measures have mostly been used to assess the patients and monitor changes in their status and not for predicting risk of adverse outcomes.

Patients with DRFs presenting to rehabilitation settings can be at risk for falls and fall-related injuries, chronic pain, and disability. An evidence-based screening procedure can be developed to identify the risk level of patients during their initial assessment. This screening procedure should be evidence based, practical in a fracture rehabilitation setting, and provide a useful mechanism to classify patients based on their extent of risk.

What Is Current Practice for Assessment of Patients With Distal Radius Fracture?

Outcomes following DRF can be broadly classified into objective clinical tests or patient-reported outcomes. Most systematic reviews of interventional studies in patients with DRFs have reported these outcomes specific to the wrist/hand area (Diaz-Garcia, Oda, Shauver, & Chung, 2011; Hoang-Kim, Scott, Micera, Orsini, & Moroni, 2009). The impairments typically measured include wrist joint range of motion (ROM) and muscle strength, and functional tests for performance and radiographs are some of the common objective measures used to gauge patients' status and recovery following DRFs. In general, rehabilitation professionals can assess these impairments using standardized procedures. Goniometry is reliable and accurate for assessing wrist ROM (Armstrong, MacDermid, Chinchalkar, Stevens, & King, 1998; Carter et al., 2009). Handheld dynamometers are reliable for assessing isometric grip strength (MacDermid, Alyafi, & Richards, 2001). Grip strength is considered an important predictor of functional recovery and patient satisfaction after DRFs (Fujii et al., 2002; MacDermid, Richards, Donner, Bellamy, & Roth, 2000) and it is extremely easy to record and follow in small rehabilitation settings. Standardized procedures for reliable assessment of grip strength have been described (Fess, 1992). These impairments focus on the injured joint, not at the person-level disability. There are multiple dexterity or hand function tests that have been used with upper extremity disorders. Measures of impairment and hand dexterity may be important indicators for the aspect of rehabilitation that focuses on restoring hand function. However, they also are unlikely to provide direction on impairments that might be contributing to future fall risk.

Obtaining patient-reported functional status following DRFs is currently recommended. Though many patient-reported outcomes have been validated for use in patients with DRFs, the Patient-Rated Wrist Evaluation (PRWE; MacDermid et al., 1998) and the Disabilities of Arm, Shoulder, and Hand (DASH; Hudak et al., 1996) have been most extensively examined and recommended for assessing functional status and disability. Recently, an international consensus group recommended that pain (assessed by either a numeric pain rating or the pain subscale of PRWE) and function (assessed either by the QuickDASH or function subscale of the PRWE) should be the minimal core measures for DRFs. These measures focus on upper extremity functions. Other outcome measures assess overall health status, such as the Short-Form 36 (Hemelaers, Angst, Drerup, Simmen, & Wood-Dauphinee, 2008; Imaeda et al., 2010); those assessing behavioral factors such as the Tampa Scale of Kinesiophobia or Catastrophizing subscale of the Coping Strategies Questionnaire have also been validated specifically in DRF patient groups. Despite this work, there has been little focus on how measures might focus on using tools as screening measures to take an active role in bone and overall health risks after a DRF.

Screening Procedures—The Evidence-to-Practice Gap?

Rehabilitation professionals are the most frequent contact for patients with DRFs and are better positioned to screen these patients for adverse outcomes. Most rehabilitation professionals treating DRFs work in a busy practice environment and require concise and easy-to-administer measurement tools for making evidence-based clinical decisions. Such tools have better uptake in clinical practice compared to those with significant administration burden. Therefore, when assessing barriers to practice we identified that a screening tool that could assist in identifying patients requiring fall prevention interventions would need to fit within this practice paradigm. This means that the outcome measures in the screening tool need to be quickly performed and easily applied without specialized equipment. At best, the screening tool should consist of one outcome measure for each of the risk factors (risk for falls, impaired balance, and risk for sustaining fall-related fractures, chronic pain, and disability). There are a number of outcome measures published in the literature for assessing these risks in conditions other than DRFs. A few studies have specifically examined some of the individual tests for a DRF population but none have looked at a menu of screening tests as means of early prevention of adverse outcomes following DRFs. Therefore, the use of existing evidence in this way should be considered indirect, because it is adapting evidence and determining its relevance and applicability for screening the DRF population. Because the impact is indeterminate we would need to insure that we evaluate its effects.

The measures used in assessing risk for falls and related injuries to lower extremities are widely available and have been routinely used across other fall-related injuries, such as hip fractures. For example, the Timed Up-and-Go Test (TUGT; Kristensen, Henriksen, Stie, & Bandholm, 2011), Single Leg Stand Test (Sherrington & Lord, 2005), and Functional Reach Test (Sherrington & Lord, 2005) are common tests for assessing impaired balance and fall risk, all have been tested for their utility in patients with hip fracture. Though the evidence for these tests is primarily for lower extremity injury patients, there are sufficient data on the reliability of the test to suggest that they might be used as indicators in evidence-based screening protocol for DRFs.

CONCEPTUALIZING THE KNOWLEDGE TRANSLATION FRAMEWORK

In the next phase of the knowledge-to-action cycle (see Figure 9-1), potential barriers to implementing evidence-based screening procedures for the DRF population need to be recognized. Few would disagree that using validated patient-based, standardized measurement is key to patient-centered, evidence-based practice. However, the barriers to implementing the use of standardized outcome measures in rehabilitation settings are known to be encountered due to multiple individual or organizational factors (Stevens & Beurskens, 2010; Swinkels, van Peppen, Wittink, Custers, & Beurskens, 2011). More often than not there is a dynamic interplay between these factors rather than a single factor contributing to the lack of adherence to using measures in clinical practice (Kay, Myers, & Huijbregts, 2001; Stokes & O'Neill, 2008; Turner, Whitfield, Brewster, Halligan, & Kennedy, 1996). In context of the DRF population, the barrier to screening the patients for type and level of risk for potential adverse outcomes emanate from the fact that screening for future fractures is not a standardized practice where the objective is to focus on rehabilitation of the acute injury. Furthermore, because DRFs typically precede life-threatening fractures by a decade (Nordell et al., 2005), the risk may not appear imminent.

Developing an entire screening protocol for each of the risk factors following DRFs "from scratch" would be both rigorous and time consuming. For this reason, we focused on making best evidence decisions using high-quality but indirect evidence. We conducted a systematic review to identify potential screening measures to assess risk for future falls, fall-related fractures, chronic pain, and disability in the DRF population. Our focus was to locate the evidence by reviewing the literature on lower extremity fall injuries and adapt the evidence for the context of the DRF population. A literature search was conducted to locate the studies where risk for future falls, fall-related fractures, and balance were examined in lower extremity fall injuries. Furthermore, we searched the literature to locate the screening measures for chronic pain and disability in DRFs by examining the common measures used for this purpose. A systematic review of high quality level was used to determine the best possible evidence for the interventional studies for fall prevention in lower extremity fall injuries or preventing pain and disability in DRFs. Following the literature search, a list of potentially appropriate screening measures was developed based on their use across the studies deemed to be the best evidence.

A few considerations informed the selection of the relevant screening measures for inclusion in the test version of the screening protocol. First, the measures were reviewed for feasibility for the patient population and for the clinical context of an outpatient rehabilitation setting. Further, the psychometric studies that established the screening rules for the selected measures as well as those that assessed the psychometric properties for these measures either in the DRF population or other fall injuries were given preference. To summarize, the frequency of use across high-quality studies, relevance to the DRF population, and feasibility of use in outpatient rehabilitation settings were the key considerations for selecting the screening measures for the test version of the screening protocol. The tentative list of outcome measures identified was as follows: TUGT for balance and fall risk (Sherrington & Lord, 2005), shortened version of the Falls Efficacy Scale for assessing perceived fall risk (Kempen et al., 2008), the Pain subscale of the PRWE for assessing risk for chronic pain (MacDermid et al., 1998), and QuickDASH for assessing the risk of disability (Gummesson, Ward, & Atroshi, 2006). We hoped to identify known subgroups (e.g., those with two or more falls in the last 6 months or no falls) when we examined the ability of these screening tests to assess the risk of adverse outcomes in the DRF population.

IDENTIFYING FURTHER STEPS

Generating New Knowledge

In the knowledge-to-action cycle, practice-based evidence leads to the next generation of the research cycle. Though we might start with identifying a tentative screening program based on adaptation of existing evidence, it will be important to test that process in a formal research study. The optimal approach would be to conduct a randomized clinical trial where some patients were randomized to receive the screening and others were not. The new knowledge would validate an evidence-based screening tool for the DRF population. The end product of these research studies will be to have a clinically applicable evidence-based screening tool that will include one test for identifying the risk for future falls, fall-related injuries, chronic pain, and disability. The tool may further be adapted to a computerized algorithm for making clinical decision rules to identify the type of risk and degree of risk (minimal, moderate, or severe).

It is acknowledged that generating new knowledge is an additive process and does not stop with one or two studies. Researchers should continue to examine better measures to assess risk of adverse outcomes following DRFs. On the same note, it is important to translate the best available knowledge to the knowledge users when there is sufficient evidence to suggest benefit.

Implementing the Screening Tool

We know that the use of standardized clinical measures in rehabilitation practice is limited (Kay et al., 2001; Stokes & O'Neill, 2008). Therefore, the knowledge translation strategy should be multipronged to ensure that it not only exposes the screening tool to as many stakeholders (rehabilitation professionals) as possible but also to ensure actions to facilitate behavior. The strategies for implementing the screening tool might be considered along with the continuum presented in Appendix H and Table 13-1, which highlights the strategies for both examples. To summarize the information in the taxonomy table, a tentative plan is outlined. Because knowledge translation is iterative, at each stage clinicians would be engaged in establishing useful next steps. Dissemination of practice surveys and information about the risk of future fracture can increase awareness of the problem. Making the screening tool available online with detailed instructions can support operationalization using best practice techniques. Rehabilitation professional associations may be supportive of sharing the tool with their membership and assist with dissemination. Rehabilitation associations may make the tool and user's guide for the tool freely available to their members on their Web sites. Furthermore, the evidence-based practice guidelines offered by these organizations can be modified to include the use of a screening tool by rehabilitation professionals in the DRF population.

Table 13-1

Using the Knowledge Translation Taxonomy to Move Evidence Into Action

LEVEL OF ACTION	TARGET AUDIENCE	
To support moving evidence into practice (action)	(Direct Knowledge User) = Clinician	
	Example 1—Facilitate Upper Extremity Motor Recovery	*Example 2—Implement DRF Screening*
Increase awareness of a problem or evidence-to-practice gap	• Systematic review of literature • Meetings with clinicians to define current practice • Presentation at conferences to highlight the disconnect between research and practice • In-services to clinicians about current research, including highlight of Web-based resources for best practice	• Publish a practice survey of rehabilitation professionals to demonstrate low use of fall prevention post-DRF, conference workshops and editorials in professional journals to highlight the problem. Involve opinion leaders
Acquire evidence-based knowledge	• Systematic review and meta-analysis to identify effective treatment methods • Design and complete a randomized controlled trial to determine effectiveness of GRASP	• Two phase research—Phase 1: Conduct a systematic literature synthesis to identify the suitable screening measures to assess falls, fall-related injuries, chronic pain, and disability in the DRF population and prepare a beta version of the screening tool with one screening test for each risk factor. • Phase 2: A clinical trial to determine whether patients who receive screening have better short- and long-term outcomes
Synthesize/evaluate knowledge	• Synthesis and appraisal of information from literature, meetings with clinicians	• Appraise results from both phases of research and prepare summary of recommendations
Make an evidence-informed decision	• Take information gained and design the intervention • Pilot GRASP and incorporate changes as necessary	• Create an algorithm for which tests should be performed for patients after DRF based on age, fracture history, and comorbid health status

(continued)

Table 13-1 (continued)

Using the Knowledge Translation Taxonomy to Move Evidence Into Action

LEVEL OF ACTION	TARGET AUDIENCE	
To support moving evidence into practice (action)	(Direct Knowledge User) = Clinician	
	Example 1—Facilitate Upper Extremity Motor Recovery	*Example 2—Implement DRF Screening*
Adaptation of evidence to context	• Meet with clinicians to obtain information about current treatment for upper limb post-stroke; determine clinician knowledge of research studies and barriers to implementation of best practice • Consideration of audience using the GRASP program. Consider current practice environment from meetings, incorporate into program design • Designed program so it can be used by a variety of users (e.g., therapists, stroke survivors, families) • Post-study meetings with study personnel to determine changes required for implementation	• Test recommendations and algorithm in clinical setting; monitor barriers and facilitators to implementation • Qualitative interviews seeking feedback of opinion leaders to obtain the barriers to behavioral change when using the screening procedures
Implement specific actions	• Meetings with key end-users of program to facilitate implementation and continued usage • Find GRASP champions to lead implementation after the study • Results from satisfaction survey completed by study participants • Designed Web page with instruction manual and exercise programs for GRASP • Developed video to outline GRASP, barriers and facilitators and tools to overcome issues	• Create a training manual for the screening testing that contains tests and training on how to perform, score, and interpret • Provide prediction rules; that is, discriminative values to determine the presence/absence of risk and the magnitude of risk • Provide the screening tool, its user's manual, and decision rules as free access online for optimal uptake by the end-users

(continued)

Table 13-1 (continued)

Using the Knowledge Translation Taxonomy to Move Evidence Into Action

LEVEL OF ACTION To support moving evidence into practice (action)	TARGET AUDIENCE (Direct Knowledge User) = Clinician	
	Example 1—Facilitate Upper Extremity Motor Recovery	*Example 2—Implement DRF Screening*
Facilitate the process of change	• See previous entry for processes in place to help change practice • Continue to be invited to present across Canada on GRASP, attendees fill out feedback forms and this information is incorporated into Web-based information on GRASP	• Share the information regarding the usefulness and availability of the screening tool via professional associations and licensing bodies; collaborate with professional organizations to advocate inclusion of the screening tool in clinical practice guidelines • Add link to change support tools in e-notifications
Process or outcome evaluation/monitoring	• Incorporation of formal and informal feedback for identification of barriers and facilitators for GRASP • Continuous contact with champions to monitor uptake and help with continued use • In process of designing surveys to track uptake and collect feedback • Best practice guidelines have included GRASP, large trial in Canada to monitor best practice uptake, will track usage of program	• Provide tracking tools that can be used by therapists to audit their own practice for process (whether screening was performed) and outcomes; that is, case identification; actions taken • Report implementation results back to team for fine-tuning of implementation

Note: This table illustrates strategies that might be undertaken to facilitate implementation of these two examples (based the process of evidence-based practice and the knowledge-to-action cycle).

Given that fracture management is an acute care paradigm, one might anticipate that professional beliefs and traditions as well as knowledge would act as barriers to implementing fracture screening. In this case, certain tools might facilitate the transition. The development of screening recommendations or a screening tool might ease this transition. The self-directed behavior facilitation for using the screening tool by rehabilitation professionals can include self-tracking tools (such as diaries or reminders) to monitor the use of the screening tool in DRF patients and readily available practice guidelines for using the tools. The external drivers to behavioral change can include reminders to use the tool by professional associations or mandating the use of such tools by the insurance providers.

Outcomes of Knowledge Translation Exercise

When monitoring the impact of change in practice it is important to consider both process and outcome. Specific methods of assessing outcomes of knowledge translation implementation are provided in the taxonomy table. The anticipated impact of the screening tool would include its administration and better identification of outcomes with respect to bone health and prevention of chronic pain. Qualitative interviews of the opinion leaders can be conducted to obtain the barriers to behavioral change. The positive, negative, or conflicting messages from the interviews can be summarized and used for developing targeted knowledge translation exercises. Misconception about the screening tool or its potential use can be eliminated by adding/removing specific information from the user's guide that creates this conflict.

CONCLUSION

Patients who present to rehabilitation settings following DRFs can be at risk for future falls, fall-related injuries, chronic pain, and disability. Early identification of such patients can help rehabilitation professionals in designing more targeted interventions to minimize such risks. This commentary identified the knowledge-to-practice gap evident in this area where no standardized tools are available for screening at-risk patients. Furthermore, potential steps for a knowledge translation exercise to generate new knowledge regarding the screening tool, disseminating the screening tool to the end-users (rehabilitation professionals), and evaluating the use of the screening tool by the end-users were outlined. The researchers involved in refining the assessment and treatment techniques in the DRF population should undertake high-quality research studies to fill the knowledge-to-practice gap to improve the management of this extremely common fall-related injury.

REFERENCES

American Academy of Orthopaedic Surgeons. (2009). *The treatment of distal radius fractures.* Rosemont, IL: Author.

Armstrong, A. D., MacDermid, J. C., Chinchalkar, S., Stevens, R. S., & King, G. J. (1998). Reliability of range-of-motion measurement in the elbow and forearm. *Journal of Shoulder and Elbow Surgery, 7,* 573–580.

Becker, C., Cameron, I. D., Klenk, J., Lindemann, U., Heinrich, S., Konig, H. H., et al. (2011). Reduction of femoral fractures in long-term care facilities: The Bavarian fracture prevention study. *PLoS One, 6,* e24311.

Berggren, M., Stenvall, M., Olofsson, B., & Gustafson, Y. (2008). Evaluation of a fall-prevention program in older people after femoral neck fracture: A one-year follow-up. *Osteoporosis International, 19,* 801–809.

Carter, T. I., Pansy, B., Wolff, A. L., Hillstrom, H. J., Backus, S. I., Lenhoff, M., et al. (2009). Accuracy and reliability of three different techniques for manual goniometry for wrist motion: A cadaveric study. *Journal of Hand Surgery, 34,* 1422–1428.

Court-Brown, C. M., & Caesar, B. (2006). Epidemiology of adult fractures: A review. *Injury, 37,* 691–697.

Diaz-Garcia, R. J., Oda, T., Shauver, M. J., & Chung, K. C. (2011). A systematic review of outcomes and complications of treating unstable distal radius fractures in the elderly. *Journal of Hand Surgery, 36,* 824–835.

Endres, H. G., Dasch, B., Lungenhausen, M., Maier, C., Smektala, R., Trampisch, H. J., et al. (2006). Patients with femoral or distal forearm fracture in Germany: A prospective observational study on health care situation and outcome. *BMC Public Health, 6,* 87.

Fess, E.E. Grip strength. (1992) In: Casanova J.S. (Ed). *Clinical assessment recommendations* (2nd ed.). Chicago, IL: Society of Hand Therapists: 41-45.

Fujii, K., Henmi, T., Kanematsu, Y., Mishiro, T., Sakai, T., & Terai, T. (2002). Fractures of the distal end of radius in elderly patients: A comparative study of anatomical and functional results. *Journal of Orthopedic Surgery, 10,* 9–15.

Gummesson, C., Ward, M. M., & Atroshi, I. (2006). The shortened Disabilities of the Arm, Shoulder and Hand Questionnaire (QuickDASH): Validity and reliability based on responses within the full-length DASH. *BMC Musculoskeletal Disorders, 7*, 44.

Hemelaers, L., Angst, F., Drerup, S., Simmen, B. R., & Wood-Dauphinee, S. (2008). Reliability and validity of the German version of "the Patient-Rated Wrist Evaluation (PRWE)" as an outcome measure of wrist pain and disability in patients with acute distal radius fractures. *Journal of Hand Therapy, 21*, 366–376.

Hoang-Kim, A., Scott, J., Micera, G., Orsini, R., & Moroni, A. (2009). Functional assessment in patients with osteoporotic wrist fractures treated with external fixation: A review of randomized trials. *Archives of Orthopaedic and Trauma Surgery, 129*, 105–111.

Hodsman, A. B., Leslie, W. D., Tsang, J. F., & Gamble, G. D. (2008). 10-Year probability of recurrent fractures following wrist and other osteoporotic fractures in a large clinical cohort: An analysis from the Manitoba Bone Density Program. *Archives of Internal Medicine, 168*, 2261–2267.

Hudak, P. L., Amadio, P. C., & Bombardier, C. (1996). Development of an upper extremity outcome measure: The DASH (Disabilities of the Arm, Shoulder and Hand) [corrected]. The Upper Extremity Collaborative Group (UECG). *American Journal of Industrial Medicine, 29*, 602–608.

Imaeda, T., Uchiyama, S., Wada, T., Okinaga, S., Sawaizumi, T., Omokawa, S., et al. (2010). Reliability, validity, and responsiveness of the Japanese version of the Patient-Rated Wrist Evaluation. *Journal of Orthopedic Science, 15*, 509–517.

Kay, T. M., Myers, A. M., & Huijbregts, M. P. G. (2001). How far have we come since 1992? A comparative survey of physiotherapists' use of outcome measures. *Physiotherapie Canada, 53*, 268–275.

Kempen, G. I., Yardley, L., van Haastregt, J. C., Zijlstra, G. A., Beyer, N., Hauer, K., et al. (2008). The Short FES-I: A shortened version of the Falls Efficacy Scale–International to assess fear of falling. *Age and Ageing, 37*, 45–50.

Kotsis, S. V., Lau, F. H., & Chung, K. C. (2007). Responsiveness of the Michigan Hand Outcomes Questionnaire and physical measurements in outcome studies of distal radius fracture treatment. *Journal of Hand Surgery, 32*, 84–90.

Kristensen, M. T., Henriksen, S., Stie, S. B., & Bandholm, T. (2011). Relative and absolute intertester reliability of the Timed Up and Go Test to quantify functional mobility in patients with hip fracture. *Journal of the American Geriatric Society, 59*, 565–567.

MacDermid, J. C., Alyafi, T., & Richards, R. S. (2001). Test–retest reliability of static and endurance grip strength tests performed on the Jamar and NK. *Physiotherapie Canada, 53*, 48–54.

MacDermid, J. C., Richards, R. S., Donner, A., Bellamy, N., & Roth, J. H. (2000). Responsiveness of the Short Form-36, Disability of the Arm, Shoulder, and Hand Questionnaire, Patient-Rated Wrist Evaluation, and physical impairment measurements in evaluating recovery after a distal radius fracture. *Journal of Hand Surgery, 25*, 330–340.

MacDermid, J. C., Roth, J. H., & Richards, R. S. (2003). Pain and disability reported in the year following a distal radius fracture: A cohort study. *BMC Musculoskeletal Disorders, 4*, 24.

MacDermid, J. C., Turgeon, T., Richards, R. S., Beadle, M., & Roth, J. H. (1998). Patient rating of wrist pain and disability: A reliable and valid measurement tool. *Journal of Orthopaedic Trauma, 12*, 577–586.

Michlovitz, S. L., LaStayo, P. C., Alzner, S., & Watson, E. (2001). Distal radius fractures: Therapy practice patterns. *Journal of Hand Therapy, 14*, 249–257.

Mitchell, R., Curtis, K., Watson, W. L., & Nau, T. (2010). Age differences in fall-related injury hospitalisations and trauma presentations. *Australasian Journal of Ageing, 29*, 117–125.

Moore, C. M., & Leonardi-Bee, J. (2008). The prevalence of pain and disability one year post fracture of the distal radius in a UK population: A cross sectional survey. *BMC Musculoskeletal Disorders, 9*, 129.

Nordell, E., Kristinsdottir, E. K., Jarnlo, G. B., Magnusson, M., & Thorngren, K. G. (2005). Older patients with distal forearm fracture. A challenge to future fall and fracture prevention. *Aging Clinical Experimental Research, 17*, 90–95.

Roudsari, B. S., Ebel, B. E., Corso, P. S., Molinari, N. A., & Koepsell, T. D. (2005). The acute medical care costs of fall-related injuries among the U.S. older adults. *Injury, 36*, 1316–1322.

Sherrington, C., & Lord, S. R. (2005). Reliability of simple portable tests of physical performance in older people after hip fracture. *Clinical Rehabilitation, 19*, 496–504.

Stevens, J. A., Corso, P. S., Finkelstein, E. A., & Miller, T. R. (2006). The costs of fatal and non-fatal falls among older adults. *Injury Prevention, 12*, 290–295.

Stevens, J. G., & Beurskens, A. J. (2010). Implementation of measurement instruments in physical therapist practice: Development of a tailored strategy. *Physical Therapy, 90*, 953–961.

Stokes, E. K., & O'Neill, D. (2008). Use of outcome measures in physiotherapy practice in Ireland from 1998 to 2003 and comparison to Canadian trends. *Physiotherapie Canada, 60*, 109–116.

Swinkels, R. A., van Peppen, R. P., Wittink, H., Custers, J. W., & Beurskens, A. J. (2011). Current use and barriers and facilitators for implementation of standardised measures in physical therapy in The Netherlands. *BMC Musculoskeletal Disorders, 12*, 106.

Turner, P., Whitfield, A., Brewster, S., Halligan, M., & Kennedy, J. (1996). The assessment of pain: An audit of physiotherapy practice. *Australian Journal of Physiotherapy, 42*, 55–62.

van Staa, T. P., Dennison, E. M., Leufkens, H. G., & Cooper, C. (2001). Epidemiology of fractures in England and Wales. *Bone, 29*, 517–522.

Watson, W., Clapperton, A., & Mitchell, R. (2011). The burden of fall-related injury among older persons in New South Wales. *Australian & New Zealand Journal of Public Health, 35*, 170–175.

SUGGESTED READINGS

Center for Evidence-Based Medicine. (2011). Levels of evidence. Retrieved from http://www.cebm.net/index.aspx?o=1025

Jebsen, R. H., Taylor, N., Trieschmann, R. B., Trotter, M. J., & Howard, L. A. (1969). An objective and standardized test of hand function. *Archives of Physical Medicine and Rehabilitation, 50*, 311–319.

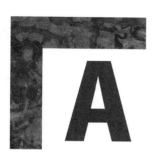

QUALITY APPRAISAL FOR
CLINICAL MEASUREMENT STUDIES
Evaluation Form and Guidelines

© MacDermid 2011. McMaster University

Quality Appraisal for Clinical Measurement Research Reports Evaluation Form

Authors: _____ Year: _____ Rater: ____

Use this form to rate the quality of a clinical measurement study. To decide which score to provide for each item on your quality checklist, pick the descriptor that sounds most like what was reported in the study you are evaluating. Items rank descriptors are provided in the guide. (Forms and guides to extract study data for evidence synthesis are available from developer at macderj@mcmaster.ca)

Evaluation Criteria	Score		
	2	1	0
Study question			
1. Was the relevant background work cited to define what is currently known about the measurement properties of measures under study, and the potential contributions of the current research question to informing that knowledge base?			
Study design			
2. Were appropriate inclusion/exclusion criteria defined?			
3. Were specific clinical measurement questions/hypotheses identified?			
4. Was an appropriate scope of measurement properties considered?			
5. Was an appropriate sample size used?			
6. Was appropriate retention/follow-up obtained? (For studies involving retesting; otherwise n/a)			
Measurements			
7. Were specific descriptions provided of the measure under study and the method(s) used to administer it?			
8. Were standardized procedures used to administer all study measures?			
Analyses			
9. Were analyses conducted for each specific hypothesis or purpose?			
10. Were appropriate statistical tests used to obtain point estimates of the measurement properties?			
11. Were appropriate ancillary analyses done to quantify in the estimates of the clinical measurement property or the confidence in the point estimate (confidence intervals, benchmark comparisons/ROC curves, alternate forms of analysis like SEM/MID, etc.)?			
Recommendations			
12. Were clear, specific, and accurate conclusions made about the clinical measurement properties and supported by the study objectives, analysis, and results?			
Subtotals (of columns 1 and 2)			
Total score (sum of subtotals ÷ 24 × 100). If for a specific paper or topic an item is deemed inappropriate then you can sum of items ÷ 2 × number of items × 100.			

Quality Appraisal of a Clinical Measurement Study Interpretation Guide

To decide which score to provide for each item on your quality checklist, read the following descriptors. Pick the descriptor that sounds *most* like the study you were evaluating with respect to a given item. If there is no documentation about any specific aspect of an item, then you must evaluate assuming that it was not done. Given the diversity in clinical measurement properties and design options, the evaluator has to make judgments using the following criteria and extend the principles to specific aspects that may not be covered in these brief exemplars. In many cases, the study will not look exactly like the descriptor so there will be some interpretation as to which level of optimal methods for clinical measurement studies have been achieved. In such cases, the evaluator can use the general approach that if this study research design and conduct is consistent with best practice (Score = 2); is acceptable but suboptimal (Score = 1); is not done/documented or is substantially inadequate or inappropriate (Score = 0).

		Descriptors
Score		
Study question		
1	2	The authors: - Performed a thorough literature review indicating what is currently known, and not known, about the clinical measurement properties of the instruments or tests under study. - Presented a critical and unbiased view of what is known about the current measurement properties. - Indicated how the current research question fills a gap in the current knowledge base. - Established a research question based on the above.
	1	All of the above criteria were not fulfilled, but a sound rationale was provided for the research question.
	0	A foundation for the current research question was not clear and the rationale was not founded on previous literature.
Study design		
2	2	Specific inclusion/exclusion criteria for the study were defined that described the patients enrolled. The subjects were described in terms of health condition/demographics, key relevant outcome mediators, and the recruitment context (setting).
	1	Some information on participants and place is provided (not all of the above). For example, age/sex/diagnosis and the name or type of the practice is listed, but no additional information.
	0	No information on type of clinical settings or study participants is provided (other than number/mean age).
3	2	Specific hypotheses or research questions are provided. The stated study purpose provides specific research questions or hypotheses that indicate which specific measurement properties will be evaluated. This should include the specific type of reliability (intra-/inter-rater or test-retest) being tested or the type of validity (construct/criterion/content, longitudinal/concurrent, or convergent/divergent) being tested. A prior hypothesis should describe the level of reliability expected, and for validity, expected relationships (strength of associations) or constructs.
	1	The types of reliability and validity being tested were apparent in the methods/title, but clear and specific research questions or hypotheses were not specified.
	0	Specific types of reliability or validity under evaluation were not clearly defined nor were specific hypotheses on reliability and validity stated. ("*The purpose of this study was to investigate the reliability and validity of...*" can be rated as zero if no further detail on the types of reliability and validity or the nature of specific hypotheses is stated.)

4	2	An appropriate scope of clinical measurement properties would be indicated by the following: 1. A detailed focus on reliability that included multiple forms of reliability (at least two of: intra-rater, inter-rater, test retest); as well as both relative and absolute reliability (e.g., ICCs and SEM/MID or limits of agreement). 2. A detailed focus on validity that included 3 or more forms of validity: content (e.g., expert review/survey, qualitative interviews, ICF linking) or structural (e.g., factor analyses or Rasch), construct (known group differences, convergent/divergent associations), criterion (concurrent/predictive), or responsiveness. Predictive, evaluative, or discriminative properties were established. 3. Three or more indicators of reliability and validity were examined concurrently and provide a rich view on measurement properties.
	1	Two or more clinical measurement properties were evaluated; however, scope was narrow and did not meet above criteria (e.g., internal consistency and one other indicator of validity or reliability).
	0	The scope of clinical measurement properties was very narrow as indicated by a narrow evaluation of only one form of reliability or validity.
5	2	Authors performed a sample size calculation and obtained their recruitment targets. Post-doc power analyses and/or confidence intervals confirm that the sample size was sufficient to define relatively precise estimates of reliability or validity.
	1	The authors provide an acceptable rationale for the number of subjects included in the study, but did not present specific sample size calculations or post-doc power analyses (or had a sample > 100 but no justification).
	0	Size of the sample was not rationalized or is clearly underpowered.
6	2	Ninety percent or more of the patients enrolled for study were re-evaluated.
	1	Seventy percent or more of the enrolled patients were re-evaluated.
	0	Less than 70% of the patients enrolled in the study were re-evaluated.
Measurements		
7	2	Documentation is provided for how the studied test is performed. This includes adequate description of the measure/test and how it is administered or scored. The authors may provide or reference a published manual/article that outlines specific procedures for administration, scoring (including scoring algorithms, handling of missing data), and interpretation that includes any necessary information about positioning/active participation of the client, any special equipment required, calibration of equipment if necessary, training required, cost, and examiner procedures/actions. If no manual is available, then the text describes key details of procedures in sufficient detail so they could be replicated.
	1	The test(s) and its administration procedures are referenced, but there is inadequate description of the test procedures.
	0	Minimal description of test procedures without appropriate references.
8	2	This item addresses the overall study procedures for administering all study measures (study measure and its comparators) in an unbiased way. Test procedures should not introduce systematic errors in the estimation of the clinical measurement properties. This includes standardized procedures for who completed or administered the measures. For self-report, this includes order of presentation, who completed at what time interval, and handling of missing items. If relevant, the paper should include how cultural literacy issues were handled (e.g., exclusion, assisted, or surrogate completion). For impairment measures, procedures would include calibration of any equipment, use of consistent measurement tools and scoring, a priori exclusion of any participants likely to give invalid results/unable to complete testing (not exclusion of after enrollment), and use of standardized instructions and test procedures. This can include order of administration of test and quality checking of scores. For reliability testing, the appropriate retest interval will depend on the nature of the condition. For acute conditions it may require retesting within 48 hours; chronic/stable conditions are commonly retested within 4 to 14 days. For estimation of clinical change, retest intervals should be ones during which a meaningful clinical change would have occurred (and from an intervention with known effectiveness). The evaluator decides overall whether this has sufficiently been addressed by the methods described.

	1	No obvious sources of bias in the study test protocol or how tests were performed/administered is apparent; however, there were suboptimal procedures or an inadequate description of the measurement protocol to be ensured control of bias or that procedures were standardized.
	0	No description of the overall procedures for administering study tests; OR an obvious source of bias in data collection methods.
Analyses		
9	2	Authors clearly defined which specific analyses were conducted for each of the stated specific hypotheses/questions of the study. This may be accomplished through organization of the results under specific subheadings or by demarcating which analyses addressed specific clinical measurement properties. Data was presented for each hypothesis/research question posed.
	1	Data was presented that addressed each of the measurement questions posed, but authors did not link specific analyses to specific research questions or hypotheses.
	0	Data was not presented for every hypothesis or clinical measurement property outlined in the purposes or methods.

10	2	<u>Tests selected.</u> Appropriate statistical tests were conducted to calculate a point estimate for clinical measurement properties. Examples are provided below; but are not exhaustive.
		1. Reliability (Relative = ICCs (Shrout & Fleiss, 1979) for quantitative, Kappa (Landis & Koch, 1977) for nominal data; absolute (SEM or plot of score differences versus average score showing mean and 2SD limit, as per Altman and Bland) (Bland & Altman, 1986; Bland & Altman, 1987).
		2. Clinical relevance: Minimal detectable change, clinically important difference (Jaeschke, Singer, & Guyatt, 1989; Beaton et al., 2001; Wells et al., 2001)
		3. Validity
		   a. Validity associations: Pearson correlations for normally distributed data, Spearman rank correlations for ordinal data; or other correlations, if appropriate.
		   b. Validity tests of significant difference: An appropriate global test like analysis of variance was used where indicated, with post-hoc tests that adjusted for multiple testing.
		   c. Validity of items scaling/responses: Rasch analysis or item response (Baylor et al., 2011; Pallant & Tennant, 2007; Kyngdon, 2006; Cipriani, Fox, Khuder, & Boudreau, 2005; Smith, Jr., Conrad, Chang, & Piazza, 2002).
		4. Responsiveness (Beaton, Bombardier, Katz, & Wright, 2001): Standardized response means or effect sizes or other recognized responsiveness indices were used.

	1	Appropriate statistical tests were used in some instances; but suboptimal choices were made in other analyses.
	0	Inappropriate use of statistical tests - incorrect tests for type of data; or a lack of analysis
11	2	The study goes beyond a single statistical point estimate of a clinical measurement property and providing supporting statistical analyses that increases confidence in the findings in terms of precision of the (key) indicator; or provide an alternate form of analysis of the clinical measurement property. The evaluator decides if these analyses are appropriate and informative. For example, with reliability, at least 2 of the following would constitute appropriate and informative analysis beyond a point estimate of a reliability coefficient: 1. Confidence intervals around the point estimate 2. Comparison to appropriate, referenced benchmarks or standards 3. SEM or MDC For correlations, tests of significance or confidence intervals were presented and indicators of the criterion benchmarks were provided. For studies involving cross-cultural validation, the analyses should compare multiple clinical measurement properties previously established for the measure and explain the extent to which the translated version is in accordance with these previously reported properties on the source measure.
	1	Either precision definition (confidence intervals) or appropriate benchmark comparison were used - NOT both. OR Some analyses were associated with indicators of precision or alternate form of analysis, but not all key indicators.

	0	Inappropriate use of benchmarks or confidence intervals; or indicators of precision or alternate form are absent.
Recommendations		
12	2	Authors made specific conclusions and clinical measurement recommendations that were clearly related to each hypotheses/question posed in the study and that were supported by the data presented. Ideal recommendations would state the estimated status of the clinical measurement property and the confidence in the estimate and the context for which those apply. To achieve a 2, the conclusion must be specific and the conclusions cannot overstate the clinical measurement properties observed the study, nor ignore suboptimal measurement properties found.
	1	Authors made conclusions and clinical measurement recommendations that were basically true (supported by study data), but vague. That is, they do not specify the extent, confidence, or context of the findings (e.g., the measure is "reliable and valid"); OR the authors made specific clinical measurement recommendations, but for only some of the study hypotheses.
	0	Authors did not make conclusions about clinical measurement; OR made recommendations that were in contradiction to the actual data presented.

REFERENCES

Baylor, C., Hula, W., Donovan, N. J., Doyle, P. J., Kendall, D., & Yorkston, K. (2011). An introduction to item response theory and Rasch models for speech-language pathologists. *American Journal of Speech-Language Pathology, 20*:243-259.

Beaton, D. E., Bombardier, C., Katz, J. N., & Wright, J. G. (2001). A taxonomy for responsiveness. *Journal of Clinical Epidemiology, 54*:1204-1217.

Beaton, D. E., Bombardier, C., Katz, J. N., Wright, J. G., Wells, G., Boers, M. et al. (2001). Looking for important change/differences in studies of responsiveness. OMERACT MCID Working Group. Outcome Measures in Rheumatology. Minimal Clinically Important Difference. *The Journal of Rheumatology, 28*:400-405.

Bland, J. M. & Altman, D. G. (1987). Statistical methods for assessing agreement between measurements. *Clinical Biochemistry, 11*:399-404.

Bland, J. M. & Altman, D. J. (1986). Statistical methods for assessing agreement between two methods of clinical measurement. *Lancet*, 1, 307-310.

Cipriani, D., Fox, C., Khuder, S., & Boudreau, N. (2005). Comparing Rasch analyses probability estimates to sensitivity, specificity and likelihood ratios when examining the utility of medical diagnostic tests. *Journal of Applied Measurement, 6*:180-201.

Jaeschke, R., Singer, J., & Guyatt, G. H. (1989). Measurement of health status. Ascertaining the minimal clinically important difference. *Controlled Clinical Trials, 10*:407-415.

Kyngdon, A. (2006). An introduction to the theory of unidimensional unfolding. *Journal of Applied Measurement, 7*:260-277.

Landis, J. R. & Koch, G. G. (1977). The measurement of observer agreement for categorical data. *Biometrics*, 33, 159-174.

Pallant, J. F. & Tennant, A. (2007). An introduction to the Rasch measurement model: an example using the Hospital Anxiety and Depression Scale (HADS). *British Journal of Clinical Psychology, 46*:1-18.

Shrout, P. E. & Fleiss, J. L. (1979). Intraclass correlations: Uses in assessing rater reliability. *Psychological Bulletin,* 86, 420-428.

Smith, E. V., Jr., Conrad, K. M., Chang, K., & Piazza, J. (2002). An introduction to Rasch measurement for scale development and person assessment. *The Journal of Nursing Measurement*, 10:189-206.

Wells, G., Beaton, D., Shea, B., Boers, M., Simon, L., Strand, V. et al. (2001). Minimal clinically important differences: review of methods. *The Journal of Rheumatology, 28*:406-412.

Data Extraction Form for Studies Evaluating the
Clinical Measurement Properties of Outcome Measures

Authors: _____ Year _____ Rater _____

Instructions

When using the data extraction form it is important to realize that the purpose of data extraction is to remove or extract the specific information reported by authors within a study, not to evaluate the validity or value of that piece of information. To make data extraction and is useful as possible and to avoid the need for repeated data extractions, it is advisable to read the accompanying guide and then be as specific as possible when extracting information.

	DATA EXTRACTED
Population studied	
Population	
Intervention	
Reliability	
Reliability (relative)	
Reliability (absolute)	
Minimum detectable change	
Content/Structural validity	
Internal consistency	
Content validity	
Floor-ceiling effects	
Factorial validity	
Item response /Rasch analyses	

Construct/Criterion validity	
Known groups	
Convergent	
Divergent	
Longitudinal validity	
Concurrent criterion	
Predictive criterion	
Responsiveness/Clinical change	
Responsiveness	
Minimally clinical important difference	
Usefulness/practicality	
Readability	
Interpretability	
Time to administer	
Administration burden	
Cultural applicability	

Data Extraction Guide for Studies Evaluating the Quality of Studies Evaluating the Clinical Measurement Properties of Outcome Measures

Instructions

Clinical measurement studies may evaluate a wide spectrum of measurement properties or evaluate aspects that relate to the implementability or interpretation of outcome measures. Individual clinical measurement studies cannot address every aspect of the measurement properties of an instrument. Ideally, systematic reviews will synthesize the quality and content of research evidence addressing the clinical measurement properties of outcome measures. The summative knowledge about the measurement properties, cultural transferability, and utility across different contexts provides the scope of information needed to select an outcome measure for a specific patient (population), purpose, and context.

This guide should facilitate extraction of data from clinical measurement studies. An explanation of the measurement property addressed in each item and how it might be measured within a given study is listed to facilitate finding and extracting that information. The accompanying extraction form can then be used to collect the specific information on these measurement or utility properties from specific studies.

The purpose of data extraction is to extract the specific information reported by authors within a study, not to evaluate the validity or value of that piece of information. Evaluation of the quality of articles (also called critical appraisal) is performed in a separate step. It is advisable to extract detailed specific information from the study, recognizing that this information may later be synthesized or subject to meta-analysis.

There is no standardized process for synthesizing clinical measurement information. Based on the findings of extraction you may elect to present the synthesize data in a descriptive way by creating a summary table of the data extracted in each category. If you find some studies with similar designs, you may be able to conduct a meta-analysis of some properties like clinically important difference (CID) or minimal detectable change (MDC)—this can be valuable as it may provide more stable estimates of these important properties.

	PROPERTY	**METHODS THAT MIGHT BE USED TO COLLECT THIS INFORMATION/ RELEVANT STATISTICS**
Population studied		
Population	A description of the study population.	Sample size, pathology/disorder, demographics, setting, acute vs. chronic, where subjects were chosen from. Report meaningful demographics and indicators of the population studied.
Intervention	Interventions (if applicable) applied during longitudinal studies.	Description of the nature, frequency, intensity of the intervention and the follow-up interval.
Reliability		
Reliability Description	The extent to which the same results are obtained on repeated administrations of the same measure when no change in status has occurred (reliability) or the precision of the scores on repeated measurements (agreement).	Test procedures or measures are typically reapplied on repeated occasions in individuals considered to have a stable condition during that time frame which repeated testing occurs. Repeated testing may be performed on different occasions (test retest) for self-report measures, OR by the same rater (intra-rater) or different raters (inter-rater) if it is an observer-based scale. In some cases different test instruments (inter-instrument) are evaluated. The most common statistic used is the intraclass correlation coefficient for quantitative data(Shrout & Fleiss, 1979) and kappa(Landis & Koch, 1977) for nominal data. Standard error of measurement is used to present a

		quantitative estimate of the reliability in the original units of measure. The retest interval should ensure that patients remained stable; but that recall does not contribute to overestimation of consistency of responses. This will be based on the nature of the condition but for acute conditions it may require retesting within 48 hours; whereas Chronic are commonly retested within 4 to 14 days. Report the type of reliability evaluated and coefficients obtained.
Reliability (relative)	The relationship (ratio) between variability in test scores when repeating the test on the same person in comparison to the overall variability (including variation between people); typically indicated by a reliability coefficient.	ICCs (Shrout & Fleiss, 1979) and their associated confidence intervals are reported.
Reliability (absolute)	The extent to which the same test scores are obtained on repeated administrations of the same measure when no change in status has occurred (reliability) or the precision of the scores are on repeated measurements (agreement). Absolute reliability is portrayed as the quantity of error that could be anticipated upon repeated testing - reported in the original units of measure.	This may be reported as the following: 1. Standard error of measurement; (in older articles you may see coefficient of variation). 2. Altman and Bland graphical technique (Bland & Altman, 1990; Bland & Altman, 1987; Bland & Altman, 1986) where the difference on repeated tests for each individual (limits of agreement) is plotted versus their mean score. The mean difference and the boundaries of 2SD are shown to define the limits of agreement.
Minimum Detectable Change	Calculated from the reliability coefficient and the level of confidence specified for error margins. This indicator reflects the amount of change required before you can be confident that change exceeds the random error that occurs in stable patients.	Extract the number and level of confidence.
Content/structural validity		
Internal consistency	The extent to which items on a test or subscale are related (an indication of the consistency of the concept measured).	Cronbach's alpha is- the inter-item correlation usually reported. Report alpha and whether it relates to the entire instrument or specific subscales.
Content Validity	The extent to which the conceptual domain or construct that a test is designed to measure is adequately reflected by the items in the measure. In assessing content validity it is important to consider the population to whom the measure applies, the completeness of the content, the relevancy and emphasis of the content assessed.	A variety of techniques can be used to assess the extent to which items on a given measure reflected the necessary content to capture the concept of interest. Some of the techniques you will find are listed. Extract what was done to determine content validity and what was found. 1) Patients and experts were involved during item selection/reduction—report how they were used and key decisions. 2) Patients were consulted for reading and comprehension—report key findings. 3) Cognitive interviews (Cibelli, 1994; Ojanen & Gogates, 2006) were done with patients to determine how items were interpreted by respondents; their perceptions of the items—report key findings. 4) Expert panels or Delphi procedures were used to select items or evaluate the validity of the instrument—report key findings in decisions. 5) During translation specific study of the meaning of the questions to another cultural or language group was studied—report key findings in decisions.

		6) ICF linking (Cieza et al., 2002) or other coding of content was performed. Report the results which may include the distribution of content across ICF domains or the distribution of specific codes.
Floor-Ceiling Effects	The measure is unable to indicated a worsening score in patients who have clinically deteriorated and/or an improved score in patients who have clinically improved.	There are a variety of potential methods so the method and conclusion should be reported. Descriptive statistics of the distribution of scores may have presented graphically or numerically may be used to indicate this. Other studies report the percentage of patients sustained a floor or ceiling effect defined by the number of people who fall in the extremes ranges. Note different studies may define the extreme ranges for floor/ceiling differently, so extract how it was defined and percentage of patients who obtained floor or ceiling category scores.
Factorial validity	The extent to which factor analysis supports assumptions surrounding constructs measured as defined by the measure or as indicated by subscale structure.	Factor analysis is may be reported as results and compared to the inherent structure of the instrument or factor analysis upon which its construction was based. Report the type of factor analysis performed (exploratory or confirmatory), rotations used and the number of factors derived, and specify whether this confirms the expected instrument structure or original factor structure.
Item response /Rasch Analyses	The extent to which items cross a range of difficulty, or a spectrum of the concept measured. The measurement scaling of the items.	Using item response theory or Rasch analysis items are fit to a model to demonstrate interval scaling and determine item difficulty (Pallant & Tennant, 2007). Analyses might address item difficulty, person's ability curves, and comparison of ability estimation. Most commonly, the item difficulty and the composition of the test that fulfills interval scaling are defined. Data to be extracted include information on the scaling of the items, whether the interval scaling has been established, and the presence or absence of differential item functioning (DIF) where items perform differently on different types of respondents.
Construct Validity		
Construct Validity - correlational	Constructs are artificial frameworks that are not directly observable. Construct validity assesses the extent to which measures perform according to a priori defined constructs. Construct validity can be cross-sectional or longitudinal (predictive). Constructed hypotheses can assess convergent validity where measures are thought to represent similar constructs or divergent validity where it is assumed they measure different constructs. For cross-cultural validation the expected relationships are those that have been reported in validation of the instrument in its original language/format.	When extracting data about correlational validity the pre-constructed hypothesis and whether it is supported should be documented. For correlational construct validity this will be the nature and strength of the prespecified relationship and the correlations that support that. Relation to other indices/constructs that are similar (convergent) or different (divergent) can be reported. Ideally, hypotheses are formulated /reported and supported by correlations that are in accordance with the hypotheses. Note that there is no consistent agreement on what subjective term should be applied to validity correlations. Note that there is no consistent agreement on what subjective term should be applied to validity correlations. Some authors use subjective

		terminology defined for reliability such as strong (>0.70) and moderate (0.40-0.70) correlations. Others use the correlations like effect size benchmarks that 0.4 indicates a moderate effect and 0.6 a large effect. For validity assessment is more important that correlations prespecified constructed hypotheses-although not all papers are written clearly with respect to this.
Convergent	The relationship between similar scales/tests. Correlations are generally expected to be moderate to strong if the relationship is one where there is confidence that they measure a similar construct.	Extract test names, prespecified expected relationship, and correlations observed.
Divergent	Divergent validity assesses the extent to which different scales/tests that are designed to measure different constructs demonstrate that they are different by a lack of correlation between them.	Extract test names, prespecified expected relationship, and correlations observed.
Construct validity-known groups	Known groups analysis supports the validity of a measure measurements by demonstrating that the measurement is able to differentiate between group's that are prespecified and <u>known</u> to be different on the construct being assessed.	Data extraction should include the nature of the subgroups and the size of the difference observed between them (and its statistical significance). Typically, statistical tests of difference are performed. Since known groups analysis can provide data that is useful in clinical practice as benchmarks for comparing these known groups, it is a more practical form of construct validity than correlational. Data extraction/presentation should reflect this by presenting the group central tendency, their margins and statistical significant in an accessible manner.
Longitudinal Validity	This form of validity supports the validity of a measure by demonstrating that the change that occurs over time onto similar instruments is correlated in a manner consistent with the nature of the relationship between the scales. It is measured over a retest interval when clinically relevant change could be expected.	Extract test names and correlations. *Note: Since longitudinal validity is based on four measures (pre-and post-test on two different measures), and since error tends to mitigate the strength of correlations, strong longitudinal correlations can be difficult to obtain.*
Criterion validity Description	Criterion validation is determined by comparing a given outcome measure to an accepted standard of measure. For subjective constructs like pain and disability it can be argued that there is no criterion since there is no external gold standard. Therefore, for self-report measures validation focuses on construct validity. For performance measures it is common to have a criterion measure that is considered to be highly precise and rigorous as the criterion comparator.	Authors will state that his or her measure is being compared against a specific instrument and report the correlation or agreement between the measures. Extract the test names and results, correlations, or other as reported.
Concurrent criterion	Concurrent validity is assessed by comparing a scale and its criterion at a single point in time.	Extract the test names and correlations.
Predictive criterion	Predictive validity is evaluated by determining the extent to which the results of administering an outcome measure at one point in time can accurately predict a future status or outcome.	Extract the test names, correlations, and time interval (and important cutoffs if those were established/reported), if diagnostic test methodology was used to examine prediction and sensitivity specificity and other diagnostic criteria reported should be extracted.

Responsiveness/Clinical Change		
Responsiveness	Does the instrument detect changes over time that matter to patients?	Extract indicators of responsiveness include effect size, standard response mean, and the method for assessing whether patients were improved, stable, or worse. (Beaton, 2000)
Clinically Important Difference (CID)	CID is the difference in scores that patients find to be observable and clinically important. It is assessed by comparing scores to an external benchmark of clinical relevance such as a global rating of change or some other method. The terminology used to rate the nature of this difference will affect the estimation process. Differences in methods include how clinically importance is framed and the metrics/process by which that is determined.	Extract the MID or CID and note the method/cut-off used to define importance. Extract how the clinically important differences were framed to respondents or determined. For example, minimal, moderate, extreme improvement, or better/not better etc.
Utility/Practicality		
Readability	The questionnaire is understandable for all patients. Authors provided specific information on the following: 1) Readability was evaluated by the target population or 2) Specific tools were used evaluate readability were applied (e.g., grade level can be assigned in some software packages).	State method and results obtained.
Interpretability (of subjective benchmarks /classifications)	The degree to which one can assign qualitative meaning to quantitative scores or define benchmarks for subgroups by scores. Authors provided information on the interpretation of the following scores: 1) Validation of subjective categories of outcome e.g., excellent/good/fair; normal/abnormal OR 2) Testing of known groups in terms of their accuracy for classification of individuals	State the type of categorization tested, relevant scores, and if appropriate the method used to validate/analyze the subgroup differences. For example, accuracy of classification can be assessed using diagnostic test methodology or agreement statistics. Extract the nature of the analysis and findings.
Time to administer	Authors provided specific information on time to administer.	Extract time.
Administration Burden	Ease of method used to administer and score the outcome measure. Authors provided specific information on the ease of scoring. For performance-based measures, equipment and training procedures should be considered.	Extract study data on scoring method burden. Report any findings about training or equipment requirements. If this is not specifically reported in the text of the study it cannot be extracted. However, during a systematic review you wish to compare scoring algorithms and administrative burden and report this. This must be done in a systematic way and the method should be documented. For example, if you wish to extract the specific scoring algorithm for an instrument and compare it to others, then multiple raters should evaluate the relative complexity of these scoring algorithms
Cultural applicability	The extent to which an instrument contains items that will be meaningful across different cultural (sub) groups; and whether the concept is measured similarly across cultures. Cross-cultural adaptation may be used to translate measures into different languages and to convert items to culturally	Extract language cultural translation performed (and relevant findings). Evaluations may address some or all of the following: Content equivalence Semantic equivalence Technical equivalence

	relevant items, if needed. In cross-cultural adaptation a number of analyses may be performed including the following: 1. A structured translation process that includes forward and backward translation and retesting clinical measurement properties of the translated version and how they compare to the original version. 2. Formal evaluation of the meaning of items in different cultures.	Criterion equivalence Conceptual equivalence Report the results of cross-cultural adaptation noting any languages/cultural adaptations that have been reported. If specific reliability and validity values are reported they can be documented in the appropriate data collection boxes above, but an annotation should be made to note that the measurement property applies to an adapted version.

Reference List

Beaton, D. E. (2000). Understanding the Relevance of Measured Change Through Studies of Responsiveness. *Spine, 25,* 3192-3199.

Bland, J. M. & Altman, D. G. (1987). Statistical methods for assessing agreement between measurements. Biochem Clin 11, 399-404.

Bland, J. M. & Altman, D. G. (1990). A note on the use of the intraclass correlation coefficient in the evaluation of agreement between two methods of measurement. *Comput Biol Med, 20,* 337-340.

Bland, J. M. & Altman, D. J. (1986). Statistical methods for assessing agreement between two methods of clinical measurement. *Lancet, 1,* 307-310.

Cibelli, K. (1994). Cognitive Interviewing Techniques: A Brief Overview. www.metagora.org/training/example/SL_1_CognitiveInterviewing_051405.pdf [Electronic version]. Available: www.metagora.org/training/example/SL_1_CognitiveInterviewing_051405.pdf

Cieza, A., Brockow, T., Ewert, T., Amman, E., Kollerits, B., Chatterji, S. et al. (2002). Linking health-status measurements to the international classification of functioning, disability and health. *J Rehabil. Med., 34,* 205-210.

Landis, J. R. & Koch, G. G. (1977). The measurement of observer agreement for categorical data. *Biometrics, 33,* 159-174.

Ojanen, J. & Gogates, G. (2006). A briefing on cognitive debriefing. Good Clinical Practice Journal 13[12], 1-29. Ref Type: Journal (Full)

Pallant, J. F. & Tennant, A. (2007). An introduction to the Rasch measurement model: an example using the Hospital Anxiety and Depression Scale (HADS). *British Journal of Clinical Psychology, 46,* 1-18.

Shrout, P. E. & Fleiss, J. L. (1979). Intraclass correlations: Uses in assessing rater reliability. *Psychological Bulletin, 86,* 420-428.

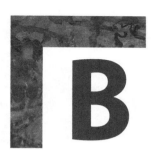

Outcome Measures Review
Form and Guidelines

Law M, MacDermid J.
*Evidence-Based Rehabilitation: A Guide
to Practice, Third Edition (pp 339–356).*
© 2014 SLACK Incorporated.

OUTCOME MEASURES RATING FORM

CANCHILD CENTRE FOR DISABILITY RESEARCH
INSTITUTE OF APPLIED HEALTH SCIENCES, MCMASTER UNIVERSITY
1400 MAIN STREET WEST, ROOM 408
HAMILTON, ONTARIO,CANADA L8S 1C7
Fax (905) 522-6095
lawm@mcmaster.ca

To be used with: Outcome Measures Rating Form Guidelines (CanChild,2004)

Name and initials of measure: _____

_____

Author(s): _____

_____

Source and year published: _____

_____

Date of review: _____

Name of Reviewer: _____

---

1. FOCUS

---

a. Focus of measurement – Using the ICF framework
   - ☐ Body Functions.................. are the physiological functions of body systems(includes psychological functions)
   - ☐ Body Structures.................. are anatomical parts of the body such as organs, limbs, and their components
   - ☐ Activities and Participation.... Activity is the execution of a task or action by an individual. Participation is involvement in a life situation.
   - ☐ Environmental Factors......... make up the physical, social and attitudinal environment in which people live and conduct their lives.

b. Attribute(s) being measured – Check as many as apply.
   This list is based on attributes cited in the ICF, 2001: WHO.

Body Functions

Global Mental Functions

□ consciousness

□ orientation

□ sleep

□ intellectual

□ global psychosocial

□ temperament and personality

□ energy and drive

Specific Mental Functions

□ attention

□ memory

□ psychomotor

□ calculation

□ thought

□ higher level cognitive

□ perceptual

□ mental functions of language

□ experience of self and time

□ mental function of sequencing complex measurements

Sensory Functions and Pain

□ seeing and related

□ hearing and vestibular

Voice and Speech Functions

□ voice

□ articulation

□ fluency and rhythm of speech

□ alternative vocalization

Functions of the Cardiovascular, Hematological, Immunological, and Respiratory Systems

□ cardiovascular

□ haematological and immunological systems

□ respiratory system

□ additional functions and sensations of the cardiovascular and respiratory systems

Functions of the Digestive, Metabolic, and Endocrine Systems

□ related to the digestive system

□ related to metabolism and the endocrine system

Genitourinary and Reproductive Functions

□ urinary

□ genital and reproductive

Neuromuscular and Movement-Related Functions

Joints and Bones

□ mobility of joint

□ stability of joint

□ mobility of bone

Muscle

□ muscle power

□ muscle tone

□ muscle endurance

Movement

□ motor reflex

□ involuntary movement reaction

□ control of voluntary movement

□ involuntary movement

□ sensations related to muscle and movement

□ gait patterns

Functions of the Skin and Related Structures

Skin
- □ protection
- □ repair
- □ other functions
- □ sensations

Hair
- □ function of the hair

Nails
- □ function of nails

Body Structures

Structures of the Nervous System
- □ brain
- □ meninges
- □ parasympathetic nervous system
- □ spinal cord and related structures
- □ sympathetic nervous system

The Eye, Ear and Related Structures
- □ eye socket
- □ eyeball
- □ around eye
- □ external ear
- □ middle ear
- □ inner ear

Structures Involved in Voice and Speech
- □ nose
- □ mouth
- □ pharynx
- □ larynx

Structures of the Cardiovascular, Immunological, and Respiratory Systems

Cardiovascular System
- □ heart
- □ arteries
- □ veins
- □ capillaries

Immune System
- □ lymphatic vessels
- □ thymus
- □ bone marrow
- □ lymphatic nodes
- □ spleen

Respiratory System
- □ trachea
- □ thoracic cage
- □ lungs
- □ muscles of respiration

Structures Related to the Digestive, Metabolic, and Endocrine Systems
- □ salivary glands
- □ oesophagus
- □ stomach
- □ pancreas
- □ liver
- □ gall bladder
- □ intestines
- □ endocrine glands

Structures Related to the Genitourinary and Reproductive Systems
- □ urinary system
- □ pelvic floor
- □ reproductive system

Structures Related to Movement

□ head and neck   □ shoulder region   □ lower extremity
□ upper extremity   □ trunk   □ pelvic region
□ additional musculoskeletal
   structures related to movement

Skin and Related Structures

□ skin   □ skin and glands
□ nails   □ hair

Activities and Participation

Learning and Applying Knowledge

Purposeful Sensory   □ watching   □ other purposeful sensing
Experiences   □ listening

Basic Learning   □ copying   □ rehearsing
                         □ learning to read   □ learning to write
                         □ learning to calculate □ acquiring skills

Applying Knowledge   □ focusing attention   □ calculating
                         □ thinking   □ solving problems
                         □ reading   □ making decisions
                         □ writing

General Tasks and Demand

□ undertaking a single task   □ undertaking multiple tasks
□ carrying out daily routine   □ handling stress and other psychological demands

Communication

□ receiving (verbal, nonverbal, written, formal sign language)
□ producing (verbal, nonverbal, written, formal sign language)
□ conversation and use of communication devices and techniques

Mobility

□ changing and maintaining   □ carrying, moving, and handling objects
   body position
□ walking and moving   □ moving around using transportation

Self-Care

□ washing oneself   □ toileting   □ eating
□ caring for body parts   □ dressing   □ drinking

Looking after one's health   □ ensuring oneself physical   □ maintaining one's health
                                comfort
                             □ managing diet and fitness

Domestic Life

Acquisition of Necessities
- □ acquiring a place to live
- □ acquisition of goods and services

Household Tasks
- □ preparing meals
- □ caring for household objects and assisting others
- □ doing housework

Interpersonal Interactions and Relationships

General
- □ general interpersonal interactions (basic and complex)

Particular Interpersonal Relationships
- □ informal social realtionships
- □ formal relationships
- □ relating with strangers
- □ family relatonships
- □ intimate relationships

Major Life Areas

Education
- □ informal
- □ preschool
- □ school

Work and Employment
- □ apprenticeship
- □ acquiring, keeping, and terminating a job
- □ renumerative employment
- □ non-renumerative employment

Economic Life
- □ basic economic transactions
- □ complex economic transactions
- □ economic self-sufficiency

Community, Social, and Civic Life

Community
- □ community life

Recreation and Leisure
- □ play
- □ sports
- □ arts and culture
- □ crafts
- □ hobbies
- □ soicalizing

Civic
- □ religion and spirituality
- □ human rights
- □ political life and citizenship

Environmental Factors

Products and Technology

- □ communication
- □ culture, recreation, and sport
- □ design, construction, and buildings for public use
- □ religion and spirituality
- □ education
- □ products or substances for personal consumption
- □ design, construction, and buildings for private use
- □ land development
- □ employment
- □ products and technology for personal use in daily living
- □ for personal indoor and outdoor mobility and transportation
- □ assets

Natural Environment and Human-Made Changes to Environment

- □ physical geography
- □ flora and fauna
- □ natural events
- □ light
- □ sound
- □ air quality
- □ population
- □ climate
- □ human events
- □ time-related changes
- □ vibration

Support and Relationships

- □ immediate family
- □ health professionals
- □ people in positions of authority
- □ acquaintances, peers, colleagues, neighbors, and community members
- □ extended family
- □ other professionals
- □ people in subordinate positions
- □ domesticated animals
- □ friends
- □ strangers
- □ personal care providers and personal assistants

Attitudes

- □ of immediate family
- □ of strangers
- □ of people in positions of authority
- □ of acquaintances, peers, colleagues, neighbors, and community members
- □ of extended family
- □ of health professionals
- □ of people in subordinate positions
- □ societal attitudes
- □ of friends
- □ of health-related professionals
- □ of personal care providers and personal assistants
- □ social norms, practices, and idealogies

Services, Systems and Policies

- □ production of consumer goods
- □ open space planning
- □ utilities
- □ transportation
- □ legal
- □ media
- □ architecture and construction
- □ social security
- □ health
- □ labour and employment
- □ housing
- □ communication
- □ associations and organizations
- □ civil protection
- □ economic
- □ general social support
- □ education and training
- □ political

---

c. Does this measure assess a single attribute or multiple attributes?

□ Single
□ Multiple

d. Check purposes that apply and indicate (*) primary purpose of the measure

□ To describe or discriminate   □ To predict   □ To evaluative

Comments:_____
_____
_____

e. Perspective - Indicate possible respondents:
   □ Client   □ Other professional
   □ Caregiver/parent   □ Other
   □ Service provider

f. Population measure designed for:
   Age: Please specify all applicable ages if stated in the manual
   □ Infant (birth - < 1 year)   □ Adult (> 18 years - <65 years)
   □ Child (1 year - < 13 years)   □ Senior (> 65 years)
   □ Adolescent (13 - < 18 years)   □ Age not specified

   Diagnosis:
   List the diagnostic group(s) for which this measure is designed to be used:
   _____
   _____
   _____
   _____

g. Evaluation context—Indicate suggested/possible environments for this assessment
   □ Home   □Education setting   □ Community
   □ Workplace   □Community agency   □ Rehabilitation centre/
                                                   health care setting

   □ Other_____

---

2. CLINICAL UTILITY

a. Clarity of Instructions: (check one of the ratings)
   □ Excellent: clear, comprehensive, concise, and available
   □ Adequate: clear, concise, but lacks some information
   □ Poor: not clear and concise or not available
   Comments:_____
   _____

b. Format (check applicable items)
   □Interview   Questionnaire: □ Self completed
   □ Task performance   □ Interview administered
   □ Naturalistic observation   □ Caregiver completed

   □ Other_____

   Physically invasive: □ Yes   □ No
   Active participation of client: □ Yes   □ No
   Special Equipment Required: □ Yes   □ No

c. Time to complete assessment: _____ minutes
   Administration: □ Easy   □ More complex   *(Consider time,*
   Scoring: □ Easy   □ More complex   *amount of training,*
   Interpretation: □ Easy   □ More complex   *and ease)*

---

d. Examiner Qualifications: Is formal training required for administering and/or interpreting?

□ Required □ Recommended □ Not required □ Not addressed

e. Cost (Cdn. Funds)
manual: $_____
score sheets: $_____ for_____Sheets
Indicate year of cost information:_____
Source of cost information:_____

3. SCALE CONSTRUCTION

a. Item Selection (check one of the ratings)

□ Excellent: included all relevant characteristics of attribute based on comprehensive literature review and survey of experts

□ Adequate: included most relevant characteristics of attribute

□ Poor: convenient sample of characteristics of attribute

Comments:_____
_____
_____

b. Weighting
Are the items weighted in the calculation of total score? □ Yes □ No
If yes, are the items weighted: □ Implicitly □ Explicitly

c. Level of Measurement □ Nominal □ Ordinal □ Interval □ Ratio

Scaling method (Likert, Guttman, etc.):_____

Number of items:_____

Indicate if subscale scores are obtained: □ Yes □ No

If yes, can the subscale scores be used alone: Administered: □Yes □ No
Interpreted: □ Yes □ No

List subscales:	Number of Items:

4. STANDARDIZATION

a. Manual (check one of the ratings)

□ Excellent: published manual which outlines specific procedures for administration; scoring and interpretation; evidence of reliability and validity

□ Adequate: manual available and generally complete but some information is lacking or unclear regarding administration; scoring and interpretation; evidence of reliability and validity

□ Poor: no manual available or manual with unclear administration; scoring and interpretaion; no evidence of reliability and validity

b. Norms available (N/A for instrument whose purpose is <u>only</u> evaluative)

         □ Yes   □ No   □ N/A

Age: Please specify all applicable ages for which norms are available

□ Infant (birth - < 1 year)   □ Adult (> 18 years - <65 years)
□ Child (1 year - < 13 years)   □ Senior (> 65 years)
□ Adolescent (13 - < 18 years)

Populations for which it is normed:

_____

_____

Size of sample: n = _____

5. RELIABILITY

a. Rigor of standardization studies for reliability (check one of the ratings)

□ Excellent: more than 2 well-designed reliability studies completed with adequate to excellent reliability values

□ Adequate: 1 to 2 well-designed reliability studies completed with adequate to excellent reliability values

□ Poor: reliability studies poorly completed, or reliability studies showing poor levels of reliability

□ No evidence available

Comments:_____

_____

_____

_____

b. Reliability Information

Type of Reliability	Statistic Used	Value	Rating (excellent, adequate or poor)

* guidelines for levels of reliability coefficient (see instructions)
   Excellent: >.80   Adequate: .60 - .79   Poor: <.60

6. VALIDITY

a. Rigor of standardization studies for validity (check one of the ratings)
   □ Excellent: more than 2 well-designed validity studies supporting the measure's validity
   □ Adequate: 1 to 2 well-designed validity studies supporting the measure's validity
   □ Poor: validity studies poorly completed or did not support the measure's validity
   □ No evidence available

   Comments:
   _____
   _____
   _____
   _____

b. Content Validity (check one of the ratings)
   □ Excellent: judgmental or statistical method (e.g. factor analysis) was used and the measure is comprehensive and includes items suited to the measurement purpose
      Method: □ judgmental   □ statistical
   □ Adequate: has content validity but no specific method was used
   □ Poor: instrument is not comprehensive
   □ No evidence available

c. Construct Validity (check one of the ratings)
   □ Excellent: more than 2 well-designed studies have shown that the instrument conforms to prior theoretical relationships among characteristics or individuals
   □ Adequate: 1 to 2 studies demonstrate confirmation of theoretical formulations
   □ Poor: construct validation poorly completed, or did not support measure's construct validity
   □ No evidence available

   Strength of Association:_____
   _____
   _____
   _____
   _____

d. Criterion Validity (check ratings that apply)
    □ Concurrent □ Predictive

 □ Excellent: more than 2 well-designed studies have shown adequate
        agreement with a criterion or gold standard
 □ Adequate: 1 to 2 studies demonstrate adequate agreement with a criterion or
        gold standard measure
 □ Poor: criterion validation poorly completed or did not support measure's
        criterion validity
 □ No evidence available

Criterion Measure(s) used: _____

_____

Strength of Association:_____

_____

e. Responsiveness (check one of the ratings)
 □ Excellent: more that 2 well-designed studies showing strong hypothesized
        relationships between changes on the measure and other
        measures of change on the same attribute.
 □ Adequate: 1 to 2 studies of responsiveness
 □ Poor: studies of responsiveness poorly completed or did not support the
        measure's responsiveness
 □ N/A
 □ No evidence available

Comments:
_____
_____

---

7. OVERALL UTILITY (based on an overall assessment of the quality of this measure)

 □ Excellent: adequate to excellent clinical utility, easily available, excellent
        reliability, and validity
 □ Adequate: adequate to excellent clinical utility, easily available, adequate to
        excellent reliability, and adequate to excellent validity
 □ Poor: poor clinical utility, not easily available, poor reliability, and validity

Comments/Notes/Explanations:
_____
_____
_____
_____
_____
_____
_____

MATERIALS USED FOR REVIEW/RATING

Please indicate the sources of information used for this review/rating:
☐ Manual
☐ Journal articles: (attach or indicate location)
    ☐ by author of measure
    ☐ by other authors
List sources:

_____
_____
_____
_____
_____
_____

☐ Books—provide reference

☐ Correspondence with author—attach

☐ Other sources:

_____
_____
_____

OUTCOME MEASURES RATING FORM GUIDELINES

FROM: CanChild Centre for Childhood Disability Research
Institute of Applied Health Sciences, McMaster University
1400 Main Street West. Room 408
Hamilton, Canada L8S 1C7
fax (905) 522-6095
lawm@mcmaster.ca

PREPARED BY: Mary Law, Ph.D. O.T.(C)

FOR FURTHER DISCUSSION OF ISSUES: Law, M. (1987). Measurement in occupational therapy: Scientific criteria for evaluation. *Canadian Journal of Occupational Therapy, 54*, 133-138.

GENERAL INFORMATION: Name of Measure, Authors, Source and Year.

---

1. FOCUS

---

a. FOCUS OF MEASUREMENT. Use the ICF framework to indicate the focus of the measurement instrument that is being reviewed. The definitions are as follows: BODY FUNCTIONS: are the physiological functions of body systems (including psychological functions). BODY STRUCTURES: are anatomical parts of the body such as organs, limbs and their components. ACTIVITIES AND PARTICIPATION: activity is the execution of a task or action by an individual. Participation is involvement in a life situation. ENVIRONMENTAL FACTORS: make up the physical, social and attitudinal environment in which people live and conduct their lives.

b. ATTRIBUTE(S) BEING MEASURED. The rating form lists attributes organized using the ICF framework. Check as many attributes as apply to indicate what is being measured by this instrument.

c. SINGLE OR MULTIPLE ATTRIBUTE. Check the appropriate box to indicate whether this measure assesses a single attribute only or multiple attributes.

d. List the PRIMARY PURPOSE for which the scale has been designed. Secondary purposes can also be listed but the instrument should be evaluated according to its primary purpose (i.e., discriminative, predictive, evaluative).

DISCRIMINATIVE: A discriminative index is used to distinguish between individuals or groups on an underlying dimension when no external criterion or gold standard is available for validating these measures.

PREDICTIVE: A predictive index is used to classify individuals into a set of predefined measurement categories... either concurrently or prospectively, to determine whether individuals have been classified correctly.

EVALUATIVE: An evaluative index is used to measure the magnitude of longitudinal change in an individual or group on the dimension of interest.
(Kirshner, B. & Guyatt G. (1985). A methodological framework for assessing health indices. *Journal of Chronic Diseases, 38,* 27-36.)

e. PERSPECTIVE. Indicate the possible respondents.

f. POPULATION for which it is designed (AGE). If no age is stated, mark as age unspecified. List the diagnostic groups for which the measure is used.

g. EVALUATION CONTEXT refers to the environment in which the assessment is completed. Check all possible environments in which this assessment can be completed.

2. CLINICAL UTILITY

a. CLARITY OF INSTRUCTIONS. Check one of the ratings. Excellent: clear, comprehensive, concise and available; Adequate: clear, concise but lacks some information; Poor: not clear and concise or not available.

b. FORMAT. Check all applicable items to indicate the format of data collection for the instrument. Possible items include naturalistic observation, interview, a questionnaire (self-completed, interview administered or caregiver-completed), and task performance.

PHYSICALLY INVASIVE indicates whether administration of the measure requires procedures which may be perceived as invasive by the client. Examples of invasiveness include any procedure which requires insertion of needles or taping of electrodes, or procedures which require clients to take clothing on or off.

ACTIVE PARTICIPATION OF CLIENT. Indicate whether completion of the measure requires the client to participate verbally or physically.

SPECIAL EQUIPMENT REQUIRED. Indicate whether the measurement process requires objects which are not part of the test kit and are not everyday objects. Examples of this include stopwatches, a balance board or other special equipment.

c. TIME TO COMPLETE THE ASSESSMENT. Record in minutes. For ADMINISTRATION, SCORING and INTERPRETATION, consider the time and the amount of training and the ease with which a test is administered, scored, and interpreted, and indicate whether these issues are easy or more complex. For ADMINISTRATION, SCORING, and INTERPRETATION to be rated as easy, each part of the task should be completed in under one hour with minimal amount of training and is easy for the average service provider to complete.

d. EXAMINER QUALIFICATIONS. Indicate if formal training is required for administering and interpreting this measure.

e. Cost. In Canadian funds, indicate the cost of the measurement manual and score sheets. For SCORE SHEETS, indicate the number of sheets obtainable for that cost. List the SOURCE and the YEAR of the cost information so readers will know if the information is up to date.

3. SCALE CONSTRUCTION

a. ITEM SELECTION. Check one of the ratings. Excellent: included all relevant characteristics of the attribute based on comprehensive literature review and survey of experts—a comprehensive review of the literature only is enough for an excellent rating, but a survey of experts alone is not enough; Adequate: included most relevant characteristics of the attribute; Poor: convenient sample of characteristics of the attribute.

b. WEIGHTING. Indicate whether the items in the tool are weighted in the calculation of the total score. If items are weighted, indicate whether the authors have weighted these items implicitly or explicitly. Implicit weighting occurs when there are a number of scales and each have a different number of items and the score is obtained by simply adding the scores for each item together. Explicit weighting occurs when each item or score is multiplied by a factor to weight its importance.

c. LEVEL OF MEASUREMENT. State whether the scale used is NOMINAL (descriptive categories), ORDINAL (ordered categories), or INTERVAL or RATIO (numerical) for single and for summary scores. Indicate the SCALING METHOD that was used and the NUMBER OF ITEMS in the measure. Indicate if SUBSCALE SCORES are obtained. Indicate whether the subscales can be administered alone and the scores interpreted alone. In some cases, the scores can be interpreted alone, but the whole measure must be administered first. List the subscales with the number of items and indicate if there is evidence of reliability and validity for the subscales so that the scores can be used on their own. *Standardization* is the process of administering a test under uniform conditions.

4. STANDARDIZATION

a. MANUAL. Check one of the ratings. Excellent: published manual which outlines specific procedures for administration; scoring and interpretation; evidence of reliability and validity. Adequate: manual available and generally complete but some information is lacking or unclear regarding administration; scoring and interpretation; evidence of reliability and validity. Poor: no manual available or manual with unclear administration; scoring and interpretation; no evidence of reliability and validity.

b. NORMS. Indicate whether norms are available for the instrument. Please note that instruments which are only meant to be evaluative do not require norms. Indicate all AGES for which norms are available, the POPULATIONS for which the measure has been normed (e.g., children with cerebral palsy, people with spinal cord injuries), and indicate the SIZE OF THE SAMPLE which was used in the normative studies.

5. RELIABILITY

Reliability is the process of determining that the test or measure is measuring something in a reproducible and consistent fashion.

a. RIGOUR OF STANDARDIZATION STUDIES FOR RELIABILITY. Excellent: More than 2 well-designed reliability studies completed with adequate to excellent reliability values; Adequate: 1 to 2 well-designed reliability studies completed with adequate to excellent reliability values; Poor: No reliability studies or poorly completed, or reliability studies showing poor levels of reliability.

b. RELIABILITY INFORMATION. *Internal Consistency*: the degree of homogeneity of test items to the attribute being measured. Measured at one point in time.

Observer: i) *intra-observer* - measures variation which occurs within an observer as a result of multiple exposures to the same stimulus. ii) *inter-observer*—measures variation between two or more observers. *Test-Retest*: measures variation in the test over a period of time. Complete the table and reliability information by filling in the TYPE OF RELIABILITY which was tested (internal consistency, observer, test-retest); the STATISTIC that was used (e.g., Cronbach's coefficient alpha, kappa coefficient, Pearson correlation, intra-class correlation); the VALUE of the statistic that was found in the study; and the RATING of the reliability. Guidelines for levels of the reliability coefficient indicate that it will be rated excellent if the coefficient is greater than .80, adequate if it is from .60 to .79, and poor if the coefficient is less than .60.

6. VALIDITY

a. RIGOUR OF STANDARDIZATION STUDIES FOR VALIDITY. Excellent: More than 2 well-designed validity studies supporting the measure's validity; Adequate: 1 to 2 well designed validity studies supporting the measure's validity; Poor: No validity studies completed, studies were poorly completed or did not support the measure's validity.

b. CONTENT VALIDITY. Check one of the ratings. *Content Validity*: the instrument is comprehensive and fully represents the domain of the characteristics it claims to measure (Nunnally, J. C. [1978]. *Psychometric theory.* New York: McGraw-Hill). Excellent: judgmental or statistical method (e.g. factor analysis) was used and the measure is comprehensive and includes items suited to the measurement purpose; Adequate: has content validity but no specific method was used; Poor: instrument is not comprehensive. METHOD. Note whether a judgmental (e.g., consensus methods) or statistical method (e.g., factor analysis) of establishing content validity was used.

c. CONSTRUCT VALIDITY. *Construct Validity*: the measurements of the attribute conform to prior theoretical formulations or relationships among characteristics or individuals (Nunnally, J. C. [1978]. *Psychometric theory.* New York: McGraw-Hill). Excellent: More than 2 well-designed studies have shown that the instrument conforms to prior theoretical relationships among characteristics or individuals; Adequate: 1 to 2 studies demonstrate confirmation of theoretical formulations; Poor: No construct validation completed.

Indicate the STRENGTH OF ASSOCIATION of the findings for construct validity by listing the value of the correlation coefficients found.

d. CRITERION VALIDITY. Check one of the ratings.
Criterion Validity: the measurements obtained by the instrument agree with another more accurate measure of the same characteristic, that is, a criterion or gold standard measure (Nunnally, J. C. [1978]. *Psychometric theory*. New York: McGraw-Hill).

Indicate whether the type of criterion validity which was investigated is CONCURRENT, PREDICTIVE, or both. Excellent: More than 2 well-designed studies have shown adequate agreement with a criterion or gold standard; Adequate: 1 to 2 studies demonstrate adequate agreement with a criterion or gold standard measure; Poor: No criterion validation completed. Indicate the STRENGTH OF ASSOCIATION of the evidence for criterion validity by listing the values of the correlation coefficients which were found in the criterion validity studies. Using the information from the assessment that has been completed on this measure, check the appropriate rating to give an overall assessment of the quality of the measure.

e. RESPONSIVENESS. Check one of the ratings (applicable only to evaluative measures).
Responsiveness: the ability of the measure to detect minimal clinically important change over time (Guyatt, G., Walter, S. D., & Norman, G. R. [1987]. Measuring change over time: Assessing the usefulness of evaluative instruments. *Journal of Chronic Diseases*, *40*, 171-178). Excellent: More that 2 well-designed studies showing strong hypothesized relationships between changes on the measure and other measures of change on the same attribute; Adequate: 1 to 2 studies of responsiveness; Poor: No studies of responsiveness; N/A: Check if the measure is not designed to evaluate change over time.

---

7. OVERALL UTILITY

Excellent: Adequate to excellent clinical utility, easily available, excellent reliability and validity. Adequate: Adequate to excellent clinical utility, easily available, adequate to excellent reliability and adequate to excellent validity. Poor: Poor clinical utility, not easily available, poor reliability and validity.

---

8. MATERIALS USED

Please indicate and list the sources of information which were used for this review. By listing sources of information and attaching appropriate journal articles or correspondence with authors, it will be easier to find further information about this measure if it is required.

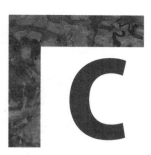

QUALITATIVE REVIEW
Form and Guidelines

© *Letts, L., Wilkins, S., Law, M., Stewart, D., Bosch, J., & Westmorland, M.,*
2007; McMaster University

Law M, MacDermid J.
Evidence-Based Rehabilitation: A Guide
to Practice, Third Edition (pp 357–373).
© 2014 SLACK Incorporated.

CITATION:

	Comments
STUDY PURPOSE: Was the purpose and/or research question stated clearly? O yes O no	Outline the purpose of the study and/or research question.
LITERATURE: Was relevant background literature reviewed? O yes O no	Describe the justification of the need for this study. Was it clear and compelling?
	How does the study apply to your practice and/or to your research question? Is it worth continuing this review?[1]
STUDY DESIGN: What was the design? O phenomenology O ethnography O grounded theory O participatory action research O other _____	Was the design appropriate for the study question? (i.e., rationale) Explain.

1 When doing critical reviews, there are strategic points in the process at which you may decide the research is not applicable to your practice and question. You may decide then that it is not worthwhile to continue with the review.

Was a theoretical perspective identified? O yes O no	Describe the theoretical or philosophical perspective for this study e.g., researcher's perspective.
Method(s) used: O participant observation O interviews O document review O focus groups O other _____	Describe the method(s) used to answer the research question. Are the methods congruent with the philosophical underpinnings and purpose?
SAMPLING: Was the process of purposeful selection described? O yes O no	Describe sampling methods used. Was the sampling method appropriate to the study purpose or research question?
Was sampling done until redundancy in data was reached?[2] O yes O no O not addressed	Are the participants described in adequate detail? How is the sample applicable to your practice or research question? Is it worth continuing?
Was informed consent obtained? O yes O no O not addressed	

DATA COLLECTION:
 	
Descriptive Clarity
Clear & complete description of
  site: O yes O no
  participants: O yes O no
 	
Role of researcher & relationship with participants:
                O yes O no
 	
Identification of assumptions and biases of researcher:
                O yes O no
	Describe the context of the study. Was it sufficient for understanding of the "whole" picture?
	
	What was missing and how does that influence your understanding of the research?

2 Throughout the form, "no" means the authors explicitly state reasons for not doing it; "not addressed" should be ticked if there is no mention of the issue.

Procedural Rigour Procedural rigor was used in data collection strategies? ○ yes ○ no ○ not addressed	Do the researchers provide adequate information about data collection procedures e.g., gaining access to the site, field notes, training data gatherers? Describe any flexibility in the design & data collection methods.
DATA ANALYSES: **Analytical Rigour** Data analyses were inductive? ○ yes ○ no ○ not addressed Findings were consistent with & reflective of data? ○ yes ○ no	Describe method(s) of data analysis. Were the methods appropriate? What were the findings?
Auditability Decision trail developed? ○ yes ○ no ○ not addressed Process of analyzing the data was described adequately? ○ yes ○ no ○ not addressed	Describe the decisions of the researcher re: transformation of data to codes/themes. Outline the rationale given for development of themes.
Theoretical Connections Did a meaningful picture of the phenomenon under study emerge? ○ yes ○ no	How were concepts under study clarified & refined, and relationships made clear? Describe any conceptual frameworks that emerged.

| OVERALL RIGOUR

Was there evidence of the four components of trustworthiness?
Credibility   ○ yes ○ no
Transferability   ○ yes ○ no
Dependability   ○ yes ○ no
Comfirmability   ○ yes ○ no | For each of the components of trustworthiness, identify what the researcher used to ensure each.

What meaning and relevance does this study have for your practice or research question? |
| CONCLUSIONS & IMPLICATIONS

Conclusions were appropriate given the study findings?
  ○ yes ○ no

The findings contributed to theory development & future OT practice/ research?
  ○ yes ○ no | What did the study conclude? What were the implications of the findings for occupational therapy (practice & research)? What were the main limitations in the study? |

Introduction

- These guidelines accompany the Critical Review Form: Qualitative Studies originally developed by the McMaster University Occupational Therapy Evidence-Based Practice Research Group and revised by Letts et al., 2007. They are written in basic terms that can be understood by researchers as well as clinicians and students interested in conducting critical reviews of the literature.
- Guidelines are provided for the questions in the left hand column of the form and the instructions/questions in the Comments column of each component.
- Examples relate to occupational therapy research as much as possible.
- These guidelines assist readers to complete critical appraisal of qualitative research articles. In recent years, there has been an increase in the number of meta-syntheses i.e., articles that examine more than one qualitative study and synthesize the data from these studies together. The approaches to conducting meta-syntheses are still emerging, and criteria for critical appraisal of meta-syntheses are not yet well-established. Over time, we anticipate that we may either revise this review form to incorporate meta-syntheses or develop another review form.

Critical Review Components

Citation

- Include full title, all authors (last name, initials), full journal title, year, volume number, and page numbers.
- This ensures that another person could easily retrieve the same article.

Study Purpose

- Was the purpose and/or research question stated clearly? - The purpose is usually stated briefly in the abstract of the article, and again in more detail in the introduction. It may be phrased as a research question.
- A clear statement of purpose or research questions helps you determine if the topic is important, relevant, and of interest to you.
- For future reference, it is useful to provide a summary of the purpose or research question in the comments section, so that you or someone else can quickly get a sense of the article.

Literature

- Was relevant background literature reviewed? A review of the literature should be included in an article describing research to provide some background to the study. It should provide a synthesis of relevant information such as previous work/research, and discussion of the clinical importance of the topic.

- The review of the literature could include both qualitative and quantitative evidence related to the study purpose.

- It identifies gaps in current knowledge and research about the topic of interest, and thus justifies the need for the study being reported. The justification for the study should be clear and compelling. Readers should be able to understand the researchers' thinking in conducting the study.

- Consider how the study can be applied to occupational therapy practice and/or your own situation before you continue with your review of the article. If it is not useful or applicable, go on to the next article.

Study Design

- <u>What was the study design?</u> There are many different types of research designs. These guidelines focus on the most common types of qualitative designs in rehabilitation research.

- The essential features of the different types of study designs are outlined to assist in determining which was used in the study you are reviewing.

- Some researchers will not describe their study using these design descriptions; they may simply refer to the research as a 'qualitative design'. In most cases, you should expect the authors to link their research to a specific research tradition, or justify why they have not done so. When reviewing articles in which the design is described only as qualitative, it can be useful to consider which of these traditions best matches the study you are reading; this will help you make a judgement about the appropriateness of the design, sampling, data collection and analyses.

- Numerous issues can be considered in determining the appropriateness of the design chosen. Some of the key issues are listed in the Comments section, and are discussed below.

Design Types

1. Phenomenology

- Phenomenology answers the question: "What is it like to have a certain experience?". It seeks to understand the phenomenon of a lived experience - this may be related to an emotion, such as loneliness or depression, to a relationship, or to being part of an organization or group. The assumption behind phenomenology is that there is an essence to shared experience. It comes from the social sciences and requires a researcher to enter into an individual's life world and use the self to interpret the individual's (or group's) experience. Phenomenology's application to occupational therapy research is discussed in detail by Wilding & Whiteford (2005).

Example: A phenomenological approach was chosen to explore the experiences of people with arthritis who were participants in two different types of arthritis education groups. Data were collected through observations of the groups, individual interviews with group participants, followed by focus groups after initial analyses were completed. Three themes are discussed by the authors: validation through connection; restructuring illness identity; and perceptions of self and disease symptoms. The themes provided insights into notions underlying transformative learning theory (Ashe, Taylor, & Dubouloz, 2005).

▌2. Ethnography

- Ethnography is a well-known form of qualitative research in anthropology, and focuses on the question: "What is the culture of a group of people, or people in a particular setting?". The goal of ethnographic research is to tell the whole story of a group's daily life, to identify the cultural meanings, beliefs and social patterns of the group, and can include the description of material culture (buildings, tools, and other objects that have cultural meaning). Culture is not limited to ethnic groups, and ethnographers study the culture of organizations, programs and groups of people with common social problems such as smoking and drug addiction. In the area of health care, Krefting (1989) described a disability ethnography, which is a strategic research approach focusing on a particular human problem and those aspects of group life that impact on the problem.

Example: An ethnographic study was conducted to explore the process and outcomes of a program of occupation for seniors with dementia within a day hospital setting, which was the culture being examined. Data from observations, interviews with patients and staff, and field notes were analyzed to discover the opportunities and barriers to conducting an occupational program in a day hospital unit (Borell, Gustavsson, Sandman & Kielhofner, 1994). Jung, Tryssenaar, & Wilkins (2005), in their ethnographic study, interviewed novice tutors and their tutor guides or mentors in order to understand the entry phase of "becoming a tutor" within the culture of problem based learning. The overarching theme was of story telling or an oral tradition within which novice tutors learned from their tutor mentors based on direct modeling and vicarious sharing of stories.

▌3. Grounded Theory

- Grounded theory focuses on the task of theory construction. The inductive nature of qualitative research is considered essential for generating a theory. The focus is on searching to identify the core social processes within a given social situation. Glaser and Strauss (1967) developed a research process that takes the researcher into and close to the real world to ensure that the results are "grounded" in the social world of the people being studied. More recently, Charmaz (2003, 2006) has argued that the ongoing work of Glaser (1978) and Strauss and Corbin (1990) has resulted in grounded theory becoming more objectivist (positivistic) and suggested that a more constructivist (interpretive) approach allows researchers to focus more on human agency, social and subjective meaning, and problem-solving practices and action. A grounded theory method is an emergent design dependent on continuous data analysis. The theory is seen as a developmental process and therefore is able to capture the nature of social interaction and its structural content.

Example: Grounded theory was used to explore the concept of playfulness in adults (Guitard, Ferland, & Dutil, 2005). Through interviews with a heterogeneous group of fifteen adults, and inductive analyses, the following components of playfulness were identified: creativity, curiosity, sense of humour, pleasure, and spontaneity. The analyses also resulted in the development of a visual model demonstrating the relationships among the components of the model.

4. Participatory Action Research (PAR)

- PAR is an approach to research and social change that can be considered a type of qualitative research. PAR involves individuals and groups researching their own personal beings, socio-cultural settings and experiences. They reflect on their values, shared realities, collective meanings, needs and goals. Knowledge is generated and power is regained through deliberate actions that nurture, empower and liberate persons and groups. The researcher works in partnership with participants throughout the research process. PAR can be time consuming because sometimes delays can occur when researchers from outside the community and community members need to negotiate phases in the research. Research describing PAR should ideally discuss the negotiation processes used in the research.

Example: Cockburn and Trentham (2002) share two examples of participatory action research projects in which they were involved. One project involved adults with mental illness working to create meaningful work experiences. The other involved older adults in a community capacity-building process related to identifying and addressing issues in their housing complex. Letts (2003) also shared a number of examples of participatory research projects that involved occupational therapists.

5. Other Designs

- These are many other qualitative research designs described in the literature. They come from different theoretical traditions and disciplines, and some are extensions of the more popular ethnographic and phenomenological designs. Some of the most frequently described designs in qualitative literature include: heuristics, ethnomethodology, institutional ethnography, hermeneutics, ecological psychology, feminism, and social interactionism. Readers interested in further inquiry of qualitative research designs are directed to the bibliography at the end of this document.

Appropriateness of Study Design

- The choice of qualitative research designs should be congruent with the following:
  - The beliefs and worldviews of the researcher i.e., the qualitative researcher usually expresses an interest in understanding the social world from the point of view of the participants in it, and emphasizes the context in which events occur and have meaning;
  - The nature of the end results desired i.e., the qualitative research is seeking meaning and understanding, which is best described in narrative form;
  - The depth of understanding and description required from participants i.e., qualitative research usually involves the exploration of a topic or issue in depth, with emphasis on seeking information from the people who are experiencing or are involved in the issue;
  - The type of reasoning involved: qualitative research is oriented towards theory construction, and the reasoning behind data analysis is inductive i.e., the findings emerge from the data.

- Crabtree and Miller (1992) suggest that the best way to determine if the choice of a particular qualitative research design is appropriate is to ask how the particular topic of interest is usually shared in the group or culture of interest. For example, if information about how clients responded to occupational therapy treatment is usually shared through discussion and story-telling among individual therapists, then a phenomenological approach may be the most appropriate way to study this experience.

- <u>Was a theoretical perspective identified</u>? The thinking and theoretical perspective of the researcher(s) can influence the study. The researcher should know something conceptually of the phenomenon of interest, and should state the theoretical perspective up front. For example, Ashe et al. (2005) presented findings from an earlier grounded theory study to explain the context of their project, and also discussed the link to adult learning theory.

Qualitative Methods

- A variety of different methods are used by qualitative researchers to answer the research question. The most common ones are described here, including the advantages and disadvantages of each.

1. Participant Observation

- A participant observer uses observation to research a culture or situation from within. There is a difference between the researcher as simply an onlooker and one who is actually participating while observing (i.e., doing what the people are doing). The observer usually spends an extended period of time within the setting to be studied and records 'fieldnotes' of his/her observations. This type of research may be called 'fieldwork', which comes from its roots in social and cultural anthropology.
- Participant observation is useful when the focus of interest is how activities and interactions within a setting give meaning to beliefs or behaviours. It fits with the assumption that everyone in a group or organization is influenced by assumptions and beliefs that they take for granted. It is therefore considered the qualitative method of choice when the situation or issue of interest is obscured or hidden from public knowledge and there are differences between what people say and what they do.
- Participant observation can be time-consuming and costly, as it can take a long time to uncover the hidden meanings of the situation/context. However, if a researcher is expecting to commit to a particular topic as part of an ongoing program of research the investment of this time can prove very valuable. The researcher should allow enough time to get at the complexity of the situation being observed.

2. Interviews

- An interview implies some form of verbal discourse. The participant provides the researcher with information through verbal interchange or conversation. Non-verbal behaviours and the interview context are noted by the researcher and become part of the data.
- Another term used frequently in qualitative research is 'key informant interviews' which refers to the special nature of the participant being interviewed - he or she is chosen by the researcher because of an important or different viewpoint, status in a culture or organization, and/or knowledge of the issue being studied. However, the method of data collection remains an interview.
- Qualitative interviews place an emphasis on listening and following the direction of the participant/informant. A variety of open-ended questions are chosen to elicit the most information possible in the time available. Frequently, the interview protocol provides

opportunities for the interviewer to probe following participant responses to open-ended questions.

- Interviews can be done relatively quickly, with little expense, and are useful when a particular issue needs to be explored in depth. However, the drawback to interviewing is related to the constraints imposed by language. The types of questions asked will frame the participants' responses, and this should be taken into account by the researcher.

3. Document Review

- Document review is often used in historical research, which involves the study and analysis of data about past events. The specific methods used are flexible and open because the purpose is to learn how past intentions and events were related due to their meaning and value. Documents are reviewed considering the context within which they were created. The historian learns about particular persons at particular times and places that present unique opportunities to learn about the topic of interest.
- It is a research method that requires the researcher to enter into an in-depth learning process, to become a critical editor of texts, such as diaries, media reports, or blogs. The researcher should explain the method used and readers should feel comfortable that the method involved adequate depth and a critical approach.

4. Focus Groups

- Focus groups are a formal method of interviewing a group of people/participants on a topic of interest.
- The same principles used for individual interviews apply with focus group interviews e.g., the use of open-ended questions, the focus on listening and learning from the participants.
- Focus groups are useful when multiple viewpoints or responses are needed on a specific topic/issue. Group members can build on one another's ideas to result in more in-depth discussions of the topic. Multiple responses can be obtained through focus groups in a shorter period of time than individual interviews. A researcher can also observe the interactions that occur among group members.
- The disadvantages of focus groups relate to the potential constraints that a group setting can place on individuals' responses. A common challenge in focus groups is to ensure that both reticent and gregarious participants have an opportunity to be heard. The facilitator of the focus group must be skilled in group process and interviewing techniques to ensure the success of the group.

5. Other

- Other forms of qualitative research methods include mapping cultural settings and events; recording, using either audio or visual techniques such as photography; life histories (biographies); and genograms.
- Some researchers consider surveys and questionnaires which are open-ended in nature to be qualitative methods if the primary intent is to 'listen' to or learn from the participants/clients themselves about the topic of interest. However, these tend to be limited, and often constrain the participants in ways that other qualitative methods do not. Answering one open-ended question at the end of a survey is not the same as participating in an in-depth interview. It is difficult to ensure that the richness of participants' experiences is really conveyed.

Researchers need to be clear about the intent of such questions, and how the results are analysed and interpreted.

Sampling

- <u>The process of purposeful selection was described</u>? - Sampling in qualitative research is purposeful and the process used to select participants should be clearly described.
- The sampling method needs to fit the study purpose or research question being explored.
- Purposeful sampling selects participants for a specific reason e.g., age, culture, experience, not randomly.
- There are numerous sampling methods in qualitative research: the sampling strategies used by the researcher should be explained and should relate to the purpose of the study. For example, if the purpose of the study is to learn about the impact of a new treatment program from the perspective of all clients involved in the program and their families, the purposeful sampling method should be broad to include maximum variation in perspectives and views. On the other hand, if the purpose is to explore an issue in-depth, such as the numerous factors and interactions that are involved in a family deciding when and where to place an elderly member in a nursing home, an individual, 'key informant' approach may be appropriate.
- <u>Sampling was done until redundancy in data was reached</u>? - The main indicator of sample size in qualitative research is often the point at which redundancy, or theoretical saturation of the data, is achieved. The researcher should indicate how and when the decision was reached that there was sufficient depth of information and redundancy of data to meet the purposes of the study.
- The sampling process should be flexible, evolving as the study progresses, until the point of redundancy in emerging themes is reached.
- The sample should be described in such a way that the reader understands the key characteristics of the participants involved. As a reader, you should then be able to consider the sample in comparison to the purpose of your critical review. You may decide at this point that the sample is different enough from your own population of interest that further appraisal of the study is not warranted.
- <u>Informed consent was obtained</u>? - The authors should describe ethics procedures, including review by a research ethics board and describing how informed consent was obtained and recorded.

Data Collection

Descriptive Clarity

- <u>Clear and complete descriptions</u>? - In qualitative research, the reader should have a sense of personally experiencing the event/phenomenon being studied. This requires a clear and vivid description of the important elements of the study that are connected with the data, namely the participants, and the site or setting.
- The researcher includes relevant information about the participants, often in the form of background demographic data. The unique characteristics of key informants help to explain why they were selected. The credibility of the informants should be explored. Particular to qualitative research, the types and levels of participation of the participants should also be

described, so it is clear what contribution each participant made to the data gathering, analysis, and interpretation of the findings.

- It is often useful to consider what information is missing. This sheds light on how the research can be understood.
- Role of the researcher and relationship with participants: Qualitative research involves the 'researcher as instrument', wherein the researcher's use of self is a primary tool for data collection. Documentation of the researcher's credentials and previous experience in observation, interviewing and communicating should be provided to increase the confidence of the reader in the process. The researcher's role(s), level of participation and relationship with participants also needs to be described, as they can influence the findings.
- Identification of assumptions and biases of researcher: The researcher should declare his/her assumptions and biases about the topic under study to make the researcher's views about the phenomenon explicit.
- A vivid but concise description of the participants, site and researcher should provide the reader with an understanding of the 'whole picture' of the topic or phenomenon of interest.

▌Procedural Rigour

- Procedural rigour was used in data collection strategies? The researcher should clearly describe the procedures used to ensure that the reader can understand the tasks undertaken to collect the data. All source(s) of information used by the researcher should be described.
- The reader should be able to describe the data-gathering process including issues of gaining access to the site, data collection methods, training data gatherers, the length of time spent gathering data, and the amount of data collected.

Data Analyses

▌Analytical Rigour

- Data analyses were inductive? - The researcher(s) should describe how the findings emerged from the data.
- Different methods are used to analyze qualitative data - the reader should be able to identify and describe the methods used in the study of interest, and make a judgement as to whether the methods are appropriate given the purpose of the study.
- Qualitative analyses are typically inductive i.e., starting with data and organizing them into "chunks" which are typically referred to as codes, categories and themes.
- You should be able to summarize the major findings of the analyses in this section.
- Findings were consistent with and reflective of data? The codes, categories and/or themes developed by the researcher(s) should be logically consistent and reflective of the data. There should be an indication that the themes are inclusive of all data that exists, and data should be appropriately assigned to codes, categories, and themes.

▌Auditability

- Decision trail developed? - The process used to identify codes, categories, patterns, themes and relationships from the data is important to understand as it is complex. This process is best articulated through the use of a decision or 'audit' trail, which tracks decisions made during the process including the development of rules for transforming the data into codes, themes etc. Researchers often confront space limitations in publishing their research, so frequently state that they used a decision trail, but may not provide all of the details. You will need to judge whether you have adequate information about the analyses, and the rationale used to describe the interpretation of the data.

- Process of analyzing the data was described adequately? - The researchers should report on how data was transformed into codes and themes and interrelationships that provide a picture of the phenomenon under study. Often a qualitative researcher will use a specific analysis method, such as an editing style or a template approach (Crabtree & Miller, 1999). The methods used should be described.
- The rationale for the development of the themes should be described.
- These steps in auditing the analysis process provide evidence that the findings are representative of the data as a whole.

Theoretical Connections

- Did a meaningful picture of the phenomenon under study emerge? The findings or discussion section should clearly describe theoretical concepts, relationships between concepts, and integration of relationships among meanings that emerged from the data in order to yield a meaningful picture of the phenomenon under study. The reader should be able to understand concepts and relationships, including any conceptual frameworks that the researchers propose.

Overall Rigour

- Rigour in qualitative studies is critical. While in quantitative research one discusses concepts such as reliability and validity, qualitative researchers argue for the use of different terminology when determining the rigour of a qualitative study (Guba & Lincoln, 1989; Krefting, 1991; Taylor, 2000). The overarching concept when considering rigour is trustworthiness.
- Was there evidence of the four components of trustworthiness? Trustworthiness ensures the quality of the findings and increases the reader's confidence in the findings. This requires that there be logical connections among the various steps in the research process from the purpose of the study through to the analyses and interpretation.

- The four components of trustworthiness are:
  - Credibility which is related to the "true" picture of the phenomenon. Are descriptions and interpretations of the participants' experiences recognizable? Ways of ensuring credibility might include:
    - collection of data over a prolonged period and from a range of participants;
    - use of a variety of methods to gather data;
    - use of reflective approach through keeping a journal of reflections, biases or preconceptions and ideas;
    - triangulation, a strategy used to enhance trustworthiness through the use of multiple sources and perspectives to reduce systematic bias. Main types of triangulation are by sources (people, resources); by methods (interviews, observation, focus groups); by researchers (team of researchers versus single

researcher) or by theories (team may bring different perspectives to research question for example a rehabilitation therapist and a sociologist); and

o the involvement of participants through member checking. Member checking may consist of the involvement of participants in a range of activities to verify data and interpretation such as returning transcriptions to participants for review of accuracy of the interview content or returning to participants at various stages during collection and analysis of data to ensure that the researcher reflects or presents the experience of the phenomenon as it is understood by the participants.

- Transferability which is related to whether the findings can be transferred to other situations. Has the researcher described participants and the setting in enough detail to allow for comparisons with your population of interest? Are there concepts developed that might apply to your clients and their contexts? Transferability is ensured through adequate descriptions of sample and setting.

- Dependability which relates to the consistency between the data and the findings. There should be a clear explanation of the process of research including methods of data collection, analyses and interpretation often indicated by evidence of an audit trail or peer review. The audit trail describes the decision points made throughout the research process.

- Confirmability which involves the strategies used to limit bias in the research, specifically the neutrality of the data not the researcher. This can be enhanced through the researcher being reflective and keeping a journal, peer review such as asking a colleague to audit the decision points throughout the process and checking with expert colleagues about ideas and interpretation of data, checking with participants about ideas and interpretation of data, and having a team of researchers.

Conclusions & Implications

- Conclusions were appropriate given the study findings? - Conclusions should be consistent and congruent with the findings as reported by the researchers. All of the data and findings should be discussed and synthesized.
- The findings contributed to theory development and future OT practice? - The conclusions of the study should be meaningful to the reader, and should help the reader understand the theories developed. It should provide insight into important professional issues facing occupational therapists. The authors should relate the findings back to the existing literature and theoretical knowledge in occupational therapy. Implications and recommendations should be explicitly linked to occupational therapy practice situations and research directions.

▌References:

Ashe, B., Taylor, M., & Dubouloz, C. J. (2005). The process of change: Listening to transformation in meaning perspectives of adults in arthritis health education groups. *Canadian Journal of Occupational Therapy, 72,* 280-288.

Borell, L., Gustavsson, A., Sandman, P., & Kielhofner, G. (1994). Occupational programming in a day hospital for patients with dementia. *Occupational Therapy Journal of Research, 14,* 219-243.

Charmaz, K. (2003). Grounded theory: Objectivist and constructivist methods. In N. K. Denzin & Y. S. Lincoln (Eds.), *Strategies of qualitative inquiry* (2nd ed., pp. 249-291). Thousand Oaks, CA: Sage.

Charmaz, K. (2006). *Constructing grounded theory: A practical guide through qualitative analysis.* Thousand Oaks, CA: Sage.

Cockburn, L., & Trentham, B. (2002). Participatory action research: Integrating community occupational therapy practice and research. *Canadian Journal of Occupational Therapy, 69,* 20-30.

Crabtree, B. F., & Miller, W. L. (1992). *Doing qualitative research: Research methods for primary care.* Newbury Park CA: Sage.

Crabtree, B. F., & Miller, W. L. (1999). *Doing qualitative research* (2nd ed.). Thousand Oaks, CA: Sage.

Glaser, B. G. (1978). *Theoretical sensitivity: Advances in the methodology of grounded theory.* Mill Valley, CA: The Sociology Press.

Glaser, B. G., & Strauss, A. L. (1967). *The discovery of grounded theory: Strategies for qualitative research.* New York: Aldine de Gruyter.

Guba, E. G., & Lincoln, Y. S. (1989). *Fourth generation evaluation.* Newbury Park, CA: Sage.

Guitard, P., Ferland, F., & Dutil, E. (2005). Toward a better understanding of playfulness in adults. *OTJR: Occupation, Participation and Health, 25,* 9-22.

Jung, B., Tryssenaar, J., & Wilkins, S. (2005). Becoming a tutor: Exploring the learning experiences and needs of novice tutors in a PBL programme. *Medical Teacher, 27,* 606-612.

Krefting, L. (1989). Disability ethnography: A methodological approach for occupational therapy research. *Canadian Journal of Occupational Therapy, 56,* 61-66.

Krefting, L. (1991). Rigor in qualitative research: The assessment of trustworthiness. *American Journal of Occupational Therapy, 45,* 214-222.

Letts, L. (2003). Occupational therapy and participatory research: A partnership worth pursuing. *American Journal of Occupational Therapy, 57,* 77-87.

Strauss, A. L., & Corbin, J. M. (1990). *Basics of qualitative research: Grounded theory procedures and techniques.* Newbury Park, CA: SAGE.

Taylor, M. C. (2000). *Evidence-based practice for occupational therapists.* Oxford, UK: Blackwell Science Inc.

Wilding, C., & Whiteford, G. (2005). Phenomenological research: An exploration of conceptual, theoretical, and practical issues. *OTJR: Occupation, Participation and Health, 25,* 98-104.

Bibliography:

Bentz, V. M., & Shapiro, J. J. (1998). *Mindful inquiry in social research.* Thousand Oaks, CA: Sage.

Burns, N. (1989). Standards for qualitative research. *Nursing Science Quarterly, 2*(1), 44-52.

Creswell, J. W. (2006). *Qualitative inquiry and research design: Choosing among five approaches* (2nd ed.). Thousand Oaks, CA: Sage.

Denzin, N. K., & Lincoln, Y.S. (Eds.). (2005). *The SAGE Handbook of qualitative research* (3rd ed.). Thousand Oaks, CA: SAGE.

de Laine, M. (1997). *Ethnography: Theory and application in health research.* Sydney, Australia: MacLennan & Petty.

Farmer, T., Robinson, K., Elliott, S. J., & Eyles, J. (2006). Developing and implementing a triangulation protocol for qualitative health research. *Qualitative Health Research, 16,* 377-394.

Patton, M. Q. (1990). *Qualitative evaluation and research methods* (2nd ed.). Newbury Park, CA: Sage.

Smith, S. E., Willms D. G., & Johnson, N. A. (Eds.). (1997). *Nurtured by knowledge: Learning to do participatory action-research.* Ottawa ON: The Apex Press.

van Manen, M. (1997). *Researching lived experience: Human science for an action sensitive pedagogy* (2nd ed.). London, ON: The Althouse Press.

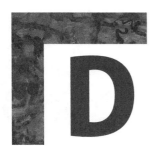

QUANTITATIVE REVIEW
Form and Guidelines

©*Law, M., Stewart, D., Pollock, N., Letts, L., Bosch, J.,
& Westmorland, M., 1998; McMaster University*

Law M, MacDermid J.
*Evidence-Based Rehabilitation: A Guide
to Practice, Third Edition (pp 375–389).*
© 2014 SLACK Incorporated.

CITATION:

| |
| |
| |

	Comments
STUDY PURPOSE: Was the purpose stated clearly? ○ Yes ○ No	Outline the purpose of the study. How does the study apply to occupational therapy and/or your research question?
LITERATURE: Was relevant background literature reviewed? ○ Yes ○ No	Describe the justification of the need for this study.
DESIGN: ○ randomized (RCT) ○ cohort ○ single case design ○ before and after ○ case-control ○ cross-sectional ○ case study	Describe the study design. Was the design appropriate for the study question (e.g., for knowledge level about this issue, outcomes, ethical issues, etc.)? Specify any biases that may have been operating and the direction of their influence on the results.

Comments

SAMPLE: N = Was the sample described in detail? ○ Yes ○ No	Sampling (who; characteristics; how many; how was sampling done?) If more than one group, was there similarity between the groups?
Was sample size justified? ○ Yes ○ No ○ N/A	Describe ethics procedures. Was informed consent obtained?
OUTCOMES:	Specify the frequency of outcome measurement (i.e., pre, post, follow-up).
	Outcome areas (e.g., self-care, productivity, leisure).　　　List measures used.
Were the outcome measures reliable? ○ Yes ○ No ○ Not addressed Were the outcome measures valid? ○ Yes ○ No ○ Not addressed	
INTERVENTION: Intervention was described in detail? ○ Yes ○ No ○ Not addressed Contamination was avoided? ○ Yes ○ No ○ Not addressed ○ N/A Cointervention was avoided? ○ Yes ○ No ○ Not addressed ○ N/A	Provide a short description of the intervention (focus, who delivered it, how often, setting). Could the intervention be replicated in occupational therapy practice?

Comments

RESULTS: Results were reported in terms of statistical significance? ○ Yes ○ No ○ N/A ○ Not addressed	What were the results? Were they statistically significant (i.e., p < 0.05)? If not statistically significant, was study big enough to show an important difference if it should occur? If there were multiple outcomes, was that taken into account for the statistical analysis?
Were the analysis method(s) appropriate? ○ Yes ○ No ○ Not addressed	
Clinical importance was reported? ○ Yes ○ No ○ Not addressed	What was the clinical importance of the results? Were differences between groups clinically meaningful? (if applicable)
Drop-outs were reported? ○ Yes ○ No	Did any participants drop out from the study? Why? (Were reasons given and were drop-outs handled appropriately?)
CONCLUSIONS AND CLINICAL IMPLICATIONS: Conclusions were appropriate given study methods and results ○ Yes ○ No	What did the study conclude? What are the implications of these results for occupational therapy practice? What were the main limitations or biases in the study?

Introduction

- These guidelines accompany the Critical Review Form for Quantitative Studies developed by the McMaster University Occupational Therapy Evidence-Based Practice Research Group (Law et al. 1998). They are written in basic terms that can be understood by clinicians, students and researchers.
- Where appropriate, examples and justification for the guidelines/suggestions are provided to assist the reader in understanding the process of critical review.
- Guidelines are provided for the questions (left hand column) in the form, and the instructions/questions in the Comments column of each component.

Critical Review Components

Citation

- Include full title, all authors (last name, initials), full journal title, year, volume and page numbers.
- This ensures that another person could easily retrieve the same article.

Study Purpose

- <u>Was the purpose stated clearly</u>? The purpose is usually stated briefly in the abstract of the article, and again in more detail in the introduction. It may be phrased as a research question or hypothesis.
- A clear statement helps you determine if the topic is important, relevant, and of interest to you. Consider how the study can be applied to occupational therapy practice and/or your own situation before you continue. If it is not useful or applicable, go on to the next article.

Literature

- <u>Was relevant background literature reviewed</u>? A review of the literature should be included in an article describing research to provide some background to the study. It should provide a synthesis of relevant information such as previous work/research, and discussion of the clinical importance of the topic.
- It identifies gaps in current knowledge and research about the topic of interest, and thus justifies the need for the study being reported.

Design

- There are many different types of research designs. The most common types in rehabilitation research are included.
- The essential features of the different types of study designs are outlined, to assist in determining which was used in the study you are reviewing.

- Some of the advantages and disadvantages of the different types of designs are outlined to assist the reader in determining the appropriateness of the design for the study being reported.
- Different terms are used by authors, which can be confusing—alternative terms will be identified where possible.
- Numerous issues can be considered in determining the appropriateness of the methods/design chosen. Some of the key issues are listed in the Comments section, and will be described below. Diagrams of different designs, and examples using the topic of studying the effectiveness of activity programs for seniors with dementia, are provided.
- Most studies have some problems due to biases that may distort the design, execution or interpretation of the research. The most common biases are described at the end of this section.

Design Types

1. Randomized (RCT)

- Randomized Controlled Trial, or Randomized Clinical Trial: also referred to as Experimental or Type 1 study. RCTs also encompass other different methods, such as cross-over designs.
- The essential feature of an RCT is a set of clients/subjects are identified and then randomly allocated (assigned) to two or more different treatment "groups." One group of clients receives the treatment of interest (often a new treatment) and the other group is the "control" group, which usually receives no treatment or standard practice. Random allocation to different treatment groups allows comparison of the client groups in terms of the outcomes of interest because randomization strongly increases the likelihood of similarity of clients in each group. Thus the chance of another factor (known as a confounding variable or issue) influencing the outcomes is greatly reduced.
- The main disadvantage of RCTs is the expense involved, and in some situations it is not ethical to have "control" groups of clients who do not receive treatment. For example, if you were to study the effectiveness of a multidisciplinary inpatient program for post-surgical patients with chronic low back pain, it may be unethical to withhold treatment in order to have a "control" group.
- RCTs are often chosen when testing the effectiveness of a treatment, or to compare several different forms of treatment.

Participants	→	Stratification	→	Randomization	↗ Experimental Group	→ OUTCOME
					↘ Control Group	

Example: The effects of two different O.T. interventions, functional rehabilitation and reactivation, were evaluated using a randomized controlled trial. 44 patients of a long-term care centre were randomly allocated to one of the two types of intervention. Outcomes were measured using a variety of psychometric tests at 3 different points in time. (Bach et al., 1995).

2. Cohort Design

- A cohort is a group of people (clients) who have been exposed to a similar situation, for example a program, or a diagnosis/disease. Whatever the topic/issue of interest, the groups of clients is identified and followed/observed over time to see what happens.

- Cohort designs are "prospective," meaning that the direction of time is always forwards. Time flows forwards from the point at which the clients are identified. They are sometimes referred to as prospective studies.
- Cohort studies often have a comparison ("control") group of clients/people who have not been exposed to the situation of interest (e.g., they have not received any treatment). One of the main differences between an RCT and a Cohort study is that the allocation of people (clients) to the treatment and control groups is not under the control of the investigator in a Cohort study - the investigator must work with the group of people who have been identified as "exposed" and then find another group of people who are similar in terms of age, gender and other important factors.
- It is difficult to know if the groups are similar in terms of all the important (confounding) factors, and therefore the authors cannot be certain that the treatment (exposure) itself is responsible for the outcomes.
- Advantages of Cohort studies are they are often less expensive and less time-consuming than RCT's.

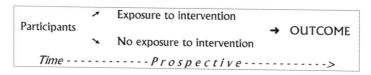

Example: Evaluation of a mental stimulation program used a cohort design to measure changes in mental status in 30 patients over a 2-month time period. The first 15 patients who were admitted to a day care centre received treatment and composed the "exposed" group. The remaining 15 admissions did not receive treatment immediately, and served as a "control" group.(Koh et al., 1994).

3. Single Case Design

- Single subject/case research involves one client, or a number of clients, followed over time, or evaluated on outcomes of interest.
- There are different types of methods used in single case designs, with different terms used such "n of 1" studies, "before-after trial in the same subject"; or single case "series" involving more than one subject/client.
- The basic feature of any single subject design is the evaluation of clients for the outcome(s) of interest both before (baseline) and after the intervention. This design allows an individual to serve as their own "control." However, it is difficult to conclude that the treatment alone resulted in any differences as other factors may change over time, for example the disease severity may change.
- It is useful when only a few clients have a particular diagnosis or are involved in a treatment that you want to evaluate. This type of study is easily replicated with more than one client. Its flexible approach makes it particularly appropriate for conducting research in clinical settings.

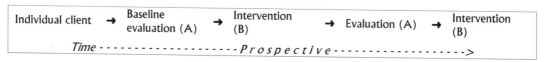

Example: A study examining the effects of environmental changes during an O.T. intervention on a psychiatric ward used a single case design to observe changes in behaviour in 10 individual patients. Observations of each patient's behaviour were made before, during, and after the intevention. (Burton, 1980).

4. Before-After Design

- Before-after design is usually used to evaluate a group of clients involved in a treatment (although as mentioned above, it is a method also used to study single cases/individuals).
- The evaluator collects information about the initial status of a group of clients in terms of the outcomes of interest and then collects information again about the outcomes after treatment is received.
- This is a useful design when you do not wish to withhold treatment from any clients. However, with no "control" group, it is impossible to judge if the treatment alone was responsible for any changes in the outcomes. Changes could be due to other factors such as disease progression, medication use, lifestyle or environmental changes.

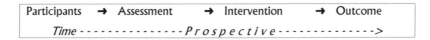

Participants → Assessment → Intervention → Outcome
Time - - - - - - - - - - - - - - *Prospective* - - - - - - - - - - - - - ->

Example: The level of caregiver strain following placement of an elderly family member with dementia in adult cay care was evaluated using a before-after design. Outcomes of caregiver strain and burden of care were measured in 15 subjects before and after the day care placement. (Graham, 1989).

5. Case Control Design

- Case control studies explore what make a group of individuals different. Other terms used are case-comparison study or retrospective study. Retrospective is the term used to describe how the methods look at an issue after it has happened. The essential feature of a case control study is looking backwards.
- A set of clients/subjects with a defining characteristic or situation, for example a specific diagnosis or involvement in a treatment, are identified. The characteristic or situation of interest is compared with a "control" group of people who are similar in age, gender and background but who do not have the characteristic or are not involved in the situation of interest. The purpose is to determine differences between these groups.
- It is a relatively inexpensive way to explore an issue, but there are many potential problems (flaws) that make it very difficult to conclude what factor(s) are responsible for the outcomes.

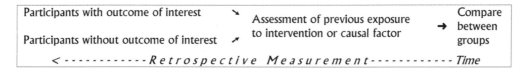

Participants with outcome of interest ⟍
               Assessment of previous exposure → Compare between groups
Participants without outcome of interest ⟋ to intervention or causal factor
  < - - - - - - - - - - - - *Retrospective Measurement* - - - - - - - - - - - *Time*

Example: If an occupational therapist wanted to understand why some clients of a day care programme attended a daily activity programme (which was optional) on a regular basis, while other clients did not attend, a case control design could be used to explore differences between the two groups of clients in relation to age, gender, interests, background and current living situation.

6. Cross-Sectional Design

- Involves one group of people, and all the evaluation of the whole group is carried out at the same time.
- This design is often used to explore what factors may have influenced a particular outcome in a group of people. It is useful when relatively little is known about an issue/outcome.
- Surveys, questionnaires, and interviews are common methods used in cross-sectional studies. They are relatively inexpensive and easy, as evaluation takes place at one point in time.
- It is impossible to know if all factors have been included in the evaluation, so it is difficult to draw cause-effect conclusions from the results beyond the group of people being studied.

Participants	➔	Measurement of outcomes and other factors at the same time
		▴ *Time: All done at one point in time* ▴

Example: Clients and their families who have been involved in a new activity programme for seniors with dementia can be surveyed or interviewed upon discharge to evaluate the impact of the programme on their quality of life, activity participation and level of satisfaction.

7. Case Study Design

- A case study is carried out in order to provide descriptive information (data) about the relationship between a particular treatment (exposure) and an outcome of interest. It is also called a descriptive study, as that is the primary purpose. There is no control group.
- It is often used to explore a new topic or treatment, when there is little knowledge. However, the results can only be considered in terms of describing a particular situation. It may generate information to support further study of the topic of interest.

Participants with condition of interest	➔	Information about clinical outcome

Example: Twelve patients on a long-stay geriatric ward were observed over a period of time to determine the effectiveness of providing individual and group activities on the ward. Engagement levels were observed and recorded at 10-minute intervals to determine any differences between no intervention, individual activities and group activities (McCormack & Whitehead, 1981).

Appropriateness of Study Design

- Some of the important issues to consider in determining if the study design is the most appropriate include:
  - Knowledge of the topic/issue: If little is known about an issue, a more exploratory method is appropriate, for example a case study or a cross-sectional design. As our level of knowledge increases, study designs become more rigorous, where most variables that could influence the outcome are understood and can be controlled by the researcher. The most rigorous design is the RCT.
  - Outcomes: If the outcome under study is easily quantified and has well-developed standardized assessment tools available to measure it, a more rigorous design (e.g., An RCT) is appropriate. If outcomes are not fully understood yet, such as quality of life, then a design that explores different factors that may involved in the outcomes is appropriate, such as a case control design.

- Ethical issues: It is appropriate to use a research design that uses control groups of people receiving no treatment if there are no ethical issues surrounding the withholding of treatment.
- Study purpose/question: Some designs are well-suited to studying the effectiveness of treatment, including RCTs, before-after designs, and single-case studies. Other designs (e.g., case control and cross sectional) are more appropriate if the purpose of the study is to learn more about an issue, or is a pilot study to determine if further treatment and research is warranted.

Biases

- There are many different types of biases described in the research literature. The most common ones that you should check for are described below under 3 main areas:
  1. Sample (subject selection) biases, which may result in the subjects in the sample being unrepresentative of the population which you are interested in;
  2. Measurement (detection) biases, which include issues related to how the outcome of interest was measured; and
  3. Intervention (performance) biases, which involve how the treatment itself was carried out.
- The reader is directed to the bibliography if more detailed information is needed about biases.
- A bias affects the results of a study in one direction—it either "favors" the treatment group or the control group. It is important to be aware of which direction a bias may influence the results.

1. Sample/Selection Biases

- a. Volunteer or referral bias:
  - People who volunteer to participate in a study, or who are referred to a study by someone are often different than non-volunteers/non-referrals.
  - This bias usually, but not always, favors the treatment group, as volunteers tend to be more motivated and concerned about their health.
- b. Seasonal bias:
  - If all subjects are recruited and thus are evaluated and receive treatment at one time, the results may be influenced by the timing of the subject selection and intervention. For example, seniors tend to be healthier in the summer than the winter, so the results may be more positive if the study takes place only in the summer.
  - This bias could work in either direction, depending on the time of year.
- c. Attention bias:
  - People who are evaluated as part of a study are usually aware of the purpose of the study, and as a result of the attention, give more favorable responses or perform better than people who are unaware of the study's intent. This bias is why some studies use an "attention control" group, where the people in the control group receive the same amount of attention as those people in the treatment group, although it is not the same treatment.

2. Measurement/Detection Biases

- a. Number of outcome measures used:
  - If only one outcome measure is used, there can be a bias in the way that the measure itself evaluated the outcome. For example, one ADL measure considers dressing, eating, and toiletting but does not include personal hygiene and grooming or meal preparation.

- This bias can influence the results in either direction; e.g., it can favor the control group if important elements of the outcome that would have responded to the treatment were missed.
- Bias can also be introduced if there are too many outcome measures for the sample size. This is an issue involving statistics, which usually favors the control group because the large number of statistical calculations reduces the ability to find a significant difference between the treatment and control groups.

- *b.* Lack of "masked" or "independent" evaluation:
  - If the evaluators are aware of which group a subject was allocated to, or which treatment a person received, it is possible for the evaluator to influence the results by giving the person, or group of people, a more or less favorable evaluation. It is usually the treatment group that is favored. This should be considered when the evaluator is part of the research or treatment team.

- *c.* Recall or memory bias:
  - This can be a problem if outcomes are measured using self-report tools, surveys or interviews that are requiring the person to recall past events. Often a person recalls fond or positive memories more than negative ones, and this can favor the results of the study for those people being questioned about an issue or receiving treatment.

3. Intervention/Performance Biases

- *a.* Contamination:
  - This occurs when members of the control group inadvertently receive treatment, thus the difference in outcomes between the two groups may be reduced. This favors the control group.

- *b.* Co-intervention:
  - If clients receive another form of treatment at the same time as the study treatment, this can influence the results in either direction. For example, taking medication while receiving or not treatment could favor the results for people in either group. The reader must consider if the other, or additional, treatment could have a positive or negative influence on the results.

- *c.* Timing of intervention:
  - Different issues related to the timing of intervention can introduce a bias.
  - If treatment is provided over an extended period of time to children, maturation alone could be a factor in improvements seen.
  - If treatment is very short in duration, there may not have been sufficient time for a noticeable effect in the outcomes of interest. This would favor the control group.

- *d.* Site of treatment:
  - Where treatment takes place can influence the results—for example, if a treatment programme is carried out in a person's home, this may result in a higher level of satisfaction that favors the treatment group. The site of treatment should be consistent among all groups.

- *e.* Different therapists:
  - If different therapists are involved in providing the treatment(s) under study to the different groups of clients, the results could be influenced in one direction—for example, one therapist could be more motivating or positive than another, and hence the group that

she worked with could demonstrate more favorable outcomes. Therapist involvement should be equal and consistent between all treatment groups.

Sample

- N = ? The number of subjects/clients involved in the study should be clear.
- Was the sample described in detail? The description of the sample should be detailed enough for you to have a clear picture of who was involved.
- Important characteristics related to the topic of interest should be reported, in order for you to conclude that the study population is similar to your own and that bias was minimized. Important characteristics include:
    - who makes up the sample—are the subjects appropriate for the study question and described in terms of age, gender, duration of a disability/disease and functional status (if applicable)?;
    - how many subjects were involved, and if there are different groups, were the groups relatively equal in size?;
    - how the sampling was done—was it voluntary, by referral? Were inclusion and exclusion criteria described?
    - if there was more than 1 group, was there similarity between the groups on important (confounding) factors?
- Was the sample size justified? The authors should state how they arrived at the sample size, to justify why the number was chosen. Often, justification is based on the population available for study. Some authors provide statistical justification for the sample size, but this is rare.
- Ethics procedures should be described, although they are often left out. At the very least, authors should report if informed consent was obtained at the beginning of the study.

Outcomes

- Outcomes are the variables or issues of interest to the researcher—they represent the product or results of the treatment or exposure.
- Outcomes need to be clearly described in order for you to determine if they were relevant and useful to your situation. Furthermore, the method (the how) of outcome measurement should be described sufficiently for you to be confident that it was conducted in an objective and unbiased manner.
- Determine the frequency of outcome measurement. It is important to note if outcomes were measured pre- and post-treatment, and whether short-term and/or long-term effects were considered.
- Review the outcome measures to determine how they are relevant to occupational therapy practice, i.e., they include areas of occupational performance, performance components ,and/or environmental components.
- List the measures used and any important information about them for your future reference. Consider if they are well-known measures, or ones developed by the researchers for the specific study being reported. It may be more difficult to replicate the study in the latter situation.
- The authors should report if the outcome measures used had sound (well-established and tested) psychometric properties—most importantly, reliability, and validity. This ensures confidence in the measurement of the outcomes of interest.

- Were the outcome measures reliable? Reliability refers to whether a measure is giving the same information over different situations. The 2 most common forms of reliability are: test-retest reliability—the same observer gets the same information on two occasions separated by a short time interval; and inter-rater reliability—different observers get the same information at the same time.
- Were the outcome measures valid? Asks whether the measure is assessing what it is intended to measure. Consider if the measure includes all of the relevant concepts and elements of the outcome (content validity), and if the authors report that the measure has been tested in relationship to other measures to determine any relationship (criterion validity). For example, a "valid" ADL measure will include all relevant elements of self-care, and will have been tested with other measures of daily living activities and self-care functioning to determine that the relationship between the measures is as expected.

Intervention

- Intervention described in detail? There should be sufficient information about the information for you to be able to replicate it.
- In reviewing the intervention, consider important elements such as:
  - The focus of the intervention—is it relevant to occupational therapy practice and your situation;
  - Who delivered it—was it one person or different people, were they trained?;
  - How often the treatment was received—was it sufficient in your opinion to have an impact? Was the frequency the same if there were different groups involved?;
  - The setting—was treatment received at home or in an institution? Was it the same for different groups of subjects if there was more than one treatment group?
- These elements need to be addressed if you want to be able to replicate the treatment in your practice.
- Contamination, co-intervention avoided? These two factors were described under Biases (see Design section). Were they addressed? If not, consider what possible issues could influence the results of the study, for example, what could happen if some of the clients in the control group received some treatment inadvertently (contamination) or if some subjects were taking medication during the study (co-intervention)? Make note of any potential influences. If there was only one group under study, mark "not applicable (n/a)" on the form.

Results

- Results were reported in terms of statistical significance? Most authors report the results of quantitative research studies in terms of statistical significance, to prove that they are worthy of attention. It is difficult to determine if change in outcomes or differences between groups of people are important or significant if only averages, means, or percentages are reported.
- Refer to the bibliography if you wish to review specific statistical methods.
- Outline the results briefly in this section, focusing on those that were statistically significant. If the results were not significant statistically, examine the reasons: was the sample size not large enough to show an important, or significant, difference; or were too many outcome measures used for the number of subjects involved.
- Were the analysis method(s) appropriate? Do the authors justify/explain their choice of analysis methods? Do they appear to be appropriate for the study and the outcomes. You need to consider the following:

- The purpose of the study—is it comparing 2 or more interventions, or examining the correlation between different variables of interest. Different statistical tests are used for comparison and correlation.
- The outcomes—if there is only one outcome measured to compare 2 different treatments, a simple statistical test such as a t-test will probably be sufficient. However, with a larger number of outcomes, involving different types of variables, more complex statistical methods, such as analysis of variance (ANOVA), are usually required.
- <u>Clinical importance was reported</u>? Numbers are often not enough to determine if the results of a study are important clinically. The authors should discuss the relevance of the results to clinical practice and/or to the lives of the people involved. If significant differences were found between treatment groups, are they meaningful in the clinical world? If differences were not statistically significant, are there any clinically important or meaningful issues that you can consider for your practice?

Drop-outs

- <u>Drop-outs were reported</u>? The number of subjects/participants who drop out of a study should be reported, as it can influence the results. Reasons for the drop-outs and how the analysis of the findings were handled with the drop-outs taken into account should be reported, to increase your confidence in the results. If there were no drop-outs, consider that as "reported" and indicate no drop-outs in the Comments section.

Conclusions and Clinical Implications

- The discussion section of the article should outline clear conclusions from the results. These should be relevant and appropriate given the study methods and results. For example, the investigators of a well-designed RCT study using sound outcome measures could state that the results are conclusive that treatment A is more effective than treatment B for the study population. Other study designs cannot make such strong conclusions, as they likely had methodological limitations or biases, such as a lack of a control group or unreliable measures, that make it difficult to "prove" or conclude that it was the treatment alone that influenced the outcome(s). In these situations, the authors may only conclude that the results demonstrated a difference in the specific outcomes measured in this study for the clients involved. The results may not be generalizable to other populations, including yours. Further study or research should therefore be recommended.
- The discussion should include how the results may influence clinical practice—do they offer useful and relevant information about a client population, or an outcome of interest? Do they warrant further study? Consider the implications of the results, as a whole or in part, for your particular practice and for occupational therapy in general.

Bibliography

Crombie, I.K. (1996). The pocket guide to critical appraisal: A handbook for health care professionals. London: BMJ Publishing Group.

 Department of Clinical Epidemiology and Biostatistics, McMaster University Health Sciences Centre (1981). How to read clinical journals: V: To distinguish useful from useless or even harmful therapy. Canadian Medical Association Journal, 124, 1156-1162.

Law, M. (1987). Measurement in occupational therapy: Scientific criteria for evaluation. Canadian Journal of Occupational Therapy, 58, 171-179.

Law, M., King, G., & Pollock, N. (1994). Single Subject Research Design. Research Report #94-2. Hamilton, ON: Neurodevelopmental Clinical Research Unit.

Mulrow, C. D., & Oxman, A. D. (Eds.). (1996). Cochrane Collaboration Handbook. Available in The Cochrane Library [Database on disk and CD-ROM]. The Cochrane Collaboration: Issue 2. Oxford: Updated Software; 1998.

Norman, G. R., & Streiner, D.L. (1986). PDQ Statistics. Burlington, ON: B.C. Decker Inc.

Sackett, D. L. (1979). Bias in analytic research. Journal of Chronic Disability, 32, 51-63.

Sackett, D.L., Haynes, R.B., Guyatt, G.H. & Tugwell, P. (1991). Clinical epidemiology. A basic science for clinical medicine (2nd ed.). Toronto, ON: Little, Brown and Co.

Streiner, D.L., Norman, G.R. & Blum, H.M. (1989). PDQ epidemiology. Toronto, ON: B.C. Decker Inc.

Articles of activity programmes for seniors with dementia (referred to in examples of study designs):

Bach, D., Bach, M., Bohmer, G., Gruhwalk, T., & Grik, B. (1995). Reactivating occupational therapy: a method to improve cognitive performance in geriatric patients. Age and Aging, 24, 222-226.

Burton, M. (1980). Evaluation and change in a psychogeriatric ward through direct observation and feedback. British Journal of Psychiatry, 137, 566-571.

Graham, R.W. (1989). Adult day care: How families of the dementia patient respond. Journal of Gerontological Nursing, 15(3), 27-31, 40-41.

Koh, K., Ray, R., Lee, J., Nair, T., Ho, T., & Ang, P.C. (1994). Dementia in elderly patients: Can the 3R mental stimulation programme improve mental status? Age and Aging, 23, 195-199.

McCormack, D., & Whitehead, A. (1981). The effect of providing recreational activities on the engagement level of long-stay geriatric patients. Age and Aging, 10, 287-291.

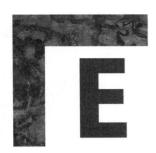

EVALUATION OF QUALITY OF AN INTERVENTION STUDY

Form and Guidelines

Law M, MacDermid J.
*Evidence-Based Rehabilitation: A Guide
to Practice, Third Edition (pp 391–400).*
© 2014 SLACK Incorporated.

Evaluation of Quality of an Intervention Study

This form is used to extract relevant data on effectiveness from your study and to rate the quality of the published study (for item interpretation see guide).

Citation: _____

Authors: _____

Title: _____

Reviewer: _____   Date: _____

Patient Characteristics (Age, sex, disorder, comorbidity/important covariates)
    1. _____
    2. _____

Sample Size _____

Interventions (Describe type, timing, frequency, equipment, provider, progression, etc.)
    1. _____
    2. _____

Outcome Measures (Type and when evaluated)
Primary: _____
Secondary: _____

Results:
Outcomes (absolute change, significance)
Primary: _____
Secondary: _____

Describe any any effect mediators (things that altered the outcomes achieved):
_____
_____

Describe any complications or adverse events that were reported:
_____
_____

Evaluation of Study Design

Evaluation Criteria	Score		
Study question	2	1	0
1. Was there relevant and sufficient background work cited that led to a clear research question?			
Study design			
2. Was a comparison group used?			
3. Was patient status at more than 1 time point considered?			
4. Was data collection performed prospectively?			
5. Were patients randomized to groups?			
6. Was allocation concealed?			
7. Were patients blinded to the extent possible?			
8. Were treatment providers blinded to the extent possible?			
9. Was an independent evaluator used to administer outcome measures?			
Subjects			
10. Did sampling procedures minimize sample/selection biases?			
11. Were inclusion/exclusion criteria defined?			
12. Was an appropriate enrollment obtained?			
13. Was appropriate retention/follow-up obtained?			
Intervention			
14. Was the intervention applied according to established principles?			
15. Were biases due to the treatment provider minimized (i.e., attention, training)?			
16. Was the intervention compared to an appropriate comparator?			
Outcomes			
17. Was an appropriate primary outcome defined?			
18. Were appropriate secondary outcomes considered?			
19. Was an appropriate follow-up period incorporated?			

Analysis			
20. Was an appropriate statistical test(s) performed to indicate differences related to the intervention?			
21. Was it established that the study had significant power to identify treatment effects?			
22. Was the the size and clinical importance of the treatment group differences reported?			
23. Were missing data accounted for and considered in analyses?			
24. Were treatment benefits, adverse events and costs/implementation considerations addressed?			
Recommendations			
25. Were the conclusions/clinical recommendations supported by the study objectives, analysis and results?			
Total Quality Score (Sum of above) =			
The total score can be reported out of 100%—total sum ÷ 25 × 100%			

© Joy C. MacDermid, 2003

Notes:

Evaluation Guidelines for Rating the Quality of an Intervention Study

This guide helps you critically appraise a published paper by assigning scores for each item of the critical appraisal checklist. Select the score where the description sounds <u>most</u> like what was done and reported in the study. In general, scores of 2 indicate strong research design, a 1 is suboptimal, and a 0 is poor research design.

Question		Descriptors
#	Score	
1	2	The authors: – Performed a thorough literature review indicating what is currently known about the problem being addressed and the intervention(s) being evaluated. – Presented a critical, but unbiased, view of the current state of knowledge. – Indicated how the current research question evolves from the current knowledge base. – Established a clear research question(s) based on the above (PICOT: patients, intervention, comparison, outcomes evaluated, and time frames).
	1	All of these above were not fulfilled, but some background literature and a clear rationale for the research question were provided; the research question was general, not specific.
	0	A foundation for the current research question was not developed and the research question was clearly stated.
		Study design
2	2	Two or more contemporary (same point in time) groups of similar patients were compared. Crossover trials which include randomization/blinding of intervention order and complete wash-out of effects equally appropriate.
	1	A comparitor group was present, but it was not clear that the groups were comparable.
	0	No comparitor group was included.
3	2	Patients were evaluated prior to the intervention and at one or more clinically relevant time points following the intervention using the same evaluation process.
	1	Patients were evaluated at more than one point in time (including case control studies) but the above criteria were not fulfilled.
	0	Patients were evaluated at only one point in time.
4	2	A standardized set of data were collected at specific pre-set intervals according to a preplanned study protocol (prospective cohort).
	1	A set of prospective data were collected from patients and later retrieved (e.g., from a database). This data was collected across multiple intervals, but the actual data collection strategy was not determined specifically for this study (retrospective cohort).
	0	Data were based on retrospective records/interpretations or recall of past events.

5	2	An appropriate randomization strategy was used to allocate patients to interventions and the specifics of randomization were described.
	1	Randomization was used but information describing the randomization process was not included or did not confirm a truly random process.
	0	Randomization was not used.
6	2	All relevant people involved in the trial including care providers, patients, study administrators, etc., are not informed about which treatment has been assigned until immediately before the treatment is administered. This includes the explicit decision and protections required to keep allocation concealed.
	1	Either treatment providers or patients are unaware of the treatment to be provided until immediately before the treatment is administered.
	0	Allocation to treatment is not blinded; providers and patients are aware of the allocation well before treatment administration.
7	2	Patients were blinded from the knowledge about which intervention they received. A thorough description of blinding procedures or a post-hoc analysis to indicate blinding indicated that blinding was effective, or it was evident that patients would be unable to distinguish which intervention they received.
	1	Blinding patients was not possible or it was unclear whether an effective blinding strategy was used.
	0	Blinding was possible, but not utilized (includes all studies without comparison groups).
8	2	Treatment providers were blinded to the intervention they were administering and this blinding was substantiated either through audits or other post-hoc analyses indicated that the blinding procedure was effective.
	1	Blinding was not possible or it was unclear whether an effective blinding strategy was used.
	0	Blinding was possible, but was not utilized.
9	2	Outcome measures were administered by an evaluator who was blind to the treatment provided or the purpose of the study. Self-report measures can be considered blinded, if provided by an independent person.
	1	Evaluators were not blinded, but were not involved in treatment of patients (were independent) or self-report forms were administered by the treatment provider.
	0	Outcome measures were obtained by unblinded treatment providers who could influence the measurements.
		Subjects
10	2	The authors explained their recruitment strategy and reported what recruitment rate was obtained from their target population. Recruitment and sampling procedures were applied equally across comparison groups.
	1	The study sample appears representative of the population of clinical interest, but adequate information on sampling procedures or description of the reference population is not provided.

	0	Sampling biases are evident, systematic differences occurred between the comparison groups, and/or selection procedures used make it impossible to determine what types of patients were included.
11	2	Specific inclusion and exclusion criteria for the study were defined.
	1	Some information on the type of patients included in the study is provided but the information is insufficient to identify a specific clinical population.
	0	No information on inclusion and exclusion criteria are stated and limited patient descriptors are provided (e.g., 3 or less, including age and gender).
12	2	Authors performed a sample size calculation to provide a minimum of 80% power on their primary outcome measure and recruited the prespecified number of subjects.
	1	The provided a satisfactory rationale for the number of subjects included in the study or the sample exceeded 100 patients/per study arm.
	0	The size of the sample was not justified.
13	2	Ninety percent or more of patients enrolled or eligible for the study were evaluated for outcomes.
	1	More than 70% of the patients eligible for study or enrolled were evaluated for outcomes.
	0	Less than 70% of patients eligible for study or enrolled were evaluated.
		Intervention
14	2	The parameters of the treatments provided (provider/equipment, frequency, duration, application process, progression, and other technical components) were sufficiently described that they could be replicated. The specific parameters used were based on published basic science or clinical evidence documenting that the specific treatment effects intended are achievable given the treatment parameters used. Treatment fidelity was considered (efforts were in place to make sure treatment was provided per study protocol [efficacy] or monitored [effectiveness]).
	1	A sound rationale and appropriate citations were provided for the treatment assignments but there was an adequate detail about dosage for application.
	0	Neither inadequate rationale nor description of the interventions was provided OR the intervention applied did not conform to present knowledge about what treatment parameters could potentially be effective.
15	2	Efforts were made to minimize sources of potential treatment provider bias as indicated by the type of study design (efficacy versus effectiveness). Blinding can minimize provider bias. Other methods for considering provider effects can include controlling or monitoring of providers' actions or training. Examples include standardizing treatment protocols, equalizing attention to groups, selecting treatment providers without vested interests in a specific intervention, training treatment providers according to a standardized process, or assuring a specific level of training when recruiting providers can be used to assure sufficient equipoise. For study designs focused on effectiveness it may be appropriate to look at the variation between providers, rather than control for it.

	1	Minimal attention was directed either in methods, analysis, or discussion for the potential impact of treatment providers having differential outcomes, but no inherent opportunity for clinically relevant bias was apparent.
	0	No attention was directed at the potential for treatment provider biases and the opportunity for bias is evident, given the nature in which interventions were applied.
16	2	An appropriate rationale was provided for the comparison intervention selected. Where no specific intervention has previously been demonstrated to be effective, placebo is an appropriate comparitor. Where a previously established effective intervention exists, this standard of care is an appropriate comparator.
	1	A clear rationale for the comparison group was not established.
	0	No comparison group was included.
		Outcome
17	2	A primary outcome measure which represents a clinically important outcome was selected and supported by evidence of appropriate psychometric properties (reliability, validity, responsiveness).
	1	A relevant primary outcome measure was evident, but was insufficient in either its clinical relevance or its psychometric properties.
	0	A primary outcome measure was not stated or did not have validity for clinical or methodological reasons.
18	2	Appropriate secondary outcome measures were identified that augmented the perspective provided by the primary outcome measure, ensuring a comprehensive view of the mechanism of intervention action and associated outcomes was obtained. These secondary outcome measures had sound psychometric properties.
	1	Secondary or multiple outcome measures were collected but were deficient either in terms of their relevance or methodological properties.
	0	Appropriate secondary outcome measures were not collected.
19	2	Patients were followed at clinically relevant time points. This may include the to measure both the early response and longer-term outcomes. A clear rationale and/or discussion of the appropriateness of these follow-up periods was included.
	1	At least one relevant follow-up evaluation was incorporated but the study did include other important clinical time points or a rationale for the specific follow-up time.
	0	The follow-up period was insufficient to establish the clinical utility of the intervention.
		Analysis
20	2	Statistical tests were performed to establish treatment effectiveness. In each case the statistical test was an appropriate option for the numerical properties of the outcome measures. The authors documented important elements on the statistical tests (e.g., software used, that statistical assumptions underlying tests were met, Alpha levels).

	1	Statistical effects of treatment effectiveness were used but it was unclear what specific analyses were performed or if data fulfilled the assumptions of the statistical tests used, or there was incomplete presentation of the findings of these tests.
	0	Statistical results for treatment effectiveness were not presented or those selected were not appropriate to the research question or data collected.
21	2	Adequate power was established. A justified sample with significant statistical differences or narrow confidence intervals can indicate this. If there was a lack of statistical difference for treatment effectiveness, a post-hoc power analysis was conducted and identified that the study was appropriately powered.
	1	The sample size was substantial (> 100/arm), but post-hoc power analyses were not conducted in response to nonsignificant results.
	0	The sample size was small and post-hoc power analyses were not conducted in response to nonsignificant results.
22	2	The authors supplemented the reporting of statistical significance with information about the size of the treatment effects observed. This could be indicated by the inclusion of confidence intervals around the mean differences between treatment groups with reference to the clinical importance of these differences and effect sizes, number-needed-to-treat, relation to clinically important differences, or other statistical methods that can be directly related to clinical significance.
	1	The relative differential treatment effects were quantified (means and confidence intervals), but the clinical significance of the treatment effect size is not specifically addressed.
	0	There was no reporting of the differential treatment effect size between treatment groups (other than critical values or P values from statistical tests).
23	2	1. Complete data collection was achieved on all subjects or 2. The rate of missing data (and whether it was random) was reported and where missing data occurred in more than 10% of cases, an appropriate imputation strategy was used.
	1	Methods around missingness were not reported (none reported and a lack of imputation strategy), but given the experimental design missing data was not likely an issue (e.g., immediate pretest post-test or complete cases selected from a database, etc.)
	0	Missing data is a relevant concern and the protocol for handling missing data was not adequately described. Imputation was used and it is not clear what percentage of data was imputed or the strategies used, or more than 20% of the data was imputed.
24	2	The study reports whether any adverse events occurred. Adverse events, costs, and implementation criteria are considered when interpreting results. Practical issues such as specific training or equipment required to achieve the effects described in the study are specified.
	1	Risks and benefits are considered, but without complete reporting of above criteria.
	0	No reporting of adverse events, costs, or practical issues.
		Recommendations

25	2	Specific conclusions and clinical recommendations are made for each of the specific objectives of the study. Specific recommendations are appropriate given the study findings with respect to risk-benefit and study limitations. Recommendations do not do any of the following:
		
		  1. Ignore observed results.
		
		  2. Overstate the generalizability or clinical impact of the study findings.
		
		  3. State that the treatment is ineffective when there was insufficient power to establish this was the case.

	1	Conclusions and clinical recommendations are incomplete, vague, or generalize to situations beyond those studied.
	0	Conclusions or clinical recommendations were not founded on the results of the study or contradict findings of the study.

© Joy C. MacDermid, 2003

Guidelines for Multiple Reviewers

1. Use the accompanying data collection sheets to extract content information from the study and your ratings of research design rigour on the 24 items above.
2. Raters should perform calibration reviews together until they feel comfortable that they understand the criteria, and have calibrated items where it may be necessary to further refine the criteria specific to the area being evaluated.
3. Raters can then independently review manuscripts and come together to compare scores. A process should be agreed upon for determining the final consensus score for each item.
   a. A potential Consensus Process Policy for Design Rigour Items is stated below (but reviewers can choose to use external reviewer for any disagreement).
      i. Reviewers will review their scores for all 25 items
      ii. Differences of 2 points on the score for any item must be adjudicated so that they are minimized by consensus to a difference of 1 point or less for any given item.
      iii. If the primary reviewers cannot agree to within 1 point, secondary reviewers will be used.
      iv. Differences of 1 point will be adjudicated and an attempt made for reviewers to assign a score by consensus; if a consensus cannot be reached, then the lower score will be assigned.

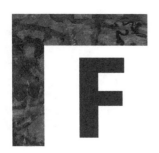

CRITICAL APPRAISAL
PROGNOSTIC STUDY
Form and Guidelines

Law M, MacDermid J.
*Evidence-Based Rehabilitation: A Guide
to Practice, Third Edition (pp 401–406).*
© 2014 SLACK Incorporated.

CRITICAL APPRAISAL: PROGNOSIS STUDY

Evaluation Criteria	Score		
Study question	2	1	0
1. Was the relevant background work cited to establish a foundation for the research question?			
Subjects / Sampling			
2. Were sample characteristics clearly stated?			
3. Were inclusion/exclusion criteria adequately defined?			
4. Was an adequate study sample size enrolled?			
5. Was the source population clearly described?			
6. Did sampling procedures minimize sample/selection biases?			
7. Were the characteristics of the refusers/acceptors stated and investigated statistically?			
8. Was appropriate retention/follow-up of subjects obtained?			
9. Is there evidence that lost-to-follow-up was adequately addressed and did not bias results?			
Exposure ascertainment			
10. Was an appropriate scope and distribution of the predictor(s) present in the sample?			
11. Was the evaluation used to measure exposure independent from treatment (if indicated)?			
12. Was the exposure (potential predictors) captured using valid and reliable instruments?			
13. If the patients received intervention during the study, was it standardized; or were intervention variations controlled for statistically?			
Outcome determination			
14. Was the outcome ascertainment independent from measurement of potential predictors and treatment?			
15. Was a valid and reliable primary outcome defined?			
16. Were appropriate secondary outcomes considered?			
17. Was an appropriate follow-up period incorporated?			
Analysis			
18. Was an appropriate statistical test performed to detect the significance of the effect of each potential prognostic variable?			
19. Were appropriate analyses used to estimate the error around the risk estimates?			
20. Was it established that the study had significant power to identify predictors?			
21. Were secondary analyses conducted to inform the understanding of the relative/absolute risk?			
22. Were the central tendency/variability of the predictive factors clearly presented?			
23. Was the distribution of the outcomes clearly presented?			
Interpretation			
24. Were clinical and practical significance considered in interpreting results?			
25. Were the conclusions/clinical recommendations supported by study objectives, analysis, and results?			
Total Quality Score (Sum of above) =			

© Joy C. MacDermid & Dave Walton, 2011

Evaluation Guidelines for Rating the Quality of an Prognosis Study

This guide helps you interpret the correct score for each critical appraisal item on your checklist. To decide which score to choose, read the following descriptors for each item. Pick the descriptor that sounds most like what was reported in the study. In general, a "2" refers to adherence to the preferred methodological standard, "1" represents partial compliance, and a "0" infers that the quality item was either not adhered to or not reported. We advise all raters to perform at least one Calibration review together to clarify how the items would be interpreted for each specific area. Following adequate calibration, a minimum of 2 independent raters complete independent appraisals. A consensus process is used to arbitrate any differences between these dependent ratings.

Question #	Score	Descriptors
		Research Question
1	2	The authors: − Performed a thorough literature review indicating what is currently known about the exposure (potential predictors) and the outcome(s) of interest. − Presented a critical but unbiased view of the current state of knowledge. − Indicated how the current research question evolves from the current knowledge base. − Established a clear research question(s) based on the above.
	1	All of these above were not fulfilled, but a clear rationale for studying for the prognostic research question was provided.
	0	An adequate rationale for the current research question was not developed.
		Subjects / Sampling
2	2	Includes: key demographics (e.g., age, gender), an indicator of the subtype or severity of the condition, and distribution of potential prognostic variables.
	1	More than two of the key descriptors above are present, but characterization of sample is inadequate.
	0	Two or less of the above descriptors are provided.
3	2	Specific inclusion and exclusion criteria for the study were defined.
	1	Some information on the type of patients included and excluded in the study was defined, but specific inclusion and exclusion criteria were not provided.
	0	No information on inclusion and exclusion criteria and limited patient's descriptors are provided.
4	2	Authors performed a sample size calculation and obtained sufficient numbers of patients to fully power each of the predictors evaluated after correcting for multiple statistical evaluations. Ssmples over 300 are assumed to be sufficiently powered except for rare exposures/outcomes.
	1	The authors performed a sample size calculation and were sufficiently powered for some of the predictors evaluated. Samples of 100 to 300 subjects can be scored as 1, except for rare exposures/outcomes or where the sample is clearly underpowered.
	0	The size of the sample is less than 100 and not rationalized or is underpowered.
5	2	The source population was described in terms of place of recruitment (geographical), time-period of recruitment, and source population (i.e., emergency room or primary care).
	1	Any two of the features of the source population are given.
	0	Less than two features of the source population are given.

6	2	The authors documented a specific recruitment strategy that was clearly an inception cohort that recruited a defined specific target population using sampling procedures that were applied equally across exposure subgroups.
	1	The study is a cohort that appears representative of the population of clinical interest, but adequate information on sampling procedures, inception criterion, or description of the reference population is not provided.
	0	Sampling biases are evident, systematic differences occurred between the exposures groups, and/or selection procedures used make it impossible to determine what types of patients were included.
7	2	1. Characteristics of the refusers were stated in terms of age, gender, and initial severity, AND 2. Refusers were shown be similar to acceptors statistically (i.e., did not differ significantly).
	1	Characteristics of refusers were: 1. Stated, but not analyzes statistically, OR 2. Statistically different than acceptors, OR 3. Anaylzed for two or fewer characteristics (age, gender, initial severity)
	0	None of the above occurred.
8	2	Ninety percent or more of the patients enrolled or eligible for study were evaluated for outcomes.
	1	Seventy to 90% of the patients eligible for study or enrolled were evaluated for outcomes.
	0	Less than 70% of patients eligible for study or enrolled were evaluated.
9	2	Characteristics of drop-outs are reported and the reasons for lost to follow-up/drop-out patients are unrelated to the outcome of recovery (complaints and disabilities).
	1	1. Characteristics of those lost-to-follow-ups are reported and appear similar but differences between completers and drop-outs are not investigated statistically, OR 2. Characteristics of those lost-to-follow-ups are shown to be significantly different than completers and this is considered in the analysis (e.g. sensitivity analysis).
	0	Dropouts are not addressed or a difference in the completers was not considered in the analysis.
		Exposure ascertainment
10	2	Subjects included a broad spectrum of the predictor variables (i.e., meaningful numbers of patients in all discrete categories or across the range of continuous responses).
	1	Either the range of exposures or the distribution of subjects across the range was limited.
	0	Both the range and distribution of subjects across the range was limited.
11	2	Exposure ascertainment was defined prior to inception of the cohort using a process or evaluator that was independent from **treatment**.
	1	Exposure was determined by a process independent from outcome ascertainment (either a factor that could be non-influenced by reporting [e.g., age]) or prospective data collected for another purpose (retrospective cohort design) but not predetermined specifically for the current study. Or exposures were self-reported, but administered by the treatment provider prior to treatment.
	0	Exposure was determined after study inception with the opportunity for recall bias/ascertainment error.
12	2	All exposure variables were determined using a process or tools that have demonstrated validity and reliability, including minimizing recall bias. For physical measures this may include inter-rater reliability; for self-report measures, test-retest reliability.
	1	At least one, but less than all, of the MAIN predictive factors (in a multi-factor study) is captured using a tool with stated evidence for validity and reliability.
	0	Reliability/validity information is not provided and exposures were determined with unvalidated tools.
13	2	One of the following conditions is met: 1. Treatment is provided according to a standardized algorithm or treatment plan that includes a description of the type/range of treatments provided and their progression, if indicated. 2. No treatment is provided (natural history). 3. Treatment is not standardized but treatment data is included as a covariate in the analysis.

	1	Subjects received different treatments subsequent to inclusion in the cohort and the treatments' type and distribution are described. BUT, the treatment effect has not been explored statistically (either as a covariate or stratification variable).
	0	Treatment is not described or controlled for OR it is unclear whether treatment was provided.
		Outcome determination
14	2	The outcome was measured by a process independent from collection of both the prognostic variables and treatment. It is explicitly stated that investigators capturing outcome were blinded to the presence/intensity of predictive factors (other than those not possible [e.g., age and gender]).
	1	Outcome was captured using self-report measures, or other measures where minimal response bias is expected (e.g., death/imaging), but blinding/independence issues were not addressed. OR outcome measurement was independent of treatment but not from assessment of prognostic variables.
	0	Outcome measurement was not blinded/independent from prognostic variables measurement or treatment.
15	2	A primary outcome measure which represented an important clinical outcome was selected and supported by evidence of appropriate psychometric properties (reliability, validity, responsiveness).
	1	A relevant primary outcome measure was evident, but was insufficient in either its clinical relevance (questionable surrogate or conceptually limited) or its psychometric properties.
	0	A primary outcome was not evident or was inappropriate because it was irrelevant or methodologically unsupported.
16	2	Appropriate secondary outcome measures were identified that augmented the perspective provided by the primary outcome measure, ensuring a comprehensive view of outcomes was obtained, and these secondary outcome measures had sound psychometric properties.
	1	Secondary outcomes were considered but were not identified as being secondary or were deficient either in terms of their relevance or methodological properties OR there was a single outcome of interest and this limitation was justified.
	0	Appropriate secondary outcomes were not considered.
17	2	Patients were followed for sufficient time to ensure the outcomes of interest had developed. A rationale and/or discussion of the appropriateness of the follow-up periods were included.
	1	At least one relevant follow-up evaluation was incorporated but the study did include other important clinical time points, or the rationale for the specific follow-up time was not specified.
	0	The follow-up period was insufficient to establish the outcome had occurred.
		Analysis
18	2	A statistical indicator of risk was calculated to determine whether exposures were statistically related to the outcome of interest. The indicator selected was appropriate to the type of data collected and the stated research objectives (e.g., RR or odds ratio in cohort or case control studies, respectively; b-coefficients for continuous outcomes). The authors documented key elements about the statistical analysis (software used, whether statistical assumptions were met, and Alpha levels).
	1	The statistical indicator used was potentially appropriate but there was insufficient documentation of data properties, whether statistical assumptions were met, or methods of calculation to be confident of its adequacy.
	0	Statistical tests were not performed or those selected were not appropriate to the research question or data collected.
19	2	Statistical analyses used appropriate methods to estimate the error around the risk estimate (e.g., confidence intervals). The authors documented important elements on how these error estimates were calculated.
	1	Confidence intervals or other error estimates were provided but were incomplete or methods unspecified.
	0	Error estimates were not calculated around the primary risk estimate.

20	2	Power was established. A justified sample with statistically significant findings on all investigative predictors OR a post-hoc power analysis that identified that the study was appropriately powered.
	1	The sample size appeared adequate (no insignificant predictors or sample >300); but power was not specifically addressed.
	0	Power was not addressed in the presence of insignificant predictors and the sample size was <300.
21	2	Supplemental statistical tests were used to examine the size or impact of the exposure using an alternative statistical method that would account for potential deficiencies in the primary statistical indicator (e.g., attributable risk or number needed to treat added to a risk ratio, a receiver operator curve to examine different risk thresholds, etc). The rationale, statistical assumptions, and methods of calculation for the supplemental tests are adequately described.
	1	Supplemental risk estimates were calculated but were inadequately described or justified.
	0	No supplemental risk estimates were performed.
22	2	The central tendency and variability for all important predictive factors were presented clearly. At a minimum, "important" predictive factors should include all factors identified as being significant in univariate or multivariate analyses. Means with estimates of variability (range, median, SD, or CI) for continuous variables and frequencies for dichotomous variables are required.
	1	The central tendency and variability for some important predictive factors were presented.
	0	The central tendency and variability of predictors were not presented.
23	2	The distribution of the main outcomes were presented clearly. This includes the number of patients who fell into good/bad or recovered/non-recovered categories or the central tendency/variability for continuous outcomes.
	1	The results for most, but not all, important outcomes were presented clearly.
	0	The results of the outcomes were either not reported, or not reported in a way that allowed pooling of results with other papers (for example, if frequencies or percentages of patients recovered/non-recovered are not presented).
		Interpretation
24	2	The authors fully addressed clinical significance by relating the observed risk/protection to established (referenced) benchmarks and considered the meaning of more than one statistical indicator of risk (e.g., relative risk and attributable risk or number needed to screen) to provide a clear indication of the overall impact of the risk/protective factor.
	1	Clinical and practical significance were addressed in the discussion of the study results but in a limited way (only conceptually or on the basis of one statistical indicator).
	0	Clinical and practical significance of the estimated risk were not considered when interpreting the results.
25	2	Specific conclusions that identify specific predictors and the nature (size and direction) of their impact on outcomes are specified. All studied predictors are addressed. Recommendations neither: 1. Ignore observed results. 2. Overstate their generalizability/clinical application. 3. State that exposures were important where this was established statistically.
	1	Conclusions and clinical recommendations were not specific, were incomplete, or generalize beyond the factors studied or results obtained.
	0	Conclusions and/or clinical recommendations were not founded on the results of the study or contradict findings of the study.

© Joy C. MacDermid, 2011

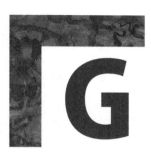

WORKSHEET FOR EVALUATING AND USING ARTICLES ABOUT DIAGNOSTIC TESTS

Law M, MacDermid J.
*Evidence-Based Rehabilitation: A Guide
to Practice, Third Edition (pp 407–412).*
© 2014 SLACK Incorporated.

Worksheet for Evaluating and Using Articles about Diagnostic Tests

Title	
Authors	
Citation	
Test(s) evaluated	
Reference Standard	☐ blinded/independent ☐ gold standard /reasonable alternative ☐ applied to all
Test methods	
Setting	

Subjects		Cases	Non- cases
	n		
	Included (Criteria/ Description)		
	Excluded (Criteria/ Description)		

Test Results	Sensitivity Specificity (see calculation appendix) Other

Evaluation	Y	N
*1. Was there an independent, blind comparison with a reference standard test ?		
* 2. Was the reference standard/ true diagnosis selected a gold standard or reasonable alternative?		
* 3. Was the reference standard applied to all patients?		
4. Did the actual cases include an appropriate spectrum of severity?		
*5. Were the non-cases patients who might reasonably present for differential diagnosis?		
6. Did the non-cases include an appropriate spectrum of patients with alternate diagnoses?		
7. Did the study have an adequate sample size?		
8. Was the description of the test maneuver described insufficient detail to permit replication?		
9. Were exact criteria for interpreting the test results provided?		
10. Was the reliability of the test procedures documented?		
11. Were the number of positive and negative results reported for both cases and non-cases?		
12. Were appropriate statistics (sensitivity, specificity, likelihood ratios) presented?		
13. If the test required an element of examiner interpretation were the qualifications and skills of the examiner described (if n/a leave blank)		
14. Were the training, skills and experience of the examiner appropriate to the test conducted? (if n/a leave blank)		

Application criteria	Y	N
1. Will I be able to accurately apply and interpreting the test in my practice setting? (Instrumentation, training, personnel)		
2. Are the results applicable to my patients? i.e., Are my patients similar in terms of the distribution of disease severity and comorbidities		
3. Will the test results influence my clinical decision-making?		
4. Will my patient benefit from the test result?		
5. Is there any potential for harm to my patient from the test or its result?		

A significant problem with any of these criteria make one question the validity and/or applicability of the study results, although the items with * are particularly important. The final decision must be made by the clinician, based on a preponderance of the information.

This form was designed by JC MacDermid based on principles of evidence-based practice described by D Sackett (1)

DIAGNOSTIC TESTS CALCULATIONS

		Target disorder		Totals
		Present	Absent	
Diagnostic test result	Positive	a	b	a+b
	Negative	c	d	c+d
	Totals	a+c	b+d	a+b+c+d

Sensitivity = a/(a+c) =
Specificity = d/(b+d) =
Likelihood ratio for a positive test result = LR+ = sens/(1-spec) =
Likelihood ratio for a negative test result = LR - = (1-sens)/spec =
Positive Predictive Value = a/(a+b) =
Negative Predictive Value = d/(c+d) =
Pre-test probability (prevalence) = (a+c)/(a+b+c+d) =
Pre-test odds = prevalence/(1-prevalence) =
Post-test odds = pre-test odds × LR
Post-test probability = post-test odds/(post-test odds +1)

For further explanation of these calculations and how to apply them in evidence-based decision making consult texts or websites that describe evidence-based practice methods

Interpretation Guidelines

A "yes" response indicates that the criterion was fulfilled. A "no" indicates that it was not fulfilled or that no documentation of the criteria being fulfilled was provided.

1. The independence of the reference standard test or gold standard diagnosis is critical to study validity and should be documented within the methods. The reference standard test should be obtained without knowledge of other test results or clinical history (blinded) .

2. The reference standard should either be a recognized gold standard or where a gold standard does not exist, a suitable best alternative. Where a gold standard does not exist, suitable justification for the alternative should be provided.

3. The same reference standard should be applied to all patients in the study (patients and controls) . Results of the test under evaluation should not influence the application of the reference standard. Nor should specific pretests be done which would affect either the application or interpretation of the reference standard.

4. The patients with the target disorder should include mild, moderate and severe cases. A description of the spectrum of disease severity should be provided.

5. Patients without the target disorder should be those for whom the test might reasonably be applied in a clinical situation - as a component of differential diagnosis. Asymptomatic controls are not appropriate. Patients with the same disorder in a different location, patients with different disorders in the same location, are examples of types of appropriate non-cases. Where the reference standard is truly a gold standard i.e. accepted to be almost perfectly accurate, then a negative test should be taken as establishing the absence of the condition; where the reference standard is known to be flawed, the actual diagnosis of the non-cases should be defined to minimize the likelihood that they are not false negatives from the reference standard testing.

6. Patients without the target disorder should include *a spectrum* of patients who might conceivably be exposed to this test in a clinical situation, i.e. a variety of appropriate alternative diagnoses or locations. The severity of illness/disability should include mild, moderate and severe cases of other competing diagnoses. The specific diagnosis determined for the controls should be documented.

7. Sample size should be justified and/or not be less than 40.

8. The test maneuver should be described in sufficient detail that it could be implemented by another clinician. This may include test instruments, calibration procedures, training

procedures, patient set-up and test application as dictated by the type of test involved.

9. The specific outcome or observation required in order for test to be interpreted as positive should be described. This may include elements of appearance, symptoms, timing or numerical cutoff's - as appropriate to the test.

10. The author should documented the reliability of the test procedures either by conducting reliability analyses themselves or referencing previous work which has done so.

11. When reporting results, the number of positive and negative cases should be reported for both cases and non-cases regardless of how these numbers are used in decision-making. Where sensitivity and specificity are reported or likelihood ratios are reported, this criterion has been fulfilled. Where raw numbers are provided that could be used in a 2 by two table to compute these values, this criterion has been fulfilled.

12. If the appropriate analyses were conducted one would expect to see sensitivity, specificity, positive/ negative predictive values and/or likelihood ratios.

13. For any test where the examiner interprets whether a score was normal or abnormal based on interpretation of a patient's response, observation or physical assessment (other than automated tests), the training and experience of the examiner is relevant to the accuracy of the test. Therefore, it it should be described so that the reader will be able to determine whether the examiners have similar training and experience to those who would be applying the test in future clinical situations. If this information is provided (regardless of whether the reader agrees that the examiner was appropriate) the item is scored as "yes". If this information is not provided, the score is "no".

14. Certain physical assessments or test interpretations are known to be reliable only with more experienced examiners or those with specific training. If this information is provided and is consistent with the training and experience required for competency in performing the test, the item is scored as a "yes". If the information is not provided or if the training and experience is inadequate, then this item is scored as a "no"

Reference List

1.   Sackett DL; Straus SE; Richardson WS; Rosenberg W; Haynes RB. Evidence-based Medicine. How to practice and teach EBM. 2nd. 2000. Toronto,ON, Churchill Livingstone.

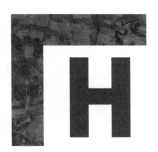

TAXONOMY OF KNOWLEDGE TRANSLATION INTERVENTIONS

Law M, MacDermid J.
*Evidence-Based Rehabilitation: A Guide
to Practice, Third Edition (pp 413–415).*
© 2014 SLACK Incorporated.

Knowledge Translation Intervention Taxonomy for Moving Evidence Into Practice

LEVEL OF ACTION To support moving evidence into practice.	TARGET AUDIENCE (Intended Knowledge User)				
	Lay public or patient population	Clinician health care provider	Policy/ decision-maker	Industry	Other
Increase awareness of a problem or knowledge gap Tools/interventions that focus on making the target audience aware of the importance/implications of a problem, or the gap between evidence and practice.					
Acquire new knowledge Tools/interventions designed to locate or access health research or research-informed information; includes push out or dissemination of evidence.					
Evaluate/synthesize new knowledge Tools/interventions that support or develop evidence synthesis (i.e., compile, appraise, or synthesize the best research information on a topic).					
Make a decision Tools/interventions that assist in the application of health research evidence to decision-making or differentiating between options (e.g. decision support tools, risk/benefit calculators, or help determine the application to a specific patient or scenario. Can include combining evidence with patient values and/or preferences).					
Adaptation of evidence to context Tools/interventions designed help users to adapt research evidence or evidence-informed information to make is relevant or useful for a given context; includes assessment of needs/barriers and modification of evidence to context.					
Implement/operationalize specific actions (implementation fidelity/scalability) Tools/interventions that focus on the operational aspects of implementing/executing specific actions that are defined by best evidence (e.g., ensure that implementation maintains intervention fidelity, scaling up from demonstration project to widespread use).					
Facilitate the process of change Tools/interventions that facilitate the general aspects of change.** These are generic strategies that help individuals or contexts to be better able to change. Tools can be designed to be self/internally initiated (by the target audience) or externally driven (applied to the target audience).					

Quality/outcome evaluation/monitoring Tools that focus on selecting or implementing processes and measures to assess the impact of evidence-informed practice changes. This can include monitoring the process, health effects, or cost-effectiveness (at the individual, group, or population level).					

This knowledge translation (KT) taxonomy is organized around the purpose of the KT intervention and is aligned with moving evidence into practice. Interventions can have more than one element or purpose. However, this taxonomy can facilitate thinking about how different strategies might be selected. Users should consult KT resources and other taxonomies to find different KT interventions and determine the supporting evidence when making these choices.

Definitions

Intervention: An action, tool, policy, or process that is used as an agent of change.

Target audience: The individual, groups, or institutions identified as the intended focus for an intervention.

Improving health outcomes through the use of new or existing research is a shared goal across all KT. The patient/public, clinicians, policy/decision-maker, industry, and other categories are used to identify the main target audiences. KT for basic scientists may be more concerned with translating research findings into new applications and hence may focus to a greater extent on industry and clinician scientists as potential target audiences. Improvements in health outcomes may be distant or indirect for this translational work. KT for clinical or population-based research focuses to a greater extent on changing behavior of individuals or systems (patients, providers, or policymakers) with the goal of implementing new practices that are expected to improve health outcomes. Improvements in health outcomes may be indirect or direct depending on the level of action/stage in the knowledge to action cycle. From a policy or health services perspective, the target may be policy makers and influence on the political environment may be the goal of the awareness.

Note: The research and scientific community is a target audience in KT; while dissemination within the scientific community falls within the field of knowledge translation, it is not specifically listed in this taxonomy which focuses on the aspects outside of KT that focus on implementation (rather than typical scientific communication).

**Interventions aimed at changing beliefs or attitudes fall under increasing awareness and are separated from interventions aimed at stimulating change in behavior. Although many KT interventions ultimately hope to change behavior (implement change in practice), the taxonomy is meant to separate interventions that have a direct focus on behavior change versus those that target precursors of change or monitor change.

© Joy C. MacDermid, 2011

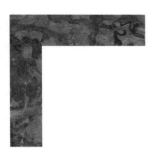

FINANCIAL DISCLOSURES

Laura Bradley has no financial or proprietary interest in the materials presented herein.

Winnie Dunn receives royalties from Pearson publishing.

Paola Durando has no financial or proprietary interest in the materials presented herein.

Jill E. Foreman has no financial or proprietary interest in the materials presented herein.

Jocelyn Harris has no financial or proprietary interest in the materials presented herein.

Mary Law has no financial or proprietary interest in the materials presented herein.

Michael Law has no financial or proprietary interest in the materials presented herein.

Jennie Q. Lou has no financial or proprietary interest in the materials presented herein.

Joy C. MacDermid has no financial or proprietary interest in the materials presented herein.

Annie McCluskey has no financial or proprietary interest in the materials presented herein.

Saurabh Mehta has no financial or proprietary interest in the materials presented herein.

Linda Tickle-Degnen has no financial or proprietary interest in the materials presented herein.

Susan L. Michlovitz has no financial or proprietary interest in the materials presented herein.

Aliki Thomas has no financial or proprietary interest in the materials presented herein.

Diane Watson has no financial or proprietary interest in the materials presented herein.

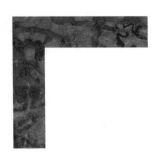

INDEX